Challenging Inequities in Health

Challenging Inequities in Health

Edited by

TIMOTHY EVANS

MARGARET WHITEHEAD

FINN DIDERICHSEN

ABBAS BHUIYA

MEG WIRTH

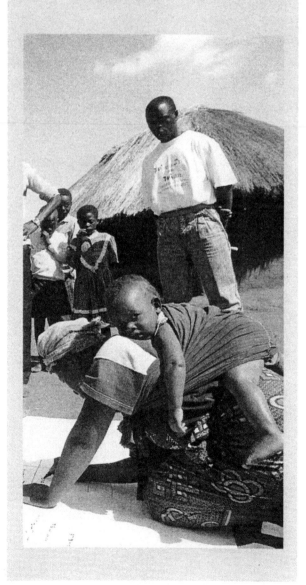

CHALLENGING

INEQUITIES

IN HEALTH

From Ethics to Action

OXFORD
UNIVERSITY PRESS

2001

OXFORD
UNIVERSITY PRESS

Oxford   New York
Athens   Auckland   Bangkok   Bogotá   Buenos Aires   Calcutta
Cape Town   Chennai   Dar es Salaam   Delhi   Florence   Hong Kong   Istanbul
Karachi   Kuala Lumpur   Madrid   Melbourne   Mexico City   Mumbai
Nairobi   Paris   São Paulo   Shanghai   Singapore   Taipei   Tokyo   Toronto   Warsaw
and associated companies in
Berlin   Ibadan

Published by Oxford University Press, Inc.,
198 Madison Avenue, New York, New York, 10016
http://www.oup-usa.org

Library of Congress Cataloging-in-Publication Data
Challenging inequities in health : from ethics to action/
edited by Timothy Evans. . . [et al.].
p. cm.   Includes bibliographical references and index
ISBN-13 978-0-19-513740-8 (pbk.)
ISBN 0-19-513739-6—ISBN 0-19-513740-X (pbk.)
1. Public health—Moral and ethical aspects—Cross cultural studies—Congresses.
2. Health promotion—Moral and ethical aspects—Cross-cultural studies—Congresses.
3. Medical ethics—Cross-cultural studies—Congresses.
I. Evans, Timothy.
RA422.C45 2001   362.1—dc21   00-062395

6 8 9 7 5

Printed in the United States of America
on acid-free paper

The health of the people is really the foundation upon which all their happiness and all their powers as a state depend.
—Benjamin Disraeli

Foreword

I am delighted that this much-needed book, *Challenging Inequities in Health,* is being published. It is the result of painstaking and cutting-edge research that has been done over the past 3 years in Bangladesh and many other parts of the world. I am proud that the conference in which the findings of these studies were presented for the first time was held in Dhaka and that I was fortunate to have had the opportunity to speak there as well. It is indeed a great pleasure and honor to write this foreword.

The question of inequity in different aspects of life is a global problem. Inequality or, more importantly, inequity, is a matter of great concern for us all. We are stunned to see the perpetuation of inequities between men and women, between urban and rural areas, and between rich and poor. At the dawn of the third millennium, the large differences in health conditions between various subgroups of the population are simply unacceptable to us. Bangladesh is one of three countries in the world where women live a shorter life than men. This is unfortunate, but it is a fact! It has to be changed.

It is essential to ensure equal rights between women and men in all spheres of life. The Constitution of Bangladesh has a provision for this. I believe that for development of any society or country the rights of both women and men have to be equally developed. A society can never be developed completely if the women are undermined and only the men are provided with education, culture, and health care services. This is particularly true in developing countries like Bangladesh, which need to take stronger measures to improve their socioeconomic conditions. Low literacy rates; malnutrition and poor health conditions, especially for women and children; rampant poverty; premature death of children; and an overall standard of living that is well below the poverty level are just a few of the conditions that these countries share. The rich and developed countries should extend their generous hands in this regard. Equal rights for men and women can help ensure balanced development of a society and country as well. The whole body cannot remain active without a limb. Similarly, the society becomes crippled and fails to be a developed one without the development of the womenfolk.

Health is the basis of all happiness. The potential for building a developed world in the new century depends crucially on equality of access to the prerequisites for health for all members of society.

Fortunately, we are moving with the rest of the world in removing health inequity from the fabric of the society in which we live. A chapter included in this volume has documented the positive impact and success of a "focused" poverty alleviation program in removing inequities in health outcome between rich and poor in Bangladesh. The world is now placing much importance on human development. In our country we have been able to remove the disparity between boys and girls in their access to primary education. We have pragmatic programs for the empowerment of women so that they can participate in the decision making along with men. These few examples show that there is light at the end of the tunnel, and we are determined to move along with the rest of the world toward a future where disparity between various groups in the population would be a strange relic of the past. In this arduous task, the joint actions of the people and governments in the North and the South, as has been successfully done in the Global Health Equity Initiative, will be of paramount importance.

Finally, I congratulate the editors and the authors of different chapters for their groundbreaking work, which I am sure will have a profound impact on the way the world thinks about equity and inequity in the future. I also thank the Rockefeller Foundation and the Swedish International Development Cooperation Agency for their support of this initiative.

Sheikh Hasina
Prime Minister of Bangladesh
Government of the People's Republic of Bangladesh
Dhaka, 12 January 2000

Preface

Motivated by a common concern about unacceptable differentials in health, what was a small initial international collaboration in 1996 evolved into the Global Health Equity Initiative (GHEI). This network links over 100 researchers from more than 15 countries who are unified by their interest in finding ways to address inequities in health. This volume, representing the combined efforts of a diverse, multidisciplinary group, presents the results of the GHEI for the first time.

Concurrent with the development of the GHEI was a burgeoning interest in inequities in health both in the literature and in policy making. In 1998, the Acheson Report on Inequalities in Health was published in the United Kingdom. In the United States, both the National Institutes of Health and the Surgeon General have declared equity in health to be a central priority. The Vietnamese Ministry of Health explicitly states equity and efficiency as dual goals for the health system. On a global level, the World Bank, UNICEF, the Pan American Health Organization, and the World Health Organization have embraced the elimination of inequalities in health as an important target and have begun to implement programs to redress health inequities. A special issue of the *Bulletin of the World Health Organization* (78(1) 2000) was devoted to inequalities in health, and the 1999 *World Health Report* includes analysis of the excess health risks experienced by the poor within each country. Furthermore, a new entity, the International Society for Equity in Health, was launched in Cuba in the summer of 2000. Thus *Challenging Inequities in Health: From Ethics to Action* is indicative of a broad global shift toward greater attention to the importance of health inequities.

The GHEI is funded by the Rockefeller Foundation and the Swedish International Development Cooperation Agency (SIDA), and its funding is a reflection of its origins. The Initiative was conceived in September 1995, when North American and Swedish researchers and policy analysts, brought together at the Harvard Center for Population and Development Studies, began to look at Swedish policy to reduce inequity. This led to wider ranging discussions, involving more countries, about the major challenge to public health that inequities in health now pose. At the same time, it was clear that the common policy response was inadequate, or even counterproductive. Much more was needed to raise awareness globally, to build capacity in countries of the South as well as the North to diagnose their own problems, and to motivate and stimulate appropriate action. The GHEI therefore represents a concerted effort to ensure that health equity research is undertaken by researchers within the countries most affected by inequities in health. As the first phase of this work, a 3-year Initiative was devised by an international group with five aims:

1. To articulate the concepts and values underlying equity in health.
2. To develop measures and tools for health research and policy to help analyze equity and inequity in health.
3. To encourage empirical research on health inequities within countries in the developing world.
4. To establish a scientific foundation for proactive advocacy, policies, and programs.
5. To stimulate action to reduce inequities in health at all levels of society, by providing decision makers with knowledge and concrete suggestions for change.

From 1996 to 2000, the first phase of the GHEI developed both conceptual and practical research agendas. During this phase, six international, interdisciplinary working groups brought an equity lens to bear on important conceptual issues: ethics, social determinants, gender, measurement, health care financing, globalization, and policy. The conceptual groups convened topic-based seminars gathering leaders in their respective fields to tackle the conceptual underpinnings of health equity. Additional publications will result from these seminars, including edited volumes on ethics and gender inequities. Forthcoming publications include *Public Health, Ethics and Equity* (Oxford: Oxford University Press) and *Engendering International*

Health: The Challenge of Equity (Cambridge: MIT Press).

Alongside the conceptual work, 12 teams, representing a range of countries in the South and the North, embarked on in-depth country analyses. The focus of these country studies was determined by the teams themselves with periodic convenings of the larger group permitting the sharing of ideas, methods, and results. Composition of the teams was also heterogeneous, ranging from researchers in diverse disciplines to policy makers and NGO providers. From Asia, there are case studies of Bangladesh, China, Japan, and Vietnam. From Africa, Kenya, Tanzania, and South Africa furnish the cases. Mexico, Chile, and two US studies represent the Americas, and Europe is represented by a chapter about Russia and a chapter providing a British-Swedish comparison. It is rare enough to see research on inequities in health in the developing world. In this volume, however, such original research is being presented in juxtaposition with inequities in industrialized and middle-income countries. There are at least three main features that make the GHEI distinctive, over and above the wide range of countries and the large number of international researchers involved:

- The participants in the Initiative share common values and concerns about equity, an interest that drew many to the Initiative in the first place.
- The country studies have been undertaken by study teams within each of the countries rather than by Northern "experts" parachuted in from outside. This is important in terms of generating ownership and ensuring relevance of the results as well as nurturing interest and capacity in health equity analysis.
- The participants in the Initiative, through a mutually supportive network, were able to engage in an ongoing dialogue on the multiple complex dimensions of health equity analysis. The meetings that facilitated these exchanges—held in various locations around the world—provided extraordinary opportunities for the diverse group to challenge their own and each other's thinking about equity in health. Although all participants benefited from such exchange, it was particularly important for those working in countries where there is little or no experience with health equity analysis.

Challenging Inequities in Health: From Ethics to Action is designed to bring the research and policy analysis of the GHEI to a wider non-specialist readership of students, professionals, and policymakers. It is the first book to give a truly global perspective on health equity, with contributors from each country of the highest caliber. Reflecting the purpose of the GHEI itself, this book aims to contribute to the building of global capacity to measure, monitor, and interpret developments in health equity at national and international levels to underpin action.

The book is organized around four key elements that structure a systematic response to inequities in health: establishing and strengthening shared values (part I), describing the health divide and analyzing causes (part II), tackling the root causes of inequities in health (part III), reducing the negative consequences of ill health and building more equitable health care systems (part IV).

This volume deals with each element in turn. Part I identifies the fundamental underpinnings of a systematic response concerned with establishing shared concepts and principles for action. Chapter 2 deals with social concepts and theories. It addresses the fundamental question of how societies generate and maintain social and health inequities and presents a unifying framework for designing research and policy development on this issue. In chapter 3, ethical concepts are clarified—What is equity in health? How is it linked to social justice? Why should we be concerned with inequities in health anyway? In chapter 4, the concept of globalization is explored and an assessment made of its potential influence on health and equity. How then are the globalizing processes that are underway to be confronted and used for, rather than against, the promotion of health equity?

Part II covers the assessment of the health divide and the analysis of its causes. It begins with an overview of fundamental measurement considerations in chapter 5, which outlines methods and indicators for making assessments in both data-poor and data-rich countries. In chapter 6, the Nobel Laureate, Amartya Sen, continues the measurement discussion with a consideration of some of the greatest challenges inherent in attempts to measure inequities in health. This is followed by six country-case studies that describe how researchers investigated the size and nature of inequities in health in their country or analyzed causes of those inequities, demonstrating how to make the best use of whatever data are available. These cases start with countries that focus on area-based analyses—China and Japan—followed by cases using individual-level (and area-based) data to analyze the health gap by race, age, education level, and cause (USA, Chile, and Russia). The final chapter in this part, presenting experiences from Tanzania, illustrates the contribution qualitative methods can make to our understanding of the nature and causes of inequities in a society.

Part III moves on to address the main determinants of inequities in health starting with an overview chapter on gender inequities. This chapter traces the complex linkages between gender, equity, and health, outlines the main policy entry points, and gives gender-related examples of each. The next four chapters analyze root causes of inequity at different policy levels: South Africa (multisectoral action to address the legacy of apartheid); Kenya (transport sector and road accidents); experiences from purposeful interventions in Matlab, Bangladesh, through microcredit schemes and other strategies to improve the economic and social status of women in their communities (thereby addressing both poverty-related ill health and gender inequities); and the Anglo-Swedish comparison (illustrating issues of the labor market and social security sectors).

Part IV focuses on policies to take care of those who are already sick by (1) reducing the socioeconomic consequences of illness and (2) building more equitable health care systems. After an introductory overview to this part, chapter 18 discusses the specific issue of how to promote greater equity in health care financing. This is followed in chapter 19 by important new analyses from Mexico, using methods to identify additional needs in geographical areas and outlining the implications for resource allocation for the provision of health care to meet those needs. Chapter 20 provides insight into the policy development approaches adopted in Vietnam, where the pros and cons of different meth-

ods of financing are being carefully weighed in light of the socioeconomic circumstances prevailing in the country.

Challenging Inequities in Health: From Ethics to Action concludes with a chapter that looks to the future and to a more structured development of the policy response. Chapter 21 provides a policy-oriented overview of the whole process from ethics to action, identifying ways of challenging inequities in health and highlighting some practical applications of the approaches advocated, drawn from the rest of the book. It suggests a way forward toward raising awareness of the issue and stimulating policy makers at various levels to take action. Given the global nature of the initiative, this incorporates an important section on how the international agencies could work together to challenge these unacceptable inequities in health. This issue deserves to be at the top of the public health agenda for the new millennium.

T.G.E.
M.M.W.
F.D.
A.B.
M.E.W.

Acknowledgments

The "seeds" of the Global Health Equity Initiative (GHEI) were sown in Bellagio in February 1996 when ten people—Sudhir Anand, Giovanni Berlinguer, Abbas Bhuiya, Lincoln Chen, Göran Dahlgren, Finn Diderichsen, Tim Evans, Max Price, Al Tarlov, and Margaret Whitehead—met to discuss concern over the growing health gap within countries around the world. The original thinkers present at that meeting laid the groundwork for the research initiative and for this volume. Eventually, four of the original ten became editors of this volume, and the Initiative grew to be over 100 strong.

The unique spirit of the GHEI springs from the enthusiasm, diversity, and caliber of its members. The periodic meetings of the GHEI allowed invaluable personal exchanges and linkages between groups not previously connected. Several institutions and their staff hosted key GHEI meetings: the Harvard Center for Population and Development Studies, the King's Fund in London, and the Bellagio Study Center in Italy (which provided an idyllic setting for both the founding meeting of the GHEI and one of the final editing sessions).

Critical initiative-wide meetings occurred over the course of 3 years to exchange ideas on study design, early results, and final drafts. These meetings were held around the globe and hosted by the Université de la Sapienza in Rome, Italy; the Ministry of Health in China; the African Medical and Research Foundation in Nairobi, Kenya; and BRAC, a rural development nongovernmental organization in Bangladesh in collaboration with the International Centre for Diarrheal Disease Research, Bangladesh. The thoughtful planning and energy expended by the hosts of these international meetings allowed in-depth exchange of ideas, as well as field visits to health centers and communities to deepen understanding of local realities.

A number of other meetings and research efforts focused on specific subcomponents of the GHEI and strengthened the conceptual underpinnings of the GHEI research: The Gender group led by Gita Sen, Piroska Östlin, and Asha George; the Ethics group led by Amartya Sen, Sudhir Anand, and Fabienne Peter; the Measurement group facilitated by Vladimir Shkolnikov, Finn Diderichsen, and Sudhir Anand; the Social Determinants meetings led by Ben Amick, Cynthia Lopez, and Jonathan Lavis; and the Finance group spearheaded by Bill Hsiao and Yuanli Liu.

Throughout its life cycle, the GHEI was shepherded smoothly thanks to the orchestration provided at first by Alison Norris and then by Meg Wirth. The funding for the initiative was provided by The Rockefeller Foundation and the Swedish International Development Cooperation Agency (SIDA). (Eva Wallstam's early support for the GHEI is especially appreciated.)

The gathering of the GHEI studies into a single volume was an immense collective effort dependent upon the work of many colleagues. Not every researcher who contributed to the GHEI is indicated in the authorship of the chapters—in many cases teams of 10 to 15 were involved in the data collection, research, and analysis of the GHEI studies. All of their efforts are recognized as critical to the final studies presented herein.

Two members of the panel of referees were asked to review each chapter. Their generous contributions of expertise and wisdom immeasurably improved the quality of the volume.

For their painstaking effort in editing, copyediting, and developing the glossary in this volume, a special debt of gratitude goes to Paula Holland and Valerie Tay. We are also appreciative of Helen Epstein's overall review of the manuscript as it neared completion.

We extend a particular debt of gratitude to the library team at The Rockefeller Foundation, specifically to Tracey Friesen for her remarkable efficiency in ensuring that reference material from the far reaches of the globe was available to us. The hard work and patience on the part of the Health Equity program colleagues is appreciated, with a particular thanks to Orneata Prawl, Henni Donnenfeld, and Di Eckerle. At the Harvard Center for Population and Development Studies, we would like to acknowledge Winifred

Fitzgerald, Sue Carlson, and Chris Cahill. Furthermore, we would like to thank Terry Fischer, Alison Strong, and Megan Klose of Communications Development, Inc., for their rigorous editing, design, and production of the figures and tables in this volume.

We are grateful to Jeffrey House of Oxford University Press for his strategic input on the flow and format of this book and for his role in making the content more accessible to a non-specialist audience. For their work in the crucial final stages of the production of this volume, we are appreciative of the attention to detail and design provided by Susan Hannan, Donna Miller, Leslie Anglin, and Edith Barry of Oxford University Press. In addition, the haven provided through the auspices of Professor Alayne Adams was critical to much of the editing process.

Finally, we owe an inestimable debt of gratitude to our families who provided support and encouragement and who withstood long absences in order to ensure this final product.

Contents

PART
I

ESTABLISHING
VALUES

Source: Sean Sprague/Panos

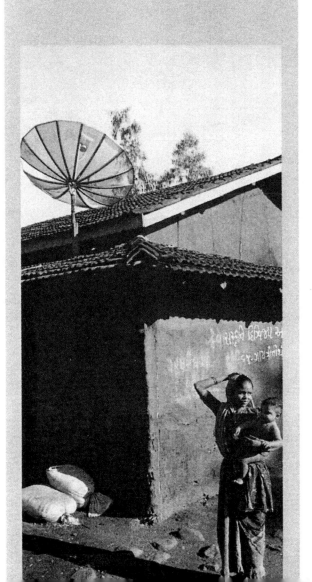

CHAPTER
1

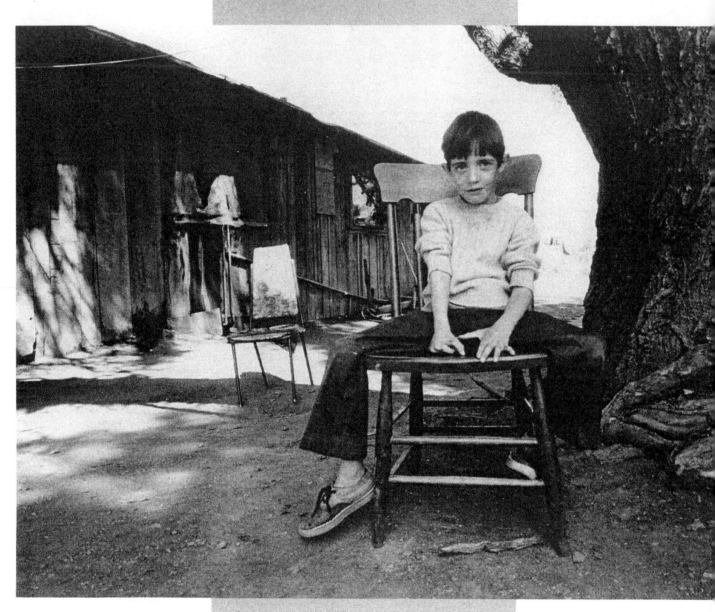

A child at a farm labor camp closed for failure to meet health code requirements. San Jose, California.
Source: Mark Ludak/Impact Visuals/Picture Quest, 1992.

Introduction

TIMOTHY EVANS, MARGARET WHITEHEAD, FINN DIDERICHSEN,
ABBAS BHUIYA, AND MEG WIRTH

Unacceptable Disparities in Health

In the last 50 years of the twentieth century, many countries have experienced gains in health status greater than at any other period in their history. Even in some of the poorest countries in the world, remarkable progress has been made with unprecedented increases in life expectancy and improvements in child survival. Although these successes in aggregate health might lead to complacency, once we scratch the surface a very different picture emerges. In some countries of sub-Saharan Africa, for example, the average age of death has declined from 5 years to 2 years in the last decade (Sen 1999). Sharp declines in life expectancy have also been recorded in countries of the former Soviet Union, including a health crisis of unforeseen proportions in the Russian Federation during the years 1993 to 1996, when life expectancy fell below 60 years for men and below 72 years for women (see chapter 11).

When national-level data are disaggregated to discern the fate of different groups within societies, similarly disturbing disparities are apparent. In post-apartheid South Africa, for example, infant mortality is five times higher among blacks than among whites, and even within each racial/ethnic population there is a "health divide" between the poor, middle-income, and rich groups (see chapter 14). In many developing economies, large differentials in health emerge between rural areas, which tend to be poorer, and the richer urban centers. The proportion of children under age 5 years who are stunted, for example, is 50% higher in rural parts of Malawi than in urban parts of the country. Even more dramatic, in Vietnam and China, rates of childhood stunting are over three times higher in the rural populations (UNICEF 1999). Maternal mortality in the poor province of Quinghai in the Chinese interior is ten times higher than in the more prosperous coastal areas such as Zhejiang Province (see chapter 7).

A similar pattern is evident in the most affluent countries in the world. In the United States, a 13 year gap in women's life expectancy and a 16 year gap for men's have been observed when comparing the counties with the lowest and highest mortality rates—patterns that closely follow the contours of poverty and ethnic minority status in the nation (Murray et al. 1998). Even in some of the healthiest countries in Western Europe—the Netherlands, Finland, and the United Kingdom included—we find a gradient in health across the social spectrum, with poorer groups dying 5 to 10 years earlier than the richer groups (Whitehead and Diderichsen 1997) and with up to a 13 year gap in disability-free life expectancy between the affluent and deprived in the same countries (van de Water et al. 1996; Valkonen et al. 1997).

Health disparities, therefore, appear to be pervasive both between and within nations across the globe.

Whether a country is rich or poor and whether it has high aggregate health or low, opportunities for good health are highly unequal.

What Is Meant by Equity in Health?

This volume reflects a growing concern for the disparities in health that are found both between and within nations. *Inequalities* in health describe the differences in health between groups independent of any assessment of their fairness. *Inequities* refer to a subset of inequalities that are deemed unfair. The unfairness qualification invokes assessments of whether the inequalities are avoidable as well as more complex ideas of distributive justice as applied to health (see chapter 3).

Characteristic of the country-case studies in this volume is a focus on equity in health outcomes. This is a deliberate point of departure and reflects the premise that disparities in health outcomes are the most important dimension of health equity. Other dimensions such as equity in access to health care, although important in their own right, need to be further understood in relation to their impact on health status. Achieving equitable access to health care is certainly desirable, but if there remain significant health disparities, then equitable health care is not a sufficient condition for health equity. Indeed, Sen (see chapter 6) argues that the assessment of health equity must extend beyond health care received to include other ways of improving health outcomes (e.g., through education) and the freedom to achieve these outcomes.

Equity in health takes intuitive ideas about what is "fair" and attempts to make them more explicit. Attaining optimal health ought not to be compromised by the social, political, ethnic, or occupational group into which one happens to fall. To the extent that disparities in health coincide with fault lines between such groups, one may make the assessment that they are unfair and thus constitute inequities. Although each of the studies in this volume focuses on a different aspect of disparities in health—child or adult health, disability, morbidity or mortality, disparities between the sexes, occupational groups, in rural and urban populations, by geographic area—in most cases, the authors are making the claim that the inequalities examined are *avoidable* and *unfair*. These claims, or value statements, may be articulated discretely through empirical descriptions of social inequalities in health or more overtly. In the Japan case, for example, the analysis sets out to assess the extent to which the cultural value of

"yokonarabi" (same to the next person) is reflected in the magnitude of geographic and occupational inequities in health (see chapter 8). Beyond empirical analyses, the credibility and integrity of these values are strengthened by engaging those most deeply affected in the definition of the dimensions of a specific inequity, as seen in the cases of Tanzania and Kenya (see chapters 12 and 15).

In addition to the moral claim about unfairness and the assessment that health inequities are avoidable, there are other dimensions of disparities in health that are important rationales for policy mobilization and action. These include arguments related to relieving pain and suffering of the least healthy, the aversion that populations feel to unequal outcomes in health for particularly vulnerable groups such as children, the threats to population health represented by residual reservoirs of epidemic infection, for example, in urban slums, and the emerging evidence that serious illness leads to impoverishment and/or acts as a constraint to economic growth.

Deep-seated imbalances generated by discrimination and power differences often underlie disparities in health. Such power discrepancies occur across a broad sociopolitical spectrum—from a state of lawlessness and corruption where a few warlords control the state and command all its resources to the other extreme of a democratic, peaceful nation with entrenched social and occupational hierarchies. Although the differences between these contexts are obvious, the fact that the broader social context influences health, whether subtle or overt, is a common phenomenon.

The aim of this volume is not to argue that the health community should tackle all instances of power differentials and conflict; nor is it our intention to address the challenging and politically unrealistic endeavor of "flattening" the social gradient. The social, economic, and political determinants that lie outside the health sector, yet that profoundly affect health status and its distribution, cannot, however, be dismissed in crafting an effective response. Similarly, a fully articulated effort to redress inequities in health must inevitably work in tandem with wider efforts toward social justice—such as the provision of safety nets; protection against medical impoverishment; provision of education, jobs training, and environmental risk reduction; and efforts to ensure peace and a political voice for all. "Health equity is best thought of not as a social goal in and of itself, but as inherently imbedded in a more general pursuit of social justice" (see chapter 3).

Securing a commitment to equity in health may be facilitated by articulating targets that take into account the distribution of health. The final chapter in this volume provides examples of two types of targets: symbolic, their main purpose being to inspire and motivate; and practical, to help monitor progress toward equity and to improve accountability in the use of resources (Whitehead et al. 1998).

How Do We Measure Inequities in Health?

Without hard evidence on trends in health equity, we can neither expose current disparities nor prove our success in narrowing these gaps over time. Hence, in many countries the lack of vital statistics and reliable health information represents a de facto statement that the health of its people does not count. "The lack of basic mortality and morbidity statistics for the black population (in South Africa) is a clear sign that their needs were simply not considered in health policy development" (see chapter 14). Even in the context of seemingly plentiful data on health, requirements for equity analysis often necessitate linkages between social and health data sets that are methodologically and logistically challenging (Krieger et al. 1997).

Despite these data constraints, each of the studies in this volume has managed to describe important health disparities that might otherwise be concealed in aggregate health indicators. It is important to recognize, however, that such descriptions of inequities in health—in terms of both their nature and magnitude—are sensitive to a number of basic considerations (see chapter 5). The myriad expressions of illness, whether disease, disability, or death, and the properties of their measurement—what Sen terms *measurability*—are primary considerations in assessing inequities (see chapters 5 and 6). Another basic consideration involves identifying a reference group or norm against which inequities in health outcomes may be assessed. Assessing gender inequities in survival, for example, may involve making judgements about the biological (or inevitable) difference in longevity between men and women (see chapter 16 on Bangladesh) or entail survival comparisons to an average for countries at a similar stage of development (see chapter 11). Values and technical considerations also underlie the discourse surrounding whether distributions of health should be assessed independent of the aggregate level of health. We maintain that it is necessary to do both—to make an assessment of aggregate health, but also to analyze differentials in health, even in data-poor settings.

These challenges or drawbacks notwithstanding, there is a wide spectrum of measures employed in this volume, ranging from the simple and intuitive to the more technically complex (see chapter 5). Despite earlier assessments in the literature (Wagstaff et al. 1991), however, it is perhaps premature to make recommendations on a single best measure. The range of issues involved in moving toward reliable and valid measures that can be compared over time and across contexts is indeed daunting, and, as Amartya Sen concludes in his chapter, "much work remains to be done" (see chapter 6).

What Are the Global Patterns of Health Inequities?

Historical analyses have indicated that although risk factors for ill health change over time, they tend to cluster disproportionately within the lower ends of the social hierarchy. In other words, the better-off, more educated, more powerful, and wealthier in society have much greater capacity to improve their health than do the less well-off—a pattern that is sustained over time and across place.

This time-tested observation is validated in this volume, which brings specific attention to the social stratification of health outcomes in a global context. It challenges the idea that disparities in health only occur above a certain level of national wealth or, alternatively, that some countries are too poor to have significant social stratification of health outcomes (Antonovsky 1979; Wilkinson 1996)—the hypothesis of absolute material deprivation. In the early 1980s in Bangladesh, one of the world's poorest countries, there was a very steep gradient in child mortality according to gender and socioeconomic status: Girls from the poorest households had the highest mortality rates, with better survival chances observed among boys and with increases in the level of household wealth (see chapter 16). The evidence from the cases supports the emerging consensus that inequities in health are found within all countries regardless of their so-called level of development and/or wealth.

A unifying element among the case studies in this volume is that they seek to document differences in health between social groups. In Chile, health disparities between educational groups are measured; in the U.S. case study, the focus is on race/ethnicity and income groups; in Russia, the indicators are sex, education, and marital status; and in Mexico and Japan, county and prefecture-level provide the focus, respectively. Below we draw on this collection of empirical evidence and summarize the most salient findings.

Poverty and Marginalization

In many of the countries respresented in this volume, poverty and marginalization are the underlying or "fundamental" causes of inequities in health. In Mexico, the highest death rates at every stage of life, from infancy to adulthood, are found in the most marginalized counties, that is, those with the lowest income, poorest household infrastructure, highest illiteracy, *and* the largest indigenous populations (chapter 19). In Tanzania, family poverty sets off a domino effect with direct consequences for adolescent health and well-being—children are forced to drop out of school and work. As unskilled labor they resort to informal sector jobs in mines or on the streets, occupations that carry disproportionately high health risks (chapter 12).

Inequities in health occur across a wide range of disease types and causes, with the vulnerability and exposure to these diseases as well as their negative consequences inevitably clustering among those at the lower end of the socioeconomic spectrum. In contradistinction to the existing orthodoxy, communicable diseases are not the only health burden borne by the poor. Accidents, injuries, and violence and many noncommunicable diseases and risk factors are disproportionately concentrated in the poorer populations.

Over a lifetime, there are cumulative adverse health effects that result from living in persistent poverty (Kuh and Ben-Shlomo 1997). Multiple, overlapping forms of discrimination or marginalization compound the effects of poverty. For example, being poor, female, and a member of an ethnic group suffering discrimination confers a magnified health risk as a result of heightened vulnerability. Likewise, although the vast majority of South Africa's poor are black, those at greatest risk are members of female-headed families, those with low education, the unemployed, and residents of former "homeland" areas (chapter 14). The cumulative health effects of poverty and marginalization, which extend across generations, are evident in the legacy of apartheid, or institutionalized racism. Furthermore, new technologies, interventions, and health opportunities tend to be more readily appropriated by the better-off (Mechanic 2000). A corollary to these observations is the fact that interventions for one specific disease will not necessarily lower the burden on the poor because their underlying vulnerability makes it likely that one risk, or disease, avoided will be rapidly replaced by another (see chapter 2).

Marginalization is often equated with poverty, but may also be defined through geographic, ethnic, or racially based exclusion or even as a result of disability and illness. The numerous forms of marginalization must be taken into account as their relative importance as stratifying variables will differ according to context. Likewise, poverty must be seen as a heterogeneous concept, a factor that inhibits well-being and multiple facets of livelihoods. As the chapters in this volume attest, part of the answer to redressing health inequities lies in meeting basic needs and eliminating structural poverty. Thus, health interventions would do well to respond to much more than just the currently expressed need, evidenced by a particular symptom or illness. Moving much further upstream to redress disproportionate risks associated with poverty—and not just the health *effects* of these risks—is critical. As shown in the Britain/Sweden comparative study, the health effects of poverty may be modified by other social policies and safety nets (see chapter 17). The fact that poverty and marginalization are so linked to ill health and yet are unfair, modifiable determinants makes these issues a health equity priority.

Urban/Rural

Rapid urbanization in many parts of the world creates an increasingly complex terrain for analysis of the disparity between rural and urban populations. Traditional "urban bias" has resulted in the preferential allocation of resources and services to the more vocal populations in cities. This bias appears to have been accentuated by China's rapid economic transition with a corresponding increase in the gap in health between urban and rural areas. Urban advantage, however, is less clear in other cases. In Russia, the mortality crisis accompanying the "shock" economic reforms was highly concentrated in urban areas. The emerging patterns of urbanization in Kenya have concentrated the risk of road traffic accidents in the more populated centers. Finally, in South Africa, "informal urban" in addition to rural and homeland dwellers had higher levels of ill health than other groups. The increasing concentration of the world's poor in urban settings presents a new field of inquiry for health equity research and intervention (Stephens 1998).

Social Status

It is commonly observed that increases in social status are paralleled by increases in health. Alternatively stated, each unit increase in education level or occu-

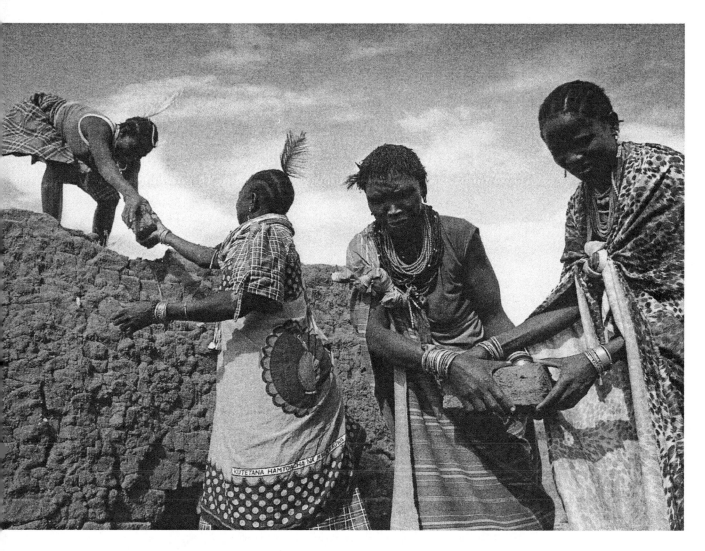

Kaabong, Karamoja, Uganda. Karamojong women unloading bricks they have made and fired as part of a WFP (World Food Programme) food for work scheme. The women are constructing premises for training women in small trades and to act as headquarters for the local Women's Club.
Source: Crispin Hughes/Panos.

pational hierarchy yields corresponding increments in health outcomes. Below we discuss two primary expressions of social status—education and employment—and their association with health and health equity.

Education

Education's role as a determinant of health has been well documented, and many of the studies in this volume provide additional evidence and new insights into this robust association. In general, survival chances are greatest in the highest educational classes. In the China and South Africa studies, greater levels of literacy or maternal education are strongly correlated with decreased rates of infant mortality (see chapters 7 and 14). In modern Japan, with very high levels of educational attainment, differentials between prefectures in education among women continue to maintain a strong association with prefecture-level life expectancy at age 40 years (see chapter 8). The important role of education may also be seen in the Chilean and Russian analyses, where education appears to act as a buffer against the adverse health effects of economic transition. Vega and colleagues argue that without a doubling of investment in education during the period of economic reforms in Chile, health inequities would be much greater than they are currently (see chapter 10). Similarly, in Russia those with higher levels of education, particularly women, were less affected in the mortality crisis than were those with lower levels of education (see chapter 11).

The weight of evidence here and elsewhere makes education a compelling policy consideration for redressing health inequities. First, higher levels of education appear to confer lower risks of ill health or death across a wide variety of causes, including cancers, cardiovascular diseases, accidents and violence, and alcohol. Second, these benefits occur across cultures and nation states and may be appreciating in the global information age (see chapter 4). Finally, the health benefits of education are not specific to age—they occur across the lifespan and spill over into future generations. As stated in the summation of the Tanzanian analysis, those who remain in school are "on the road to health," a path that leads to a life of opportunities (see chapter 12).

Employment or livelihoods

At the most basic level, the link between employment and health lies in whether individuals can generate an income sufficient to sustain well-being. In Russia, the unemployed have the highest mortality rates in the adult population. Furthermore, job security has an ef-

fect on life expectancy—in Russia, high job turnover rate is strongly correlated with decreased life expectancy. Also important is the extent to which unemployment coincides with poverty or with lower socioeconomic status. There is evidence of a health benefit in the provision of employment as seen in Bangladesh, where health benefits for both women and their children are correlated with increasing women's income-generating opportunities through microcredit.

Within the employed workforce health is stratified by job-related factors such as exposure to specific health hazards and the degree of labor regulations. In Tanzania, the most destitute adolescents are forced to eke out their livelihoods in the highest risk occupations—working in unsafe mines and engaging in commercial sex work (see chapter 12). Labor conditions affect not only the workers themselves, but the public at large. In Kenya, the increasing health burden attributable to road traffic accidents is seen to stem, in part, from an unregulated, corrupt *matatu* (bus) industry (see chapter 15). Even in contexts where the majority of employment is in the formal sector, there are important health gradations across occupations. In Japan, death rates among male service and agricultural workers are one-third higher than death rates among managers, professionals, clerks, and salesmen (see chap-ter 8). In both Sweden and Britain, there are striking stepwise gradients in health across the hierarchy from semiskilled/unskilled manual workers to high-level professionals and managers (see chapter 17). Such occupational health gradients have been demonstrated in many other settings and represent one of the primary lines of inquiry into the social determinants of health.

Gender

Inequity in health stemming from gender-related determinants can be thought of in two distinct ways. First, biologically specific health needs of men and women may not be fairly accommodated by health and social systems. Perhaps the starkest example of this type of gender inequity is seen in international differences in maternal mortality: In the poorest countries of the world women's chances of dying in childbirth are 1 in 16, whereas in the richest countries the risks are 1 in 2000. Second, differentials in health between men and women may arise from societal constructions of gender and not from biological differences between the sexes. Differences in the roles societies accord males and females stratify their opportunities for good health. For example, intrahousehold allocation of food is often male biased, leading to greater undernutrition for girls. This cultural preference for sons in some countries of Asia has led to a disproportionate number of males relative to females, a phenomenon Amartya Sen has labeled "missing women" (Sen 1992; Das Gupta 1998).

Gaps in health outcomes between sexes are observed in most of the cases in this volume. Most striking, perhaps, are the mortality or survival differentials. In Russia, women now outlive men by 13 years on average, among the widest within country gender gaps in life expectancy recorded (see chapter 11). In contrast, in China since 1987, the gender gap in infant mortality rates (IMRs) has grown steadily due to ongoing improvements in male IMRs and a disturbing absence of improvements among females (see chapter 7). When direct mortality comparisons are made between men and women, their underlying biological differences in survival must not be overlooked. Adjusting the comparison of child mortality in Bangladesh according to male and female norms revealed the persistence of a significant gender inequity, whereas the unadjusted comparison indicated gender equality (see chapter 16). The analysis of gender differentials in health provides some revealing insights into the fundamental distinction between equity and equality. Namely, it is entirely conceivable that there may be equality of outcomes that are inequitable and, conversely, unequal outcomes that are equitable.

The cases in this volume suggest that gradients in health may have significantly different expressions for men and women. The chapter on gender and health equity provides examples of how poor women fare compared with poor men in terms of adult mortality—with the relative sex advantages varying across countries (see chapter 13). The analysis in Bangladesh showed that socioeconomic inequities in female child survival were more pronounced relative to those for males in the early 1980s. In contrast, the observation that social gradients in health for adult men are generally more pronounced or steeper than for women (Macintyre 1998) is supported in the analyses of education inequalities in Russia and Chile, income and race differentials in the United States, occupational inequalities in Britain and Sweden, and county marginality in Mexico. It is important to note, however, that the comparison of such social gradients between men and women may be compromised by the gender insensitivity of the classification system itself—for example, specific occupational differences within levels of a job hierarchy and women's dual burden in the home may not be reflected in a straightforward comparison of existing measures of social class (Sacker et al. 2000).

Above all, the evidence herein supports the need for sex disaggregation of health data. Not only are the pat-terns of inequality in health different, the underlying causes, the pathways through which the social context stratifies health, and the specific diseases through which these social processes are manifested are likely to differ based on gender. Furthermore, the explicit role of policies both within and outside of the health sector must be assessed for their role in exacerbating gender inequities (see chapters 12 and 13).

Social Context and Social Policies

Social policies and social context represent a broad set of determinants encompassing political, cultural, social, and economic factors. As articulated in the South Africa chapter, the nature of the political system, its values and processes for participation, define the frontiers of opportunity for health equity. Systems characterized by the absence of democracy, pervasive corruption, violence, endemic racism, and gender discrimination are breeding grounds for inequities in health (and in other social spheres). In contrast, societies with flourishing democracies, respect for human rights, transparency, and opportunities for civic engagement—high social capital—are more likely to be equity-enhancing.

Reflecting this underlying context, macroeconomic, labor, and social policies may either limit or enhance health opportunities for different groups in the population. In the era of liberal macroeconomic policy "pro-growth" strategies tend to provide enhanced opportunity to those with resources and high levels of education while large segments of the population without these assets are unlikely to be beneficiaries and may—as seen as Russia—even become casualties of economic transition. Unfortunately, less attention has been paid to education and labor policies, which not only modify the effects of macroeconomic policies but are fundamental determinants of human agency, and ultimately health, in all contexts. Regulation of the transport industry, the promotion or subsidization of substances such as tobacco and alcohol, and the government's approach to domestic violence are among the spectrum of policies that have a bearing on health and health equity. Insofar as all of these aspects of the social context are seen as key determinants of health, they must increasingly become an inherent part of public health strategies. As Gilson and McIntyre acknowledge, "health policy makers . . . have a vital role in signaling when other policies may undermine efforts to promote health equity" (see chapter 14).

One critical component of social policy is the health or medical care system. Although it is well established and increasingly acknowledged that health care is but one determinant of health outcomes (Bunker et al. 1999), it is nevertheless quite an important one. Despite remarkable progress in medical knowledge and technologies, access to health care remains highly skewed both within and between countries. In addition to financial, geographic, and cultural barriers to accessing care, widespread health sector reforms promoting privatization of health care and regressive health care financing schemes figure prominently in the generation of health inequities. In China, where the health care system is undergoing such reforms, up to one-third of the poor are unable to access hospital care due to its prohibitive costs. For those who are able to access care, the costs of doing so may be impoverishing, leading households into a downward spiral of indebtedness and further poor health. Beyond these two stratifying effects of health care lies the more general tendency of health systems—even those offering free and universal health care—to disproportionately cater to the needs of healthier and wealthier groups. In Mexico, in the highly marginalized counties where health needs are greatest, public hospital beds, physicians per capita, and the percentage of deliveries in hospitals are the lowest.

A Global Response

Several global trends over recent decades have made the need to challenge health inequities a matter of greater urgency. First, an increasing number of countries have been going through periods of intense economic transition. When coupled with economic growth policies that pay no attention to social investments or to compensatory educational and labor policies, these transitions have exacerbated the extent of inequity in health. In this respect, a number of the case studies in this volume—those on Russia, Chile, and China—bear witness to these adverse effects.

Second, there has been a transition in the burden of disease in many countries, which is not, as was previously thought, simply a matter of a switch from communicable to noncommunicable disease as countries develop. Rather, in many countries, the poor now carry a disproportionate triple burden—communicable, noncommunicable, and sociobehavioral. Thus, death and disability due to violence, substance abuse, and road traffic accidents take a greater toll on the poor in many contexts. The sweep of globalization will likely exacerbate the sociobehavioral threats, with a predicted disproportionate impact on the poor (see chapter 4).

Third, globalization is rapidly emerging as an important stratifier of health outcomes. Whether its potential is effectively harnessed or its threats duly delivered remains to be seen. The global health community, however, cannot afford to stand by idly and watch what happens. Rather, health concerns and opportunities must be actively voiced in global debates and institutional settings (chapter 4). As Jonathan Mann presciently noted in the mid 1990s—not only is the risk of AIDS global but so too is the response (Mann 2000). The litmus test of a new era for global health equity lies in the world's response to the AIDS epidemic.

Fourth is the evidence of a worsening situation, with more countries reporting growing disparities in health between different groups in their populations as socioeconomic inequalities widen. An overriding message in this volume, articulated by Whitehead and colleagues in Chapter 21, is that we need not, and must not, tolerate these adverse developments. Although disparities in health between social groups exist in all societies, it is imperative to emphasize that such disparities can be modified by specific policies: They are not inevitable. This requires a refocusing of effort to

- Become more sensitive to our propensity to *generate* disparities through the health and social sectors
- Recognize inequities in health as a critical reflection of social injustice
- Promote distribution in health as a legitimate focus of health policy and health research
- Generate evidence on how to monitor and redress inequities

The challenge before us, therefore, is not merely the promotion of health, but a fair chance for all to achieve it.

References

Antonovsky A. 1979. Social class, life expectancy and overall mortality. *Milbank Memorial Fund Quarterly* XLV(2):31–72.

Bunker J.P., Frazier H.S., Mosteller F. 1995. The role of medical care in determining health: creating an inventory of benefits. In: Amick C., Levine S., Tarlov A.R., Walsh D.C., (eds), *Society and Health*, New York: Oxford University Press, pp. 304–341.

Das Gupta M. 1987. Selective discrimination against female children in rural Punjab, India. *Population and Development Review* 13:77–100.

Krieger N., Williams D.R., Moss N.E. 1997. Measuring social class in public health research. *Annual Review of Public Health* 18:341–378.

Kuh, D., Ben-Shlomo Y. (eds). 1997. *A Life Course Approach to Chronic Disease Epidemiology*. Oxford: Oxford University Press.

Macintyre S. 1998. Social inequalities and health in the contemporary world: comparative overview. In: Strickland S.S., Shetty P.S. (eds), *Human Biology and Social Inequality*. 39th Symposium volume of the Society for the Study of Human Biology. Cambridge: Cambridge University Press, pp. 20–33.

Mann J. 2000. The transformative potential of the HIV/AIDS pandemic. *Reproductive Health Matters* 7(14):164–173.

Mechanic D. 2000. Rediscovering the social determinants of health. Book Review Essay. *Health Affairs* May/June:269–276.

Murray C.J.L., Michaud C.M. McKenna M.T., Marks J.S. 1998. *U.S. Patterns of Mortality by County and Race: 1965–1994.* Cambridge: Harvard Center for Population and Development Studies

Sacker A., Firth D., Fitzpatrick R., Lynch K., Bartley M. 2000. Comparing health inequality in women and men: prospective study of mortality 1986–1996. *British Medical Journal* 320:1303–1307.

Sen A. 1992. Missing women: social inequality outweighs women's survival advantage in Asia and north Africa. *British Medical Journal* 304:587–588.

Sen A. 1999. *Development as Freedom.* New York: Alfred A. Knopf.

Stephens C. 1998. The policy implications of health inequalities in developing countries. In: Strickland S.S., Shetty P.S. (eds), *Human Biology and Social Inequality.* 39th Symposium volume of the Society for the Study of Human Biology. Cambridge: Cambridge University Press, pp. 288–307.

UNICEF. 1999. *The Progress of Nations 1999.* New York: UNICEF.

Valkonen T., Sihvonen A.-P., Lahelma E. 1997. Health expectancy by level of education in Finland. *Social Science and Medicine* 44:801–808.

van de Water H., Boshuizen H., Perenboom R. 1996. Health expectancy in the Netherlands 1983–1990. *European Journal of Public Health* 6: 21–28.

Wagstaff A., Paci P., van Doorslaer E. 1991. On the measurement of inequalities in health. *Social Science and Medicine* 33:545–577.

Whitehead M., Diderichsen F. 1997. International evidence on social inequalities in health. In: Drever F., Whitehead M. (eds), *Health Inequalities—Decennial Supplement.* DS Series No. 15. Office for National Statistics. London: The Stationery Office, pp. 45–69.

Whitehead M., Scott Samuel A., Dahlgren G. 1998. Setting targets to address inequalities in health. *Lancet* 351:1279–1282.

Wilkinson R. 1996. *Unhealthy Societies: The Afflictions of Inequality.* London, Routledge.

CHAPTER
2

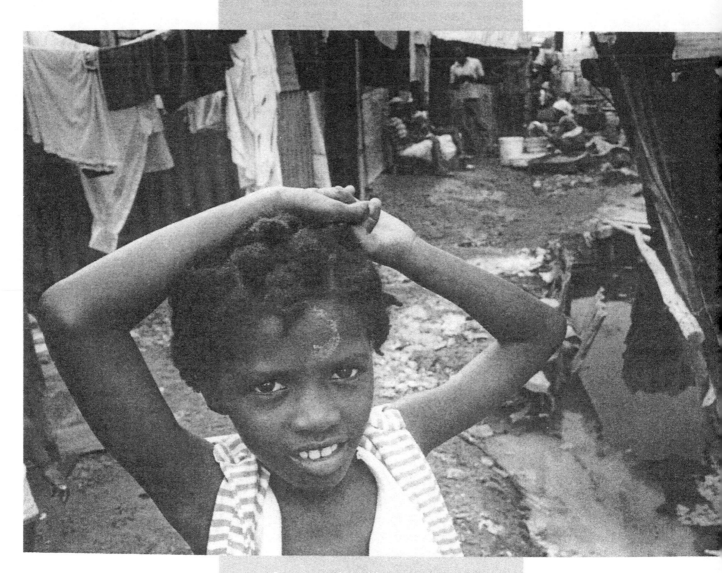

A community with open sewers,
Port-au-Prince, Haiti.
Source: Marc French/Panos.

The Social Basis of Disparities in Health

FINN DIDERICHSEN, TIMOTHY EVANS, AND MARGARET WHITEHEAD

No variation in the health of the states of Europe is the result of chance; it is the direct result of physical and political conditions in which nations live.

—William Farr, 1866

William Farr's insight into the nonrandom nature of health variations between nation-states is as valid at the beginning of the twenty-first century as it was in the mid-nineteenth century—perhaps even more so. Despite the growing capabilities of societies to extend longevity and to combat disease, variations in health between and within countries remain worryingly omnipresent. Some might try to lay blame on the trend in health care and medical research toward an excessive focus on individuals—their biological and behavioral risks of illness—to the relative neglect of population groups and the societal forces that create health divides. This view has provoked lively debates among health researchers, with some arguing for more clinically relevant research on the proximate causes of illness (Rothman et al. 1998), while others point to the health gains that might be achieved by a better understanding of more distal or upstream determinants of health (McKinlay 1993; Krieger 1994).

This chapter takes the view that if we want to understand and intervene against social inequities in health, we will have to look both upstream into the mechanisms of society and downstream into the mechanisms of human biology and the clinical issues of how people cope with disease and disabilities. This is by no means a radical thought. In the nineteenth century, wherever there existed the combination of critical epidemiological thinking, available health data, and a well-organized public health movement, there was a growing interest in the social, physical, and biological causes of epidemic diseases (Beaglehole and Bonita 1997). We posit that a similar combination of clear thinking, good data, and policy mobilization are key ingredients for progress in redressing today's inequities in health.

The burgeoning literature on the social determinants of health (Marmot and Wilkinson 1999; Blane et al. 1994; Kuh et al. 1997) points to substantial differences in health between different population groups that challenge our sense of justice and provoke our scientific curiosity. Although the field is in rapid evolution, there are a number of emerging generalizations worth highlighting.

1. Social gradients in health are pervasive within all countries of the world and not just within rich societies. The "ubiquity, both over time and space, of the observed pattern of systematically poorer health and a shorter life span is associated with each successively lower position in any given system of social stratification" (Macintyre 1998). This challenges earlier think-

ing that the existence of widespread, severe material deprivation in some societies meant that most of the population would suffer from poor health, and there would thus be little differentiation between groups (Antonovsky 1967). It also contrasts with the idea that absolute poverty is the major determinant of inequities in health. A gradient exists in countries and across groups, even in areas where material deprivation is less prevalent. Indeed, health inequities do not go away with the achievement of survival for all (Stephens 1998).

2. There is little understanding of the physiological mechanisms that link social factors to health outcomes although there are a number of exciting areas of inquiry that may shed some light, such as socio-neuroendocrine/immune pathways (Karasek and Theorell 1990) and biological programming (Barker 1998). What is the importance of "stress biology" relative to health-related behaviors (Brunner and Marmot 1999)? What are the precise effects on human biology of prolonged social isolation, social disruption, low social status, job strain, and job insecurity? Initial evidence of physiological mechanisms involving altered functioning of the main neuroendocrine stress pathways indicates that the psychosocial pathway to ill health is not only plausible, but that it should be a significant social policy consideration.

3. The conceptualization of the social determinants of health is limited but evolving rapidly. Traditionally, social determinants have been identified as a characteristic of the individual, such as a person's social support network, income, or employment status. Populations are not merely collections of individuals, however; the causes of ill health are clustered in systematic patterns, and in addition, the effects on one individual may depend on the exposure and outcome for other individuals. The way we organize communities, workplaces, and our societies on the larger national and global scale cannot be understood or measured by looking solely at individuals. Community attributes not specific to individuals, such as social capital and cohesion, and processes such as "globalization" are challenging the individual characterization of social factors (Kawachi and Kennedy 1997; Waitzman and Smith 1998).

These important findings from the social determinants literature have greatly influenced—and will continue to be critical to—our growing understanding of inequities in health. There is now increasing interest in a more explicit investigation of the complex issues about the fairness of disparities in health—thinking about how to differentiate variations in health from inequities in health (see chapter 3, on ethics). Part of making this distinction entails looking at the factors that cause these differentials in health. Insofar as these causes are related to modifiable social arrangements such as access to health care or opportunity for employment, they may be considered unjust. An accurate analysis of the social origins of differentials in health, therefore, may reveal policy entry points for effective action to redress inequities. This chapter presents one such framework for thinking about the social basis of inequities in health.

A Framework for Understanding Social Origins of Health Inequities

The pervasive clinical orientation of epidemiology has resulted most often in the identification of "individual" attributes that differentiate health risk. Such factors include age, sex, dietary habits, smoking, alcohol intake, weight, and blood pressure. The burgeoning literature on social determinants of health emphasizes that many of these individual risk factors cluster around (or are strongly associated with) an individual's *social position* as well as characteristics of the broader *social context* such as place of residence (urban or rural), work environment, or wider social and economic policies of society. For example, social positions measured by levels of education, occupation, or income are frequently found to be associated with a set of individual health risks such as smoking and poor quality diet. Furthermore, the social context and social position may also play an important role in buffering or predisposing different population groups to the "social consequences" of disease or injury. Any practical framework must capture the idea that the physiological end-pathways leading to an individual's ill health are inextricably linked to the social setting.

Furthermore, the articulation of effective actions to redress health inequities is contingent on elucidating the pathways through which social context and position are linked to health outcomes and social consequences of disease. To this end we draw on a framework developed by Diderichsen and Hallqvist (1998). The framework delineates four main mechanisms—social stratification, differential exposure, differential susceptibility, and differential consequences—that play a role in generating health inequities. For each mechanism, the possible policy entry points for interventions are identified. In the following sections, each of the components is dealt with in turn, as illustrated in Figure 1.

Figure 1 A framework for elucidating the pathways from the social context to health outcomes and for introducing policy interventions

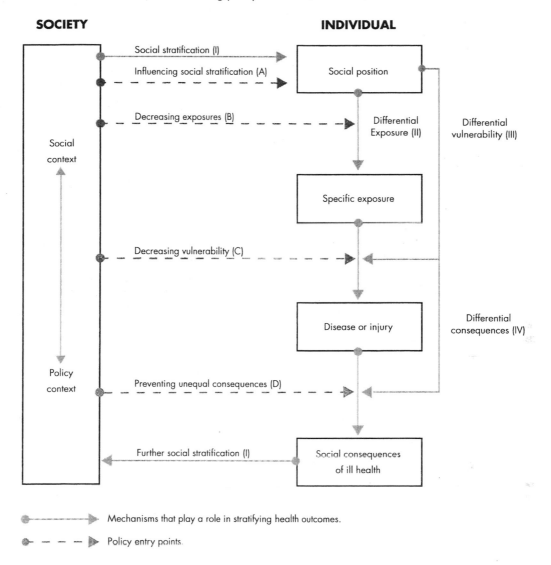

Source: Adapted from Diderichsen and Hallqvist 1998

Social Stratification—
Mechanism I

Social context is a deliberately broad, catch-all phrase used to refer to the spectrum of factors in society that cannot be directly measured at the individual level. Context therefore encompasses the structure, culture, and function of a social system. Although there is no sociological or epidemiological definition of social context, there are four reasons for making links to health and the distribution of health.

First, there is a measurement issue—certain risks for illness are not characteristics of individuals and can only be measured at the group or societal level. Often indicators of context can be measured as aggregates of the characteristics of individuals in a population such as average income or unemployment rates. In other instances, we have to use integral measures such as legislation, cultural norms, and institutional arrangements to capture aspects of the social context that are not simply a function of aggregating individual characteristics (Diez-Rouz 1998).

Second is a conceptual issue—that a population cannot be seen merely as a collection of independent individuals. Rather, a population must also be viewed as a social system in which the distribution and clustering of both exposures and health outcomes are important and in which the contacts between "susceptible" and "contagious" individuals are crucial for the transmission of both biological/infectious agents and social behaviors (Koopman and Longini 1994).

Third, from an etiological point of view, the structure and culture of the social context—the social environment—might be a contributing cause of disease and injury. There are neighborhoods where norms allow violence to prevail, and there are industries and workplaces where organizational behaviors induce stress with its consequent patho-physiological effects (Syme 1994; Hallqvist et al. 1998).

Fourth and finally, the social context encompasses those central engines in society that generate and distribute power, wealth, and risks. Examples include the educational system, labor policies, gender norms, and systems of political representation. These mechanisms exist on local, regional, national, and global levels. Many would argue that the global engines are stronger now than ever before, while the national level is weakened (see chapter 4, on globalization). Global resource flows, human migration, debt payments, and the reach of multinational companies are but a few examples of aspects of social context that have a great influence on the health-related conditions for populations in many countries.

Individuals in a society are defined in part by their relationship to the social context. We refer to the concept of "social position" to describe a person's "place" or social standing within the society in which they live. These social positions (or classes), identified by a person's occupation, for example, exist, to a certain extent, independent of the individuals who fill them (Sørenson 1994). In some countries gender, race, or religion plays a major part in what social position a person occupies. Social positions are derived from, or generated by, a particular social context, meaning that classifications of social position will therefore vary in societies with differing economic or industrial structures. In highly industrialized societies with a finely graded labor market, detailed occupational classifications may be an appropriate measure of social position, while in largely rural, agrarian societies engaged in myriad income-generating activities, land ownership or size of dwelling may reflect social position more effectively than occupation. In many countries ethnicity may be a salient marker of social position, with ethnic origin, for example, governing people's chances of employment, their income, and where they are likely to live. The concept of "socioeconomic status" is often used in a similar way to "social position," but tends not to be linked explicitly to a theory of the political and economic forces generating inequality (Sørensen 1994).

The social context may lead to equalization of opportunities for individuals through, for example, equal rights of citizenship or universal access to health care (Mechanism I, Fig. 1). Conversely, it may lead to widening inequalities between members of society, as when the level and form of social benefits depend on citizenship or occupation. In all societies, valued resources are distributed unequally to different social positions (Grusky and Takata 1992). Typically, those individuals or families in the most privileged positions enjoy a disproportionate share of the valued resources (e.g., property, power, or prestige). In this sense, the process of social stratification is an inevitable characteristic of the social context—it both allocates power and wealth to social positions and allows individuals into different positions. Furthermore, the different dimensions of social positions may cluster or move in the same direction. Thus a person from a minority ethnic group may be more likely to have, on average, lower educational attainment, fewer employment opportunities, and less income than a person of the majority ethnic group. In the United States this process has resulted in the concentration of African Americans in urban neighborhoods with high levels of poverty and little opportunity (either educational or employment) (Wilson 1987).

The relationship between the social context and the way in which individuals are sorted into certain social positions is central to the issue of social differentials in health. Drawing the line between inequalities and inequities in health is linked to whether the underlying social arrangements determining opportunities for health (and other social outcomes) are fair or unfair (see chapter 3). Fairness, in turn, is linked both to how power and wealth are sorted or "matched" to certain social positions and how individuals are matched to positions. Before the associations between risk factors or health outcomes and a particular social position are examined, it is possible to evaluate the fairness of social contexts. The structure and function of certain institutions and social arrangements might be simply judged "unfair," for example, restricted mobility for women, institutionalized racism, or limited access to primary education based on ability to pay. Stephens (1998: 302) argues that structural inequities in distribution of control over resources and opportunities to gain control are at the heart of inequities in health. For example, in many developing countries, the poor have the least access to potable water and pay higher prices than the wealthy for poorer quality water (Stephens 1998).

Conversely, a social context may be judged "fair"—a minimum wage, progressive taxation, and universal access to care. There may be social contexts in which an intrinsic ordering is deemed fair or tolerable, for example, job grade or educational attainment level, but where its association with disadvantage in other important outcomes like health status raises equity concerns. A good example emerged in the Whitehall Study of health in the British civil service (Marmot et al. 1978). The fact that there is a clear occupational hierarchy with top civil servants being paid a salary higher than those in the next levels down may not, of itself, stir much sense of unfairness; yet the robust association between descending job grade and poorer health may seem highly unfair. Such revealed inequities in health, strongly related to social position and social context, are sobering reflections on the multiple expressions of injustice.

Differential Exposure—Mechanism II

Ideally, a clear and cogent theory of social stratification, complemented by shared ideas of what is equitable, should inform the selection of appropriate indicators of social context and social position for studying health inequities. The theory should then extend to postulating potential mechanisms by which the social contexts and positions link to health outcomes. The question is "how social forces, ranging from political violence to racism, come to be embodied in individual pathology" (Farmer 1999). One striking finding is that so many diseases, each with different established risk factors, show similar social patterns—a phenomenon referred to as the *hypothesis of generalized susceptibility* (Berkman and Syme 1976). A crucial feature of the theory linking social inequities to health is the mechanism of "differential exposure": the idea that each social position encounters specific patterns of health risks (Mechanism II, Fig. 1).

Exposures may vary between social groups by type, amount, and duration. Other things being equal, these exposure differentials may explain excess risk of ill health associated with lower social positions across a wide range of specific diseases. For example, unskilled service workers usually earn low incomes and often have limited control over their work and less liberty to choose healthy lifestyles. Given the likelihood that their parents were also poor, they might even have been exposed to adverse early childhood conditions such as

poor nutrition. In the United States, a growing body of literature demonstrates the link between environmental exposures and social class. The findings, across a wide range of pollutants, demonstrate that low social position is associated with occupations and housing that lead to greater risk of toxic exposure, which in turn leads to toxic insults and disability (Schell and Czerwnyski 1998). In the developing world, the exposures associated with living in an impoverished setting include air- and water-borne diseases such as diphtheria, tuberculosis, cholera, typhoid, infectious hepatitis, yellow fever, and malaria.

The findings about differential exposures are deepened by an emerging "life course" perspective that notes that advantages and disadvantages accumulate over a lifetime, implying that a single snapshot evaluation of inequities in health will not suffice (Bartley et al. 1997). The accumulation of health risks, and even the intergenerational transfer of socially produced health risks (such as the transfer of accumulated lead from mother to child via the placenta), necessitates a wide-angle lens for the study of differential exposures in order to capture the life-long risks associated with exposure at all ages (Power et al. 1996; Holland et al. 2000; Schell and Czerwnyski 1998).

Differential Vulnerability—Mechanism III

The clustering of health-damaging exposures along social gradients is closely related to the third mechanism, "differential vulnerability." The health impact of a specific exposure depends on whether other contributory causes or risk factors are present. Because individuals in lower social positions are often exposed to many different risk factors, and these may interact, the vulnerability to the effect of one specific cause might be higher than in more advantaged social groups (Hallqvist et al. 1998). In essence, this theory posits that even when a given risk factor is distributed evenly across social groups, its impact on health may be unevenly distributed due to underlying differences between social groups in their vulnerability or susceptibility to that factor (Mechanism III, Fig. 1).

This vulnerability may also reflect differences between social groups in their biological defenses against health-damaging factors. Thus in more vulnerable members of the population—children and the elderly—the host defenses of certain social groups may be so worn down, or overwhelmed to such an extent, that for a given exposure the impact on their health is magnified or accentuated. A similar concept is inherent in the idea of biological programming whereby adults appear at increased risk of chronic disease due to deprivation during critical periods of organ development in utero (Barker 1998). The various theories of susceptibility may play a part in explaining the dramatic rise in the level of ill health across chronic causes among men with lower socioeconomic status in Central and Eastern Europe at the time of economic crisis (Kristenson et al. 1998).

The concept of vulnerability can be extended from the biological to the social context. Vulnerability to ill health among African women, it is claimed, stems from their lack of access to education, greater burden of work, and minimal income-generating possibilities and from the likelihood that some will turn to commercial sex work (Kalipeni 2000). Some argue that despite living in absolute poverty, parental psychosocial control over even very scant resources has an important influence on child morbidity and mortality from childhood infection (Leon and Walt 2000). Thus issues of control, social support, and psychosocial well being are strongly linked to ideas of differential vulnerability to ill health.

It is important to note that these theories linking social position to inequities in health are not mutually exclusive. Both differential exposure and differential vulnerability are likely to contribute to the inequities in health that are observed across the social scale. Furthermore, they reflect a conceptual basis for understanding differential risk and as such are not substitutes for research on pathways underlying specific gradients. For example, in the Chilean case in chapter 10, there is a strong relationship between educational status and mortality. To explain the relationship one must understand how education affects an individual's living conditions, behaviors, and psychological status. The effect of education, for example, has been hypothesized as resulting from one or more of the following pathways: (1) labor market, economy, and household conditions allow more educated individuals to obtain less hazardous and higher paying jobs; (2) more educated people are more likely to avoid health risks such as smoking and engage in preventive behaviors such as health check-ups and prenatal care; and (3) more education may also lead to more resilient social psychological status—sense of control or self-efficacy (Levine et al. 1994).

Differential Social (and Economic) Consequences of Ill Health—Mechanism IV

Just as Amartya Sen makes a case for thinking beyond income for income's sake (Sen 1999), the social consequences of disease extend thinking beyond health for health's sake. Events such as accidents or the onset of chronic illnesses often alter an individual's life dramatically. The loss of a limb may make certain types of manual labor impossible, while impaired speech due to a stroke may severely diminish social interactions. Ill health may initiate a downward spiral linked to excessive expenditures on health care and to the loss of work-related income which in turn increases risks for further ill health. Therefore, "social consequences" refer to the impact a certain health event may have for an individual's or a family's socioeconomic circumstances.

The underlying social context and social stratification may lead to an inequitable distribution of the social consequences of ill health. In a system without social safety nets such as universal health care or unemployment or disability insurance, the direct costs of health care and income forgone due to inability to work are absorbed by individuals and their families. Although this is the case for people from all social positions, there is a tremendous range in the ability of individuals to cope with these costs depending on their socioeconomic circumstances. In general, individuals in wealthier groups are more able to absorb costs, often have access to private insurance mechanisms, and are unlikely to pass costs on to other family members or to incur significant debt. Poorer groups correspondingly have less of a financial cushion, are less likely to be able to afford or invest in private insurance, and are often forced to find new income sources, often through other family members or through crippling debts (Mechanism IV, Fig. 1).

These four differentials in ability to withstand external shocks will lead to a skew in the costs and consequences of illness against lower socioeconomic strata. Even when the social context provides strong or pro-equity safety nets, for example, universal health care insurance, the thinness of "reserves" among poorer groups in terms of minimal disposable income and few assets leads to a high probability of a further falling behind the better endowed groups. The adverse welfare consequences often extend beyond the individual to the family. In particular, household income for children's food, education, and health care is reduced when a parent or breadwinner falls ill (Pryor 1989; Evans 1989). The cost of health care itself can push people into poverty when individuals with severe or chronic illness have to meet a substantial portion of this cost themselves. The importance of catastrophic health costs as a primary cause of impoverishment was corroborated in a global study of 60,000 poor persons entitled *Voices of the Poor* (Narayan et al. 1999).

On a larger scale, the prevalence of impoverishing illness may overwhelm the coping abilities not only of the more marginal groups in the population but also of the entire system. This is perhaps nowhere more evident than in Africa today where acquired immunodeficiency symdrome (AIDS) has risen to such proportions that it threatens the development of the entire continent. In Tanzania, for example, it is estimated that due to the existence of human immunodeficiency virus (HIV)/AIDS, gross domestic product is between 14% and 24% lower than it would have been without the epidemic (World Bank 1993). In Zimbabwe, by the year 2005, it is predicted that HIV/AIDS will consume 60% of the health budget (UNICEF 1999). In the Ivory Coast one schoolteacher is lost every day due to AIDS (Piot, personal communication 2000). Thus, the impoverishing effects of illness are evident on a global scale, with entire populations and nations crippled by the catastrophic costs of the AIDS pandemic, and, as a consequence, further global stratification of nations is a likely effect.

Identifying Policy Entry Points

In sum, therefore, we have identified four conceptual mechanisms relating social context to the emergence and entrenchment of health inequities: social stratification, differential exposures, differential vulnerability, and differential social consequences. The intent of this analysis is to hcighten awareness of the inextricable link between pervasive social hierarchy and inequities in both health outcomes and the consequences of ill health. The rationale of this line of thinking is twofold: to incorporate social factors more explicitly and adequately into scientific research design and to provide a strong link to the policy world in recognition that social inequities are largely avoidable, preventable, and unjust. A number of entry points for policy to reduce health inequities can be identified from the above framework, as discussed below. Chapter 21 provides more in-depth analysis of policy options for redressing health inequities.

Influencing Social Stratification—Policy Entry Point A

An important starting point for policy to reduce inequities in health is recognizing the importance of the social context and the hierarchical effects of social position. Although perhaps the most critical area in terms of diminishing disparities in health, social stratification is often seen as the domain of "other" policy concerns and not central to health policy making, given the rigid distinctions between sectors.

Two general policy approaches can be considered. First is the promotion of policies that diminish social inequalities (Entry Point A, Fig. 1). Labor market, education, and family welfare policies, for example, may influence the opportunities people have to improve their welfare and indeed can influence how wide the gulf is between people in different social positions. Likewise, policies aimed at diminishing gender disparities will influence the position of women relative to men. In particular, providing greater social and economic opportunities to poor women is likely to have positive equity consequences (see chapter 16, on Bangladesh). Second is an impact assessment of social and economic policies to mitigate their effects on social stratification. In the Mexico study in chapter 19, for example, national macroeconomic and social policies are shown to exacerbate social inequalities as expressed by a measure of county-level "marginalization" leading to increasing intercounty inequities in health. Likewise in the South Africa study, the authors recommend greater vigilance over macroeconomic readjustment policies given their propensity to accentuate rather than diminish systemic underlying racial disparities (see chapter 14).

Given the large body of research linking poverty to health through specific individual pathways (specific exposures), a focus on best options for reducing social inequities can be undertaken without extensive data collection on individual health to replicate findings in the literature. Further research can improve policy effectiveness by identifying particular types of processes or mechanisms of social stratification that cause health inequities. Those advocating a life-course approach argue that policies that prevent an accumulation of risk in the critical biological and social periods—such as prenatal development, the transfer from primary to secondary school, entry to the labor market, and exit from the labor market—should be especially important in protecting the most vulnerable (Bartley et al. 1997; Blane 1999).

Decreasing Exposures and Vulnerability—Policy Entry Points B and C

Beyond efforts to alter the social stratification process, policy makers might focus more specifically on reducing the excess exposures to health hazards of those occupying lower social positions (Entry Point B, Fig. 1). In general, most health policies do not differentiate exposure or risk reduction strategies according to social position. Anti-tobacco efforts, for example, have mostly

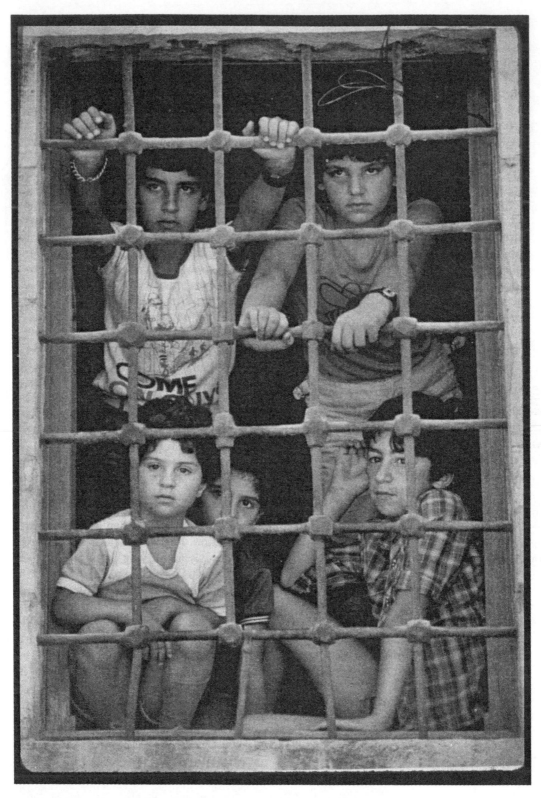

Lebanese children looking out from behind bars.
Source: Bill Foley/Stock South/Picture Quest, 1992.

targeted the smoking population as a whole, not the poor smokers specifically. The unintended result has been encouraging decreases in smoking prevalence among the rich and better educated and no change among the poor, thereby increasing social inequality in tobacco consumption (Townsend et al. 1994).

There is increasing experience, however, with health policies aiming to combat inequities in health that target the specific exposures of people in disadvantaged positions such as unhealthy housing, dangerous working conditions, and with nutritional deficiencies (Marmot and Wilkinson 1999). In the case of HIV/AIDS, explanations of HIV transmission that focus on the social production of the disease would recommend surveillance that emphasizes the link between increased risk of HIV infection and membership in groups defined by economic deprivation and racial discrimination (Krieger and Zierler 1999). Success in these policies is measured by a disproportionate benefit accruing to the target or disadvantaged groups. The size of this benefit, however, is contingent on the constellation of other exposures and perhaps more importantly on the macro social and economic forces (Policy Entry Point A) all of which may be worsening, that is, moving in the other direction. This awareness of the larger picture may help explain why documentation of significant changes in the exposure profiles of disadvantaged populations is hard to find. It also brings up a larger policy issue of whether intervening in a single exposure is sufficient.

An alternative way of thinking about this modification of the effect of exposures is through the concept of differential vulnerability. Intervention in a single exposure may have no effect on the underlying vulnerability of the disadvantaged population. Reduced vulnerability may only be achieved when interacting exposures are diminished or relative social conditions improve significantly. A wide literature has pointed to the benefits of female education as one of the most effective means of mediating women's differential vulnerability (Kalipeni 2000; Mehrotra 1997). Diminishing one key exposure, such as lack of education, might reduce the vulnerability of women to the effects of other risks (Entry Point C, Fig. 1).

Preventing Unequal Consequences of Ill Health and Further Social Inequalities—Policy Entry Point D

Given inequities in health, how can the system stem unfair differentials in the consequences of ill health and prevent the further widening of social inequalities and differentiation of health outcomes? This area of policy

is the intervention point where the great bulk of health care resources are currently concentrated. Typically, the health care equity literature argues for care according to need (Wagstaff and van Doorslaer 1993). One critical issue therefore is the definition of need. If need is defined with no sensitivity to the special needs of disadvantaged populations, for example, all post-heart attack patients should have a standard regimen of care, then it is likely that inequities will be accentuated. Despite having the same diagnosis, disadvantaged patients may have more difficulties recovering and surviving and therefore require more time with caregivers and ancillary supports such as home help workers in order to achieve similar post-heart attack rehabilitation (Entry Point D, Fig. 1). Without special consideration, they may be prone to prolonged disability and more complications.

Hence, secondary and tertiary care of patients has a strong propensity to follow the inverse care laws even when prescribed according to an equity principle of care based on need (Tudor Hart 1971). As such, policy options must demand evidence for the range of interventions—disease specific and related to the broader social environment—that will reduce the likelihood of unequal consequences of ill health. Most of the recent thinking on equity in resource allocation has gone further in emphasizing that it is not just a question of matching health care resources to need but also a question of whether they can be allocated specifically to reduce differentials in health outcomes. Additional resources for rehabilitation, for example, might be allocated to reduce the social consequences of illness. In 1998, the U.K. government set the British National Health Service a new resource allocation objective of this nature—to apply health care funds to contribute to the reduction in inequalities in health (United Kingdom Department of Health 1999).

The social context plays a large role in the stratification of social opportunity for people who are sick. As discussed earlier, a system with accessible and functioning safety nets can do much to prevent the social differentiation induced by ill health. Another critical component of this (discussed in further detail in chapter 18) is equitable health care financing. This involves protection from the impoverishment arising from catastrophic illness as well as an understanding of the implications of various public and private financing mechanisms and their use by disadvantaged populations. Equitable public financing of health care is of little use if poor patients access usurious private health care services.

In summary, the conceptual framework identifies four socially based components that must be considered in understanding and redressing inequities in health: (*1*) factors affecting social stratification, (*2*) differential exposures to health-damaging factors, (*3*) differential vulnerabilities leading to unequal health outcomes, and (*4*) differential social consequences of illness. The question of which of these mechanisms is important in a particular society can be tested empirically within this framework. These conceptual areas also help to frame policy options (A to D, Fig. 1) and to make health equity impact assessments of those options, as illustrated in the European analysis in chapter 17. It is likely that research in each of these four areas would yield important insights and guidance to policy makers. Given that "a society's understanding of the determinants of health has an important influence on the strategies it uses to sustain and improve the health of its population" (Mustard 1996: 303), heightened awareness of the social production of ill health and disability is a critical component of the health equity agenda. The larger challenge is to assess the range of policy entry points along the continuum of the social basis of health inequities in order to identify effective synergies and comparative advantages of policies within a particular societal context.

References

Antonovsky A. 1967. Social class, life expectancy and overall mortality. *Milbank Memorial Fund Quarterly* 45(2):31–73.

Barker D.J.P. 1998. *Mothers and Babies, and Disease in Later Life*, 2nd ed. Edinburgh: Churchill Livingstone.

Bartley M., Blane D., Montgomery S. 1997. Health and the life course: why safety nets matter. *British Medical Journal* 314(7088):1194–1196.

Beaglehole R., Bonita R. 1997. *Public Health at the Crossroads: Achievements and Prospects*. Cambridge: Cambridge University Press.

Berkman L.F., Syme S.L. 1976. Social networks, host resistance and mortality: a nine-year follow-up of Alameda County residents. *American Journal of Epidemiology* 109:186–204.

Blane D. 1999. The life course, the social gradient and health. In: Marmot M., Wilkinson R.G. (eds), *Social Determinants of Health*. Oxford: Oxford University Press, pp. 64–80.

Brunner E., Marmot M. 1999. Social organization, stress and health. In: Marmot M., Wilkinson R.G. (eds), *Social Determinants of Health*. Oxford: Oxford University Press, pp. 17–43.

Diderichsen F., Hallqvist J. 1998. Social inequalities in health: some methodological considerations for the study of social position and social context. In: Arve-Parès B. (ed) *Inequality in Health—A Swedish Perspective*. Stockholm: Swedish Council for Social Research, pp. 25–39.

Diez-Rouz A.V. 1998. Bringing context back into epidemiology: variables and fallacies in multilevel analysis. *American Journal of Public Health* 88(2):216–222.

Evans T.G. 1989. The impact of permanent disability on rural households: river blindness in Guinea. *IDS Bulletin* 20(2):41–48.

Farmer P. 1999. *Infections and Inequalities: The Modern Plagues*. Berkeley: University of California Press.

Farr W. 1865 report in: Humphreys NA (ed.). *Vital statistics: a memorial volume of selections from the reports and writings of Willard Farr*. London, The Sanitary Institute of Great Britain, 1885.

Grusky D.B., Takata A.A. 1992. Social stratification. In: Borgatta E.F., Borgatta M.L. (eds), *Encyclopedia of Sociology*, 1955–70. New York: Macmillan.

Hallqvist J., Diderichsen F., Theorell T., Teuterwall C., Ahlbom A. 1998. Is the effect of job strain on myocardial infarction risk due to interaction between high psychological demand and low decision latitude? *Social Science and Medicine* 46:1405–1415.

Holland P., Berney L., Blane D., Davey Smith G., Gunnell D.J., Montgomery S.M. 2000. Life course accumulation of disadvantage: childhood health and hazard exposure during adulthood. *Social Science and Medicine* 50:1285–1295.

Kalipeni E. 2000. Health and disease in southern Africa: a comparative and vulnerability perspective. *Social Science and Medicine* 50:965–983.

Karasek R., Theorell T. 1990. *Healthy Work: Stress, Productivity, and the Reconstruction of Working Life*. New York: Basic Books.

Kawachi I., Kennedy B. 1997. Health and social cohesion—Why care about income inequality? *British Medical Journal* 314:1037–1040.

Koopman J.S., Longini I.M. 1994. The ecological effects of individual exposures and nonlinear disease dynamics in populations. *American Journal of Public Health* 84:836–842.

Krieger N. 1994. Epidemiology and the web of causation—Has anyone seen the spider? *Social Science and Medicine*. 39:887–902.

Krieger N., Zierler S. 1999. What explains the public's health? A call for epidemiologic theory. In: Beauchamp D., Steinbock B. (eds), *New Ethics for the Public's Health*. New York: Oxford University Press, pp. 45–49.

Kristenson M., Orth-Gomér K., Kucinskienë Z., Bergdahl B., Calkauskas H., Balinkyniene I., Olsson A.G. 1998. Attenuated cortisol response to a standardized stress test in Lithuanian vs. Swedish men: the Livicordia Study. *International Journal of Behavioral Medicine* 5(1):17–30.

Kuh D., Power C., Blane D., Bartley M. 1997. Social pathways between childhood and adult health. In: Kuh D., Ben-Shlomo Y. (eds), *A Life Course Approach to Chronic Disease Epidemiology*. Oxford: Oxford University Press. pp. 169–198.

Leon D., Walt G. 2000. Poverty, inequality and health in international perspective: a divided world? In: Leon D., Walt G. (eds), *Poverty, Inequality and Health*. Oxford: Oxford University Press.

Levine R.A., Levine S.E., Richman A., Tapia Uribe M.F., Correa C.S. 1994. Schooling and survival: the impact of maternal education on health and reproduction in the third world. In: Chen L.C., Kleinman A., Ware N. (eds), *Health and Social Change in International Perspective*. Cambridge, MA: Harvard University Press. pp. 303–338.

Macintyre S. 1998. Social inequalities and health in the contemporary world comparative overview. In: Strickland S.S., Shetty P.S. (eds), *Human Biology and Social Inequality*. 39th Symposium volume of the Society for the Study of Human Biology. Cambridge: Cambridge University Press. pp. 20–35.

Marmot M.G., Rose G., Shipley M.J., Hamilton P.J. 1978. Employment grade and coronary heart disease in British civil servants. *Journal of Epidemiology and Community Health* 32:244–249.

Marmot M.G., Wilkinson R.G. (eds). 1999. *Social Determinants of Health*. Oxford: Oxford University Press.

McKinlay J.B. 1993. The promotion of health through planned sociopolitical change: challenges for research and policy. *Social Science and Medicine* 36(2):109–117.

Mehrotra S. 1997. Social development in high-achieving countries: common elements and diversities. In: Mehrotra S., Jolly S. (eds), *Development with a Human Face: Experiences in Social Achievement and Economic Growth*. Oxford: Clarendon Press.

Mustard J.F. 1996. Health and social capital. In: Blane D., Brunner E., Wilkinson R. (eds), *Health and Social Organization: Towards a Health Policy for the 21st Century*. London: Routledge, pp. 303–313.

Narayan D., Chambers R., Shah M., Petesch P. 1999. Global Synthesis: Consultations with the Poor. Prepared for Global Synthesis Workshop, September 22–23, 1999. Poverty Group, PREM, World Bank. Washington, DC: World Bank.

Power C., Mathews S., Manor O. 1996. Inequalities in self-rated health in the 1958 birth cohort: life time social circumstances or social mobility? *British Medical Journal* 313:449–4523.

Pryor J. 1989. When breadwinners fall ill. *IDS Bulletin* 20:49–57.

Rothman K.J., Adami H.O., Trichopoulos D. 1998. Should the mission of epidemiology include the eradication of poverty? *Lancet* 352:810–813.

Schell L.M., Czerwnyski S.A. 1998. Environmental health, social inequality and biological differences. In: Strickland S.S., Shetty P.S. (eds), *Human Biology and Social Inequality*. 39th Symposium volume of the Society for the Study of Human Biology. Cambridge: Cambridge University Press, pp. 114–131.

Sen A.K. 1999. *Development as Freedom*. New York: Alfred A. Knopf, pp. 114–131.

Sørensen A. 1994. Women's economic risk and the economic position of single mothers. *European Sociological Review* 10:173–188.

Stephens C. 1998. The policy implications of health inequalities in developing countries. In: Strickland S.S., Shetty P.S. (eds), *Human Biology and Social Inequality*. 39th Symposium volume of the Society for the Study of Human Biology. Cambridge: Cambridge University Press, pp. 288–307.

Syme S.L. 1994. The social environment and health. *Daedalus* 12(4):79–86.

Townsend J., Roderick P., Cooper J. 1994. Cigarette smoking by socioeconomic group, sex, and age: effects of price, income and health publicity. *British Medical Journal* 309(6959):923–927.

Tudor Hart J. 1971. The inverse care law. *Lancet* i:405–412.

UNICEF. 1999. *The Progress of Nations 1999*. New York: UNICEF.

United Kingdom Department of Health. 1999. Saving Lives: Our Healthier Nation. Command White Paper 4386. London: The Stationery Office.

Wagstaff A., van Doorslaer E. 1993. Equity in the finance and delivery of health care: concepts and definitions. In: van Doorslaer E., Wagstaff A., Rutten F. (eds), *Equity in the Finance and Delivery of Health Care: An International Perspective*. Oxford: Oxford University Press, pp. 7–19.

Waitzman N.J., Smith K.R. 1998. Separate but lethal: the effects of economic segregation on mortality in metropolitan America. *Milbank Quarterly* 76(3):304, 341–373.

Wilkinson R. 1994. The epidemiological transition: from material scarcity to social disadvantage? *Daedalus* 123(4):61–77.

Williams W.J. 1987. *The Truly Disadvantaged: The Inner-City, the Underclass and Public Policy*. Chicago: University of Chicago Press.

World Bank 1993. *Investing in health. World Development Report 1993*. Washington, D.C.: World Bank.

CHAPTER
3

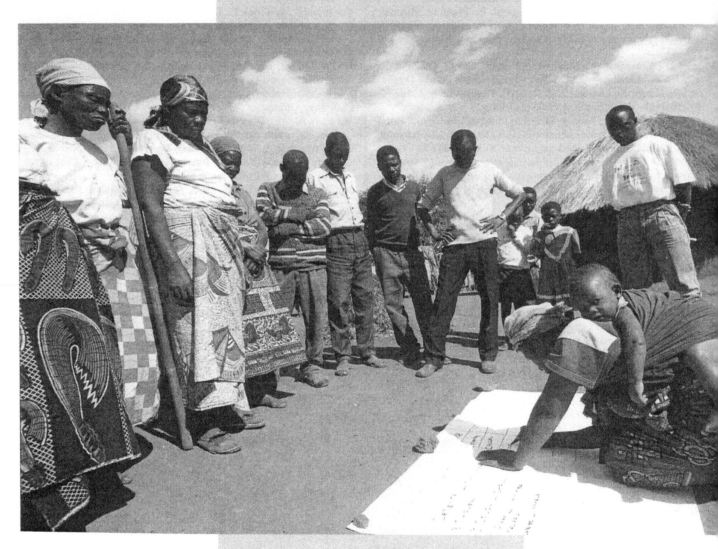

Community meeting to identify village
sanitation needs, Zambia 1998.
Source: Giacomo Pirozzi/Panos.

Ethical Dimensions of Health Equity

FABIENNE PETER AND TIMOTHY EVANS

Vast disparities in health status, whether between global regions, nations, social groups, or genders, are an affront to basic intuitions of fairness. The current concern with health equity underlines the fact that, rather than being simply an individual problem related to biological makeup and behavior, health is affected by social circumstances and a wide range of public policies. The finding that, more often than not, a more privileged social position is linked to better health has drawn attention to health and social inequalities in health as a problem distinct from, but related to, other policy issues, such as poverty, income inequality, or unequal opportunities. It is in this terrain that ethical discourse on social justice may inform the field of health equity.

At first glance, health equity as a social goal may seem an obvious idea: Health is important to most people, and society should ensure that people have equal chances to enjoy good health. Underlying such a common sense proposition, however, is a maze of complex issues related to the multidimensionality of the concept of health, its sociobiological constitution, and a limited understanding of the factors that affect the distribution of health status within and across populations.

Turning to the literature on moral and political philosophy, one finds few direct efforts to deal with health equity. Theories of social justice are generally silent on the topic of health. Insofar as the topic of health equity is addressed at all, the focus has tended to be on access to health *care* (Fried 1975; Daniels 1985). Similarly, bioethics—a field of applied moral philosophy—has tended to focus on medical care and the rights of individual patients while failing to address fairness in the population or the social patterning of health. This is linked to the criticism that the whole field of medicine can be accused of ignoring the social basis of health. In an analysis of the broader social and economic forces leading to the poor health of the Haitian poor, Farmer and Bertrand comment critically on the lacunae of physician training: "we study vitamin deficiencies, but not land reform—we learn about pathophysiology, but never the embodiment of the social forces that set in motion a series of events leading, ultimately, to a critical somatic process" (Farmer and Bertrand 2000: 87).

Slowly, the situation is changing, and the ethical dimensions of health equity and related themes are beginning to receive more attention (Marchand et al. 1998; Beauchamp and Steinbock 1999). Wikler (1997) maintains that bioethics is now ready to move to a new phase that embraces ethical analysis of population health issues. The pervasiveness of social gradients in health status has piqued the curiosity of eminent philosophers and public health practitioners alike, leading to fresh discourse and new writings (Marchand et al. 1998; Beauchamp and Steinbock 1999; Daniels et al. 1999; Anand et al. Forthcoming). Similarly, in the context of the literature related to the *new public health* (Mann 1995; Krieger and Birn 1998), there is a renewed emphasis on the link be-

25

tween the pursuit of public health and the pursuit of social justice.

This chapter is but one contribution to this emerging literature exploring the link between social justice and health. It discusses some of the main issues and challenges in assessing the fairness of social inequalities in health. Starting with a brief discussion of the idea of health itself, it proceeds by identifying two fundamental types of judgments that help to determine what is equitable and inequitable in the distribution of health. Insofar as the basis for making these judgments is unclear, the third section of the chapter critically reviews a variety of philosophical approaches to justice that might inform such assessments. While the chapter provides an overview of these fundamental questions, it also pursues a line of argument of its own. The premise is that health equity cannot be an apolitical, acultural, "technocratic" concept restricted to the domain of health care and public health. The chapter suggests that health equity is best thought of not as a social goal in and of itself, but as inherently imbedded in a more general pursuit of social justice. As such, it attempts to provide support to those who invite us to "resist the hubristic belief that, as public health professionals, we have all the answers or can by ourselves improve the public's health without efforts to ensure social and economic justice" (Krieger and Birn 1998: 1603).

The Concept of Health: Its Causes and Its Distribution

Inevitably, the concept of health—its definition and measurement—is a fundamental starting point in the discussion of health equity, about which there are many important ethical issues. Perhaps most important is the recognition that although inextricably linked to biology and nature, health can never be a purely descriptive, value-free concept (Canguilhem 1991 [1966]; Toulmin 1975). Value judgments are required in order to make distinctions between normal and abnormal, healthy and pathological, and even medical disease versus deviation from some other nonmedical social norm (Engelhardt 1975; Margolis 1981; Hare 1986). Health is thus not simply a biological norm but the product of complex social and biological valuations. Neglecting either aspect of health will hinder the assessment of health equity. A view of health as solely a matter of biomedical factors tends to minimize the social basis of health and may obscure distributional issues. For example, variations in serum cholesterol levels may be considered only in terms of dietary intake of fats without recognizing

the social patterning of diet. On the other hand, too broad a social view may unduly camouflage the biological basis of health.

One consequence of viewing health as the product of complex social and biological assessments is that there may be different perspectives on health and illness and on their meaning in people's lives. In this context, Sen (chapter 6) discusses the necessity of combining the perspectives of "external" observers, such as public health experts, with the "internal" perspectives of those afflicted by illness and disability to ensure an adequate informational basis for assessments of health equity. A related issue, as discussed in Chapter 5, is that different metrics for health measurement can dramatically alter the direction and magnitude of health inequalities.

Health is a state of being over which an individual has only partial control throughout the life course. We are born with a social and biological heritage that leaves an indelible imprint on the health projections of our lives (Barker 1994). We have little choice in our preadult years during which we are exposed to physical and social environments that have a large bearing on our current and future health. As adults we theoretically exercise greater choice and therefore control over our health, for example, regular exercise, low fat diets, and avoidance of toxic substances such as tobacco; however, it is clear too that these behaviors are strongly influenced by social context and only partly volitional. Moreover, as we age, our biological susceptibilities emerge, many of which we are powerless to alter at this time. Finally, while it has been possible to extend longevity, the lifespan is clearly bounded.

Although there are biological limitations and many adverse impacts of social factors on health, there are also vast opportunities for social policies to improve health. Improvements in nutrition and living standards in the last three centuries have contributed enormously to better population health (McKeown 1976; Fogel 1994). Universal education, particularly of women, may be the single greatest contributor to health globally in the last century. The discovery of antibiotics and vaccines for infectious killers, new technologies to dramatically lower the fatal risks of child bearing, and new drugs to lower the risks of chronic diseases are but a few of the giant strides in medical care that have contributed significantly to health potential in the last 50 years. Similarly a burgeoning understanding of the modifiable behavioral risks arising from the study of public health, for example, smoking cessation and physical activity, are also nontrivial components of improvements in health achievement. Nutrition, living standards, education, health care, and public health, therefore, provide a powerful armamentarium with which societies can improve their population's health.

It is the unequal opportunity of subgroups in the population to participate in these health and other social benefits that underlies our concern with equity. Particularly disturbing is the danger of vicious cycles: relative or absolute deprivation as a factor that causes ill health, and ill health as a cause of impoverishment. For example, in the recent study by the World Bank (1999), *Voices of the Poor*, ill health and its consequences emerged from interviews with over 60,000 poor persons as the primary reason for impoverishment. As such, health is a critical building block, or capability (Sen 1980, 1985, 1993), to a better and more meaningful life and ill health a huge threat to social and economic well-being.

At the same time, health is unlikely to ever be equally distributed across individuals. Individual biological variation, certain environmental exposures, free and informed choice, and pure chance are among the less modifiable factors that differentiate individual health outcomes. At an individual level, therefore, health will always be unequally distributed. In evaluating the fairness of the individual distribution of health, therefore, this baseline variation must be acknowledged. The inevitability of variations in health at the individual level may be acceptable insofar as they are randomly distributed across social groupings such as gender, occupation, and race/ethnicity and not associated with education, income, or access to health care. Evidence of a skew in the distribution of health across these or other social strata may raise fundamental questions about social justice.

Distinguishing Health Inequities from Health Inequalities

How, beyond identifying and analyzing these social inequalities in health, should we make judgments about health equity? For Brian Barry (1990 [1965]), equity is a *comparative* principle, a judgment about how a person or a group of people is situated relative to others. Equity requires that "equals be treated equally and unequals be treated unequally" (Barry 1990 [1965]: 152). This is analogous to the concepts of horizontal and vertical equity in health care analysis (Culyer and Wagstaff 1993), which ensure that the principle of equality is preserved while the diverse health needs of individuals are recognized. Barry identifies two fundamental types of judgments to identify what is equitable. The first is to identify existing standards of distribution, which define in what ways people should be viewed as equals

or unequals, and to then analyze whether these standards are applied consistently. The second encompasses the development of standards where none exist.

Addressing the first scenario, if the standard is universal immunization for children, then inequity exists if certain groups in the population are not being immunized. Similarly, standards for equity may involve identifying a minimum or basic level of health attainment, for example, all regions of a country achieve a life expectancy at birth of at least 70 years. Equity is achieved if all regions achieve this minimum, even though there may continue to be considerable inequality between regions above this threshold.

Often, however, there are no clear standards against which to assess equity. In most comparisons of social groups (rural vs. urban, men vs. women, rich vs. poor, and so forth) there may not be an obvious criterion for when and how people count as equals and what inequalities are appropriate and/or required—the standards themselves need to be developed first. For example, in comparing the health of women and men, how do we weigh the fact that women often tend to have longer life expectancy but higher morbidity? Furthermore, even when standards exist, these may be contestable, as when it is argued that norms of health that were developed for men do not apply to women. In assessments of health equity of this second type, broader considerations of social justice and of the social good will have to be taken into account and judgments of equity become interlinked with judgments of social justice and fairness.

A similar reasoning underpins Margaret Whitehead's proposal (1992) for distinguishing between social inequalities and inequities in health: that inequalities which are avoidable and unfair constitute health inequities. Whitehead (1992) develops a list of seven determinants of health differentials and suggests that those related to biological variation and free informed choice are more likely to be unavoidable or fair inequalities. Those differentials arising from determinants where individuals have less choice in lifestyle, work conditions, or access to health care and other public services are more likely to be considered avoidable and unfair and thus inequities. As Figure 1 suggests, judgments about justice and fairness presuppose that health inequalities are at least in principle avoidable. Admittedly, judgments about avoidability may be highly intricate because they have to be understood in a broad sense and not just with regard to the status quo. For example, tropical diseases should not be interpreted as unavoidable just because the public health problems they generate have failed to register as research and development priorities for the global phar-

Figure 1 Judging the equity of health outcomes

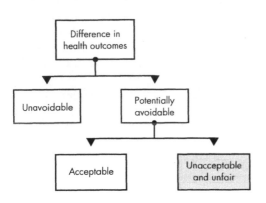

Note: Adapted from Whitehead 1992

maceutical industry. The bottom line is that when premature death, illness, or disability is unavoidable, judgments of fairness and justice do not apply—which is not to deny, of course, that such instances may be sad or tragic. The fundamental question for assessing health equity is, then, how to decide which social inequalities in health are unfair and hence constitute inequities.

Can Moral Philosophy Inform Judgments About Health Equity?

Evaluation of the fairness of health inequalities will, in each case, inevitably be very complex, and one should not hope for facile solutions. Nevertheless, one may seek guidance from existing theories of social justice (Marchand et al. 1998; Pereira 1993). Here we discuss how various philosophical approaches might consider the fairness of social inequalities in health.

In the literature on social inequalities in health and health equity, there is often an underlying assumption that social inequalities in health are "unjust" because they prevent the population from attaining its maximum health potential. There is a parallel between this view and the philosophical doctrine of *utilitarianism*, which states that we should maximize the sum of individual well-being. Under the additional assumption that everybody's capacity for health is equal, maximizing population health entails bringing everybody up to the highest possible level of health. Before that level is reached, however, a maximizing approach to population health implies that we are indifferent between health benefits to, say, the poor and the rich, as long as these benefits have the same impact on overall pop-

ulation health. Indeed, a common critique of utilitarianism is its inability to address issues of distributive justice (Williams 1973). The problem is even more acute when health losses are weighted by the income lost due to illness and disability, thus attaching greater value to the health of a rich person than to the health of a poor person.

Egalitarian theories, in contrast, emphasize distributive considerations independently of aggregate population health and may, for that reason, be better suited to making health equity judgments. There are many different egalitarian theories, and, depending on what egalitarianism is perceived to entail, the theories vary in the extent to which they endorse a social obligation to secure individual health or to provide health care. The primary issue to be clarified is, as Sen (1980) puts it, "equality of what?" Some egalitarian theories emphasize equality of *outcomes*, which, in the context of health, would translate into equality of health status. A possible application would be to argue that it is more just if everyone in a population has a life expectancy of 60 years rather than if the average life expectancy is 70 years but half the population can only expect to live to 50 years while the other half can expect to live to 90 years.

It should be emphasized, however, that egalitarianism does not necessarily imply strict equality, and indeed many would not want to go as far. For the bioethicist Robert Veatch (1991: 83), for example, egalitarianism in the context of health "requires that persons be given an *opportunity* to have *equal health status* insofar as possible." Veatch and others (Sen 1980) thus stress equality of *opportunity*. It should be noted that equality of opportunity generally requires disproportionate efforts toward disadvantaged groups to overcome social barriers to health.

The requirement of equality may also be seen as satisfied if everybody is above a certain threshold. Sen's idea (1985) of "basic capabilities" reflects such a view. Furthermore, egalitarian principles may be weighted. John Rawls' theory of justice as fairness (1971) is often interpreted as requiring the giving of priority to the worst off groups in society—in the case of health, to improve the health of the poorest in society (Marchand et al. 1998).

Not all forms of egalitarianism privilege health. A case in point is Ronald Dworkin's approach (1981) to equality of resources. Dworkin (1993) argues that justice requires no more than equality of general resources (e.g., earning opportunities, access to education). Once equality of resources is achieved, it is up to people to decide how they want to make use of these resources, for instance, how much they want to invest in their health. In his view, in a society that guarantees equality of resources, there would be no need to give particular weight to health. We shall come back to this argument below.

Derek Parfit (1997) criticizes egalitarian theories, arguing that it is misleading to treat equality as in itself valuable. To make his point, he quotes approvingly from Joseph Raz (1986: 240):

"what makes us care about various inequalities is not the inequality but the concern identified by the underlying principle. It is the hunger of the hungry, the need of the needy, the suffering of the ill, and so on." What is relevant is "that their hunger is greater, their need more pressing, their suffering more hurtful, and therefore our concern for the hungry, the needy, the suffering, and not our concern for equality, makes us give them priority."

The so-called priority view thus constitutes a third approach to health equity. It may be seen as a weighted utilitarian principle. While maximization requires that health benefits be allocated in a way that produces the greatest overall improvement, the priority principle requires that they should be given to the sickest. Just like the maximization principle, the priority view entails that differences in health outcomes between social groups matter only derivatively; what counts are health outcomes and the severity of illness, not who is afflicted and through what pathways. This view corresponds with the arguments being put forward by the World Health Organization for an interindividual assessment of health distribution that is independent of social groups (Gakidou et al. 2000). Put another way, such an approach emphasizes those with the poorest health and not necessarily the health status of the poorest. For this reason, the priority view may have more relevance within the health care system than a broader "society and health" perspective.

What all three approaches thus far discussed have in common is that they focus on the distributive *pattern* of health outcomes. An alternative approach to health equity interprets what is ethically wrong with social inequalities in health as linked to the *causes* of these inequalities. To answer the question of what constitutes health inequities, therefore, it is necessary to move beyond information about health status to an understanding of the underlying social processes and their fairness.

Rooted in Rawlsian justice (Rawls 1971, 1993a), this type of approach to health equity starts from an ideal of society as a *fair system of cooperation*. The goal of social justice is to ensure that basic social, economic, and political institutions (the "basic structure of society") work in a way that is not exclusive. This fundamental ideal has been well expressed by Onora O'Neill (1993: 315), who argues that social arrangements are unjust if they "hinge on victimizing some, so on destroying, paralyzing, or undercutting their capacities for action for at least some time and in some ways." The upshot of Rawls's principles of justice is that inequalities in society are justifiable as long as society's main economic, social, and political institutions do not require sacrifices from the worse-off groups purely to the benefit of the better-off groups. Because of its emphasis on the *processes* that bring about certain outcomes, rather than on the outcomes themselves, such an approach to justice is called "procedural."

How can Rawlsian justice be applied to making health equity judgments? This approach points to the particular weight of health inequalities that can be traced to the working of society's main political, social, and economic institutions and that are the result of social arrangements that do not fulfill the requirement of a fair system of social cooperation. This is to say, it identifies as unjust those class, gender, race, regional, and other inequalities in health that originate in the basic structure of society and seem to be the result of a social division of labor that is to the benefit of the better-off groups only at the (health) expense of the worse-off groups.

At the same time, research on social inequalities in health and their underlying causes may tell us something about whether social arrangements do or do not entail a fair system of social cooperation. An understanding of how cultural, social, and economic forces affect health outcomes can thus supplement economic and sociological information about the achievements of different social arrangements and their changes over time and our assessment of overall social justice. In other words, social inequalities in health may be seen as a sensitive barometer of the fairness of the underlying social order. This point is frequently overlooked—typically it is only asked how assessments of justice apply to health, not how health problems may affect our assessments of justice. It is overlooked, for example, in Dworkin's argument (1993) that health need not be singled out if equality of resources (i.e., equality with respect to goods such as income and education, but not health) is achieved. Because of the complex entanglement of individual health outcomes and the influence of social arrangements, it is not possible to assess the justice of these arrangements without taking their effects on health into account.

There is thus a two-way relationship between the requirements of Rawlsian justice and the concern with social inequalities in health. On the one hand, our evaluation of health equity will depend on the link between health inequalities and injustices in society. On the

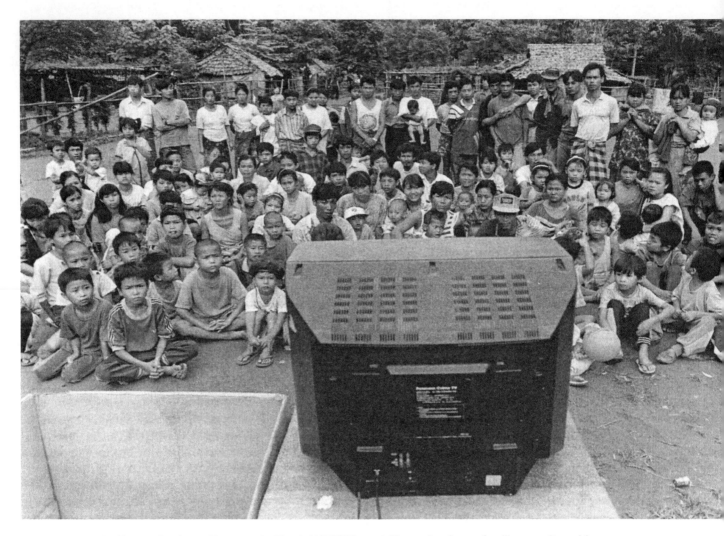

All Burma Students Democratic Front (ABSDF) and Karenni refugee families await a video screening on the anniversary of the democratic uprising in Burma. Nu Pu Ah refugee camp, Thailand.
Source: Dean Chapman/Panos.

other hand, information about health achievements and social inequalities in health may contribute to our evaluation of the justice of social arrangements.

It seems that this approach captures many of our intuitions about what is wrong with social inequalities in health. After all, empirical research on social inequalities in health does not partition a society into random groups. Instead, research is guided by preconceptions of social institutions as hierarchical and as imposing inequalities of different kinds. This is the rationale for looking at racial inequalities, or at inequalities between occupational groups, in the first place. The approach proposed here attempts to make such judgments explicit. The main premise is that social inequalities in health are unfair because they are the result of a division of labor in society that puts certain groups of people at a disadvantage, not only economically, socially, and politically, but in terms of their possibilities to be healthy as well.

The Rawlsian approach has important policy implications. Other approaches that consider health outcomes alone may exaggerate the potential for remedies in the sphere of medicine and traditional health promotion (e.g. education about health behavior). In contrast, if the emphasis of a conception of health equity is on the broader social causes underlying inequalities in health, then the search for remedies has to extend to social policies at large. An example are policies that address the empowerment of women and other marginalized groups. The goal becomes one of inducing social change toward social arrangements that do not—in O'Neill's language—victimize certain social groups.

Admittedly, viewing health equity as part of a broader pursuit of social justice may complicate assessments of health equity, for it requires balancing health goals against other goals on the grounds of social justice. In an assessment of female garment workers in Bangladesh, the adverse occupational health effects have to be balanced with a wide range of benefits including delayed age of marriage and childbearing, increased wages, greater freedom, and independence. How we decide about such tradeoffs is again linked to the question of whose perspective of the fairness of health inequalities we consider: that of the person or groups with the health problem versus that of an external observer (see chapter 6).

Concluding Remarks

A comprehensive theoretical framework for health equity analysis faces the challenge of bridging moral and political philosophy and epidemiology, the basic science of public health. Epidemiological studies of social inequalities in health and their causes need to take into account concepts and tools from other social sciences and cannot bracket explicit considerations of social justice. Applying moral and political philosophy to the complex issue of social inequalities in health requires that we address the tension between the influence of social factors and of biological relations. As the first section of this chapter argues, this issue arises in the very idea of health itself.

The chapter presented four different approaches to health equity. The first three—based on utilitarianism, egalitarianism, and the priority view—provide perspectives on health equity as a separate social goal. The last approach, in contrast, drawing on the Rawlsian ideal of society as a fair system of cooperation, places the pursuit of health equity in the context of the larger pursuit of social justice. Although it is argued that this last ethical approach is the most appealing, there is nothing to say that these approaches are mutually exclusive. Despite the different approaches, there may be substantial consensus about when a social inequality becomes an inequity. Moreover, different types of judgments about fairness may help identify what is at stake and which issues deserve priority, especially given the likelihood of incomplete knowledge of the root causes of social inequalities in health.

Regarding assessment of the relative importance of health problems and aligning priorities for action, measures of inequalities in health will provide a sense of the magnitude of an inequality, which may be one of many criteria by which one ranks the importance or priority of inequities. As Sen notes (see chapter 6), a simple accounting approach may be problematic, and the fourth approach suggested here entails rating the importance of health inequities according to their respective causes. Inequities that arise from deliberate discrimination may be judged as most pernicious and therefore deserving most attention compared with those that arise from passive neglect (although this may be disguised willful neglect) (see also Pogge 1999). Alternatively, specific types of social inequities in health, for example, those affecting the particularly vulnerable group of children or mothers, may take precedence over health disparities among other age and sex groups. Similarly, social inequalities in the distribution of certain diseases that are highly stigmatized or risk outbreak epidemics may be less likely to be labeled as inequities than, say, unequally distributed chronic or noncommunicable diseases. Given the pervasiveness of resource constraints, much further work needs to be undertaken to improve understanding and provide some guidance.

There has been insufficient attention in this chapter to the issue of who is making health equity assessments.

As Arthur Kleinman argues when discussing the complexities of suicide in China, the ethical discourse must be enlightened by local realities, and ethnographically informed evaluations of "local knowledge and local moral processes" must be made "as salient as are the issues in global ethical discourse" (Kleinman 1999: 3). In an anthropological analysis of Tibetan theories of medicine, Adams notes the centrality of cultural freedom to health. She poses the following question for the international health equity community: How do we "accommodate non-secular, non-Western epistemological claims in a fair way?" (Adams 1999: 27). Such grounding of ethical principles might be facilitated through inclusive, participatory, democratic policy evaluation and decision making. It can be pointed out, in this context, that methods of participatory research and policy evaluation are becoming more mainstream and have the potential to bring to the fore concerns that have not yet received sufficient attention on the health equity agenda. In this regard, ethical theories may provide broad guidelines; however, specific standards and criteria for health equity should emerge from local discourse.

The imperative of participatory democratic assessments is linked to a further issue that was not dealt with in this chapter and that represents a major challenge for health equity analysis. From a global perspective on health equity, one major drawback of the ethics literature is the paucity of theories of international justice. Rawls (1993b) has suggested the idea of extending a fair system of cooperation to the international context. In like fashion, we may expand on the idea that inequalities in health are unjust if they are caused by unjust (international) social arrangements. Thomas Pogge (1999: 3) suggests such an approach when he rejects "the moral significance of compatriotism—belonging to the same state—with respect to the prevention and mitigation of health problems in whose production we are involved." In addition, the transnationalization of health risks (see chapter 4) arising from environmental threats, communicable disease, social change, and so forth make clear the importance of a global ethical framework for assessing inequalities in health. Such a framework would have to address the proper scope of such assessments and identify international institutions that can promote an inclusive discourse on health equity.

References

Adams V. 1999. Equity of the Ineffable: Cultural and Political Constraints on Ethnomedicine as a Health Problem in Contemporary Tibet. Working Paper Series. Cambridge, MA: Harvard Center for Population and Development Studies.

Anand S., Peter F., Sen A. (eds). Forthcoming. *Public Health, Ethics, and Equity*. Oxford: Oxford University Press.

Barker D. 1994. *Mothers, Babies and Disease in Later Life*. London: BMJ Publishing Group.

Barry B. 1990 [1965]. *Political Argument*. Berkeley: University of California Press.

Beauchamp D., Steinbock B. 1999. *New Ethics for the Public's Health*. New York: Oxford University Press.

Canguilhem G. 1991 [1966]. *On the Normal and the Pathological*. New York: Zone Books.

Culyer A., Wagstaff A. 1993. Equity and equality in health and health care. *Journal of Health Economics* 12:431–457.

Daniels N. 1985. *Just Health Care*. Cambridge: Cambridge University Press.

Daniels N., Kawachi I., Kennedy B. 1999. Is social justice good for our health? *Daedalus*. 128(4):215–251.

Dworkin R. 1981. What is equality? Part 2: equality of resources. *Philosophy and Public Affairs* 10:283–345.

Dworkin R. 1993. Justice in the distribution of health care. *McGill Law Journal* 38:883–898.

Engelhardt H.T. 1975. Concepts of health and disease. In: Engelhardt H.T., Spiker S. (eds), *Evaluation and Explanation in the Biomedical Sciences*. Dordrecht: D. Reidel, pp. 125–141.

Farmer P., Bertrand D. 2000. Hypocrisies of development and the health of the Haitian poor. In: Kim J.Y., Millen J.V., Irwin A., Gershman J., et al. (eds), *Dying for Growth*. Monroe, ME: Common Courage Press, pp. 65–90.

Fogel R. 1994. *Economic Growth, Population Theory, and Physiology: The Bearing of Long-Term Processes on the Making of Economic Policy*. Cambridge, MA: National Bureau of Economic Research.

Fried C. 1975. Rights and health care: beyond equity and efficiency. *New England Journal of Medicine* 253:241–245.

Gakidou E.E., Murray C.J.L., Frenk J. 1999. Defining and measuring health inequality. *Bulletin of the World Health Organization* 78(1):42–54.

Hare R.M. 1986. Health. In: Hare R.M. (ed.) *Bioethics*. Oxford: Clarendon, pp. 31–49.

Kleinman A. 1999. Ethics and Experience: An Anthropological Approach to Health Equity. Working Paper Series. Cambridge, MA: Harvard Center for Population and Development Studies.

Krieger N., Birn A.E. 1998. A vision of social justice as the foundation of public health: commemorating 150 years of the spirit of 1848. *American Journal of Public Health* 88(11):1603–1606.

Mann J.M. 1995. Human rights and the new public health. *Health and Human Rights* 1(3):229–233.

Marchand S., Wikler D., Landesman B. 1998. Class, health, and justice. *Milbank Quarterly* 76:449–468.

Margolis J. 1981. The concept of disease. In: Caplan A., Engelhardt H.T., McCartney J. (eds), *Concepts of Health and Disease*. Reading, MA: Addison-Wesley.

McKeown T. 1976. *The Modern Rise of Population*. London: Edward Arnold.

O'Neill O. 1993. Justice, gender, and international boundaries. In: Nussbaum M.C., Sen A. (eds), *Quality of Life*. Oxford: Clarendon, pp. 303–323.

Parfit D. 1997. Equality or priority. *Ratio* 10:202–221.

Pereira J. 1993. What does equity in health mean? *Journal of Social Policy* 22:19–48.

Pogge T. 1999. Justice in Health Care: Reflections on the Foundations of Health Equity. Working Paper Series. Cambridge, MA: Harvard Center for Population and Development Studies.

Rawls J. 1971. *A Theory of Justice*. Cambridge: Harvard University Press.

Rawls J. 1993a. *Political Liberalism*. New York: Columbia University Press.

Rawls J. 1993b. The law of peoples. In: Shute S., Hurly S. (eds), *On Human Rights: The Oxford Amnesty Lectures*. New York: Basic Books, pp. 41–82.

Raz J. 1986. *The Morality of Freedom*. Oxford: Clarendon.

Sen A. 1980. Equality of what? In: McMurrin S. (ed), *The Tanner Lectures in Human Values*, vol 1, Salt Lake City: University of Utah Press, pp. 195–220.

Sen A. 1985. *Commodities and Capabilities*. Amsterdam: North Holland.

Sen A. 1993. Capability and well-being. In: Nussbaum M.C., Sen A. (eds), *Quality of Life*. Oxford: Clarendon, pp. 30–53.

Toulmin S. 1975. Concepts of function and mechanism in medicine and medical science. In: Engelhardt H.T., Spiker S. (eds), *Evaluation and Explanation in the Biomedical Science*. Dordrecht: D. Reidel.

Veatch R.M. 1991. Justice and the right to health care: an egalitarian account. In: Bole T.J., Bondeson W.B. (eds), *Rights to Health Care*. Dordrecht: Kluwer, pp. 83–102.

Whitehead M. 1992. The concepts and principles of equity and health. *International Journal of Health Services*. 22(3):429–445.

Wikler D. 1997. Bioethics, human rights, and the renewal of Health for All: an overview. In: Bankowski Z., Bryant J.H., Gallagher J. (eds), *Ethics, Equity and the Renewal of WHO's Health for All Strategy*, Geneva: Council for International Organizations of Medical Scientists, pp. 21–30.

Williams B. 1973. A critique of utilitarianism. In: Smart J.J.C., Williams B. (eds), *Utilitarianism; For and Against*. Cambridge: Cambridge University Press, pp. 75–150.

World Bank. 1999. *Voices of the Poor*. Washington, DC: World Bank.

CHAPTER

4

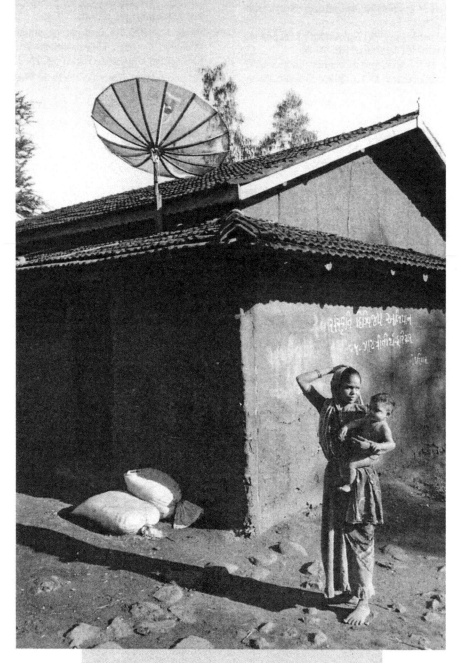

Gujarat, India.
Source: Sean Sprague/Panos.

Health Equity in a Globalizing World

LINCOLN C. CHEN AND GIOVANNI BERLINGUER

At the beginning of the new millennium, there is much talk about "globalization"—of international finance and trade, of real-time information, of science and technology, of labor standards, and environmental safety. A common misperception is that globalization is simply the integration of the world economy as highlighted by the Asian financial crisis or the protests during the World Trade Organization conference in Seattle. Another misunderstanding is that globalization may be a variant or derivative of such longer term trends as internationalism, modernization, or interdependence (Schoettle and Grant 1998).

Accelerating since the 1980s, globalization is quantitatively and qualitatively different from the past. It involves the multidimensional integration of the world economy, politics, culture, and human affairs, and it is fundamentally changing world health dynamics. This is marked by unprecedented health risks, the emergence of new diseases, and new challenges to global health institutions. Examples of these globalizing health phenomena are fresh environmental health threats, new and re-emerging infectious agents, and changing modes in the production and distribution of drugs and other health technologies.

Facilitated by a scientific revolution in information and biological technology, globalization is generating global "connectivity"—a dramatic compression of time and distance worldwide. Advances in digital technology are moving communications toward an integration of the computer, Internet, telephone, and television. Breakthroughs in genome research are likely to alter profoundly our capacity to control life and death. Some claim that the new information age will produce social changes as profound as the agricultural (10,000 years ago) and industrial (200 years ago) revolutions (Wriston 1992). The velocity of change is also very rapid. "Moore's law"—that digital capacity in computing power, speed, and miniaturization will double every 18 months—has held up well since it was formulated in in 1965 (Lucky 1998). Virtual information and communications mean that geographic and physical boundaries—nation states, communities, and neighborhoods—are increasingly transcended. Faraway actions can affect ordinary people in distant places. The linkages between global and local are increasingly more direct and powerful.

In this chapter we do not argue whether globalization is intrinsically good or bad or whether we should nurture or impede it. Nor do we explicitly praise or criticize it. Rather, we accept that globalization is a reality, not a choice. Globalization is here and inescapable because it corresponds to the present phase of historical development and because it has the power to fulfill many human wants.

A more pertinent question concerns the direction of globalization. What type of globalization is good or bad for human health? Toward which ends should the power of globalization be directed? To address these questions, we begin by reviewing the health dimensions of globalization. We then consider growing concerns about the impact of globalization on inequities in health. Finally, we argue that globalization generates new risks and offers unprecedented opportunities to meet the global equity agenda. How these opportunities are seized, we believe, is the premier global health challenge of our time.

Global Health Dynamics

Globalization in History

Health and disease have shaped human history, including trade, migration, and conflict (McNeill 1976). One of the most significant events in the globalization of disease dates back to 1492 with the discovery of the New World. European conquest forever altered the epidemiological pattern of disease in isolated populations of the Americas. Before Columbus landed, American populations had never encountered smallpox, measles, or yellow fever (just as syphilis was unknown in Eurasia and Africa) (Berlinguer 1992). The initial exposure was so devastating to nonimmunized populations that America's indigenous peoples experienced a virtual "health genocide." Massive declines of these immunologically unprepared populations followed the microbial assault, which was compounded by sociopolitical factors—war and conflict, slavery and enforced labor, disrupted food and nutrition, and psychological breakdown due to the loss of cultural identity, confidence, and security (Diamond 1999).

It took three centuries after global microbial unification in the sixteenth century for the world to recognize the mutualism of global health risks and interests. During the industrial revolution of the nineteenth century, governments recognized that free markets driving economic progress could not be all-embracing. Human health, safety, and dignity required social protection. By the end of the nineteenth century, the three preconditions for the control of infectious diseases were systematically put into place—knowledge of causation, development of effective preventive and curative tools, and mobilization of the requisite political will for social action.

In all three areas, international cooperation played a critical role. Smallpox immunization entered Europe from Turkey, where traditional female healers had developed the practice of transferring serum from healed smallpox blisters to induce attenuated disease and subsequent protection. The same empirical knowledge developed in Africa and was used by African Americans when smallpox struck North America in the eighteenth century. For generations Western physicians had rejected this alien advance until Edward Jenner reinvented it, improved it, and demonstrated its effective-

ness in European populations. A century ago many microbes were discovered (e.g., tuberculosis, plague, and *Vibrio cholerae*); their transmission became understood (John Snow identified contaminated water from the Broad Street pump as the cause of cholera even before the vibrio was discovered); and protective sera and vaccines were developed. These technical advances were accompanied by social legislation to regulate working hours, to prohibit the cruelest forms of child labor, and to protect pregnant women. Governments assumed formal responsibility for national health, and social insurance was introduced for collective health protection. The imperative of international cooperation was recognized and acted on, culminating in an International Sanitary conference, the original world health organization (Zacher 1999).

The historian Arnold Toynbee observed that "The 20th century shall be essentially recalled not so much as an epoch of political conflicts and technical inventions, but rather as the time when human society dared to think about health care of the whole human species as a practical objective within its reach" (Toynbee 1992).

Another Round?

Today, one century later, globalization is again fueling dynamics in the pattern of disease worldwide. The traditional typology of disease is tripartite—communicable diseases, noncommunicable diseases, and injury. A first generation of diseases is linked to poverty—common infections, malnutrition, and reproductive health hazards mostly affecting women and children. These predominantly communicable diseases are overwhelmingly concentrated among the poor in low-income countries. A second generation of primarily chronic and degenerative diseases—such as cardiovascular disease, cancer, stroke, and diabetes—predominate among the middle-aged and elderly in all countries. Susceptibility to these noncommunicable diseases is linked to changing environment, lifestyle, and health-related behavior. To these two groups of diseases may be added injuries, caused by both violence and accidents, which are also prevalent in both rich and poor countries.

This classification system appears to be breaking down in our globalizing world (Chen 1998). New health threats are being superimposed on traditional diseases, driven at least in part by the forces of globalization. Globalization, thus, is generating epidemiological diversity and complexity. Three examples, discussed below, are emerging infections, environmental hazards, and sociobehavioral pathologies.

Emerging Infections

Our complacency over the successful conquest of infectious diseases (except for common childhood infections among the poor in developing countries) has been rudely disturbed. Since the global spread of the human immunodeficiency virus (HIV) began in the early 1980s, more than 29 new bacteria or viruses have been identified, many capable of global spread. With more than 1 million travelers flying across national boundaries every day, many of these pathogens have the capacity to reach anywhere in the world within 24 hours (Lederberg 1997). Moreover, many infectious agents are not new but rather well-known pathogens rekindled by changing conditions.

Rapid urbanization with urban poverty and squalor, for example, created conditions conducive to recent epidemics of dengue fever in Jakarta, Indonesia, and Mexico City and a plague outbreak in Surat, India (Institute of Medicine 1997). Tuberculosis has seen a resurgence in part because of the acquired immunodeficiency syndrome (AIDS), which compromises the human immune system (Farmer 1999). The acceleration of international trade has precipitated new epidemics (cholera in Latin America), sparked local epidemics in previously protected populations (cyclospora in the United States, where one-third of fruits and vegetables are imported), and generated unprecedented health fears ("mad cow disease" or bovine spongiform encephalitis in Europe). At the same time, one of our most powerful defenses against infection, antibiotics, may be rendered impotent by the emergence of antibiotic resistance—for example, multidrug resistant tuberculosis or chloroquin-resistant malaria (Committee on International Science, Engineering, and Technology 1995).

Environmental Threats

Environmental health damage results from the pollution of air, water, and soil along with the depletion of nonrenewable natural resources. Traditional conceptions of environmental health are of two types—the challenges of providing clean water and sanitation still unavailable to the poor in low-income countries and a second generation of industrial exposures to chemical and other pollutants among high-risk individuals, families, and local communities. Superimposed on these hazards is another round of fresh environmental threats.

In a manner paralleling infectious diseases, many new environmental health hazards are associated with globalization due to unhealthy production and consumption patterns in a globalizing economy. The negative health effects of ozone depletion, global warming, and the disposal of toxic wastes have transnational reach. No single community or nation can escape their health consequences fully. The air pollution in Southeast Asia in 1997, caused by the burning of Indonesian forests and exacerbated by El Niño, vividly demonstrates the regional implications of atmospheric change. The projected impact of global warming (coastal flooding, population displacement, and spread of disease vectors) underscores the permeability of national borders to the health implications of global climate change (McMichael and Haines 1997).

Sociobehavioral Pathologies

Sociobehavioral pathologies include mental illness, the abuse of addictive substances, the hazards of unsafe sexual behavior, and the toll of violence and injury. Mental illness accounted for 10% of the disability-adjusted life years (DALY) lost in the 1990 global burden of disease analysis and it is projected to increase to 15% by 2020 (Murray and Lopez 1996). This growing burden is magnified by the lack of public recognition linked to the marginal position of mental health in the hierarchy of medical care and continuing social stigmatization of those suffering from mental illness (Desjarlais et al. 1995). Furthermore, many believe that treatment for mental illness is a "luxury" the poor cannot afford when in fact depression, anxiety, and alcohol abuse are common among the poor (Patel et al. 1999). Linked to this ignorance is the inattention paid to the rapid sociocultural and demographic dynamics fueling the epidemic. Accelerated urbanization, being uprooted from traditional cultural socialization, joblessness, and homelessness are common social determinants underlying depression, substance abuse, and violence.

The dynamics of violence—which is the primary cause of death among adolescents and young people, especially men, in almost all countries—exemplifies the globalization of disease. Because of limited data and insufficient research, the taxonomy of violence has yet to be firmly established. Violence in our globalizing world can be "real" (with physical or mental damage) or "virtual" (with psychological and social damage through violent content in computers, television, and films). Violence can also be intentional or without malice of forethought. Industrial and road violence are customarily considered "accidental," but our standard ideas of negligence, imprudence, or lack of compliance with regulations seem insufficient to account for clear epidemi-ological evidence of modifiable risk factors (such as poor road conditions, lack of seat belts, or car engines built to exceed reasonable speed limits). Intentional or willful violence may be perpetrated on the weak, against children, women, or the elderly. Recent studies underscore the global prevalence of gender-based violence, including sexual abuse and sexual harassment against women (World Health Organization 1997; Heise et al. 1994). In many statistical systems, intentional violence may also be disguised as "accidental," as suggested by the disproportionately high death rate due to "accidental fires" among recently married Indian women that many attribute to purposeful "bride burning" for dowry (Kumari 1989). Suicide or self-inflicted violence is a growing problem in many societies—among young Chinese women, Scandinavians especially during dark winters, and reportedly among Asians after the recent financial crisis (see chapter 7, on China).

Finally, there is organized violence in contrast to informal violence. Informal violence usually comes from individual acts, ranging from hooliganism, to petty crime, to the loss of behavioral control (e.g., road rage). Organized criminal violence, in contrast, is aimed at advancing illegal activities. Global connectivity is facilitating the spread of organized criminal activities worldwide. Government is the only institution to which citizens have ceded legitimacy in the use of violence for public safety. Among some nations, even legitimately organized violence by the state can be abusive, for example, among some military or oppressive rulers.

What Links Globalization and Health?

The examples cited earlier raise a fundamental question. What links a particular disease to globalization? As globalization itself is in its early stages, why would some diseases be included while others excluded? The answer necessarily must link specific diseases to core globalization processes (Chen et al. 1999). Three or more interactive linkages may be proposed.

First is the clear transmissibility of health determinants and risks. Enhanced international linkages in trade, migration, and information flows have accelerated the cross-border transmission of disease and the international transfer of behavioral and environmental health risks. Emerging infections are diseases of globalization because of accelerating world travel and trade and also changing microbial–host interactions—human penetration into virgin forests, intensive domestication of livestock, artificial change of cows from herbivores to carnivores, and the ecology of unprecedented urbanization due to migration. It is increasingly recog-nized that violence, like infectious diseases, may be transmissible—not only through the illegal activities of international criminal organizations (and sometimes also the behavior of nation states) but also via material and cultural paths—by imitation, suggestion, and normative endorsement. Rapid social change can be psychologically destabilizing, expanding tensions that can produce ripples of violence among individuals, social groups, and whole nations. Competition between social groups for economic opportunity or environmental resources can escalate into intranational conflict. Wherever violence breaks out in the world—due to gender, ethnic group, race, religious beliefs, organized crime, political oppression—the challenge is the social response. Because violence has no vaccines or drugs (because violence is anthropogenic), counteracting it requires social and cultural "antibodies" that are constantly being shaped by globalization processes. Faced with violence, the attitudes of societies may be selective rejection or acceptance, depending on prejudice or bias. Modifying social attitudes is an essential precondition for a global approach to violence.

A second criterion is shared risks and consequences worldwide and over time. Intensified pressures on common-pool global resources of air and water have generated shared environmental threats. Environmental damage due to global warming, ozone depletion, chemical pollution, and the unsafe disposal of toxic wastes are examples. While local and regional contexts may shape the health dimension of environmental insults, many new threats are genuinely global in scale. In other words, no one can escape fully the risk or the consequences incurred. Although some environment and health linkages are scientifically uncertain, two considerations are in order. The first is practical. Even when damage is unpredictable, we may already have the knowledge of the potential health risks involved. Is it possible to avoid action when, even if there is uncertainty, much of the damage will undoubtedly become irreversible? The second consideration is ethical. Environmental damage often has an impact far away in distance and time from the originator. Under such circumstances, standard risk–benefit analyses are inoperable. The asymmetry is that the benefits accrue to some while risk or damage must be borne by others. Even the golden rule of ethics here seems insufficient. We may rather have to apply Hans Jonas' "responsibility principle" (1990: 12) involving both an ethics of proximity and an ethics of distance in which the frame of reference is the entire world space and the time is of future generations. Such an ethical underpinning can only operate across time on a global scale, requiring profound changes in governance and public policies.

A final dimension is health change associated with the technological and institutional transformations of globalization. The technological advances underpinning globalization are profoundly altering the landscape of global health. Some examples are the market-driven priorities of private pharmaceutical companies, the penetration of private markets into health services, the neglect of research and development against "orphan diseases" afflicting the poor, and iatrogenesis due to inappropriate application of new and often expensive health technologies. As globalization transcends national boundaries, the institutional performance of key actors like national governments and international agencies is also undergoing transformation. "Although responsibility for health remains primarily national, the determinants of health and means to fulfill that responsibility are increasingly global" (Jamison et al. 1998). The revitalization or stagnation of diverse health institutions, therefore, may be also considered linked to core globalization processes.

Looming Health Inequities

Will globalization improve or worsen world health equity? A lively debate is currently underway over the social impact of globalization. On the one hand are those who believe that globalization accelerates economic progress and expands personal liberties. A rising tide of wealth lifts all boats, leading to health advancement and equity. Indeed, despite marked disparities in life expectancy among countries (40 years in Sierra Leone vs. 80 years in Japan), national mortality trends in the past half century exhibit growing convergence. Lower income countries have achieved a faster pace of longevity gain than high-income countries, in part because of effective application of health technologies among the former and biological ceilings slowing the pace of gain among the latter. Why should the secular convergence of national mortality trends not continue during this era of globalization?

On the other hand, concerns about social inequity and human insecurity have been voiced in these times of rapid change. Left unattended, the forces of globalization could significantly worsen inequities in health. Continuing the analogy, a rising tide could lift big yachts, but capsize small dinghies. As health is knowledge based, the production, distribution, and utilization of knowledge can have significant distributive implications. Unconstrained or inadequately regulated private markets driven by commercial interests are not likely to be equity enhancing. As only small groups are able to capture the benefits of globalization, many could be left behind, thereby worsening inequities in health. Some trends in the 1990s underscore these health equity concerns— the world's worst health indicators are in countries racked by conflict, mortality improvements have been reversed in regions affected by the AIDS pandemic, especially sub-Saharan Africa, and life expectancy has declined sharply in Russia during its massive political and economic transition.

Our understanding of inequities in health should be nuanced by understanding several distinctive types of inequities. First of all, there is international disparity— that is, between nation states. Within all countries, rich and poor alike, intranational disparities may also be found. Global disparity recognizes both international and intranational disparities. Truly global disparities consider the health of each person regardless of the health dynamics and population size of any particular country. Computation of global disparities would require comprehensive data on both international and intranational disparities with global estimates weighting the countries according to population size. Sen (1999) has also introduced the concept of inequalities and social justice between groups that are neither defined as individuals nor nation states but by social affinity, identity, and relationships. Moreover, added to these "horizontal disparities" are changing dynamics over time among all types of disparities. Widening or narrowing gaps over time may be as important as the absolute or relative differences at any single point of time.

As data are not available, we can only hypothesize the changing dynamics of these different types of health disparities among population groups and across time. One penetrating analysis proposed by Paul Streeten (1998) is that globalization is worsening inequity and social exclusion both within and across countries. Those with education, knowledge, capital, and enterprise in all countries have an opportunity to join the global mainstream, thereby reaping the benefits of globalization. Many if not most of the world's people in both rich and poor countries are left behind. The formation of a world elite is based on the development of cosmopolitan identity, associations, and affinity across national and cultural boundaries. To this transnational elite, Miami becomes the financial and cultural capital of Latin America just as Paris serves this role for the Francophone world. An outcome is that rather than investing in social cohesion within one's own community or nation state, an exclusionary process is set off, with the privileged becoming less responsive or obligated to the socially underprivileged within their own communities and countries. Equity and social cohesion, therefore, lie beyond weakened nation states, requiring global social action.

There are thus legitimate concerns over global inequities in health (Walt 1998). Although the evidence is not conclusive, some mechanisms for worsening of health equity may be hypothesized, as described below.

Economics and Trade

Wealth and income are among the most important social determinants of health. Not only does the relationship depend on the use of income to command a basket of material goods (food, clothing, housing, and so forth) necessary for good health but also income distribution itself may reflect an independent health effect (Wilkinson 1996; Kawachi et al. 1997). Early evidence suggests that economic globalization is worsening income distribution and income stability. Private markets may generate efficiency in resource allocation, but also skew wealth and income distribution and exacerbate fiscal instability and volatility. These inequitable effects seem to be relevant to both intranational as well as international disparities. Indeed, the recent Asian financial crisis has precipitated a historically unprecedented process of mass impoverishment, where tens of millions of Indonesian families were pushed below the poverty line. Other world regions, like sub-Saharan Africa, feel excluded from or exploited by these global processes, while still others, as in Eastern Europe, journey on a rocky road in attempts to join the global flows. Even in wealthy countries like the United Kingdom and the United States, empirical data confirm worsening income distribution (Whitehead and Diderichsen 1997).

These inequities are global in scope among and between northern and southern countries. The dynamics operate directly on many distributive dimensions beyond income. Two examples are the health conditions of low-paid workers and environmental health hazards. The World Trade Organization conference in Seattle encountered fierce protests over lax, nonexistent, or unenforceable labor standards in poor countries as low-wage industries increasingly shift from northern to southern countries. Child or forced labor, lack of minimum wage, and deplorable working conditions—all with health implications—are among the issues at stake. The distributive impact of globalization of labor may become more complicated as fears emerge that shifting production may drive wages upward in low-income countries and downward in high-income countries. Some argue that foreign investment in low-wage labor in low-income countries may have beneficial equity impact, by, for example, providing income-generating opportunities for women and thereby enhancing socioeconomic empowerment. There are few data to support this positive outcome. Similar divisiveness surrounds environmental hazards where health-damaging production is shifted to countries with weak environmental standards. In addition to international equity concerns, most environmental hazards disproportionately affect the poor within countries—for example, toxic waste dumps near low-income neighborhoods.

Trade in addictive substances between northern and southern countries underscores the disconnection between health equity and international ground rules. Indisputable is the fact that consumption of heroin, cocaine, and tobacco is health damaging, especially among the young. The negative health impact is both direct as well as indirect (e.g., HIV transmitted through contaminated needles). So too are the many deleterious aspects of illegal drug movement—organized crime, recycling of profits into legal business, and the use of money to corrupt political processes. In terms of equity, it is important to recognize that the global movement of addictive substance is bidirectional: south to north for heroin and cocaine and north to south for tobacco. An objective assessment of policies by governments and agencies highlights inequitable policies in these international flows.

The United Nations has set up a special agency to control opium and cocaine grown in the south for export to the north. No such international agency exists for control of the reverse flow, mediated by multinational corporations, of tobacco from the north to the south. The World Health Organization (WHO) recently launched a global tobacco program that may over time help correct these imbalances. But WHO efforts to regulate world advertising and trade in cigarettes has run into charges of interference with free trade. Yet, it would be ludicrous to legitimize advertising for the reverse flow of addictive drug from the south into the north. These imbalances are generated in part by the self-interests of national powers. Even as the European Union announced a $2 million fund in its fight against cancer, it simultaneously invested more than $2 billion to subsidize tobacco production in Europe, much for export to other countries. Similarly, the United States donated tobacco seeds worth $700 million to poor countries with a pledge to buy leaves for cigarette production under its foreign aid "Food for Peace" program (Berlinguer 1996: 18). At the same time, the U.S. government threatened trade sanctions against four Asian nations unwilling to give market access to cigarettes manufactured in the United States.

Private Markets in Health Services

Private markets, unconstrained and inadequately regulated, are perhaps the most powerful globalizing force driving inequities in health. Particularly disturbing is the commercialization and commodification of health, for example, the sale of body parts, such as kidneys (sometimes even from live donors) (Berlinguer 1999). Penetration of private markets into health services comes at a time when the state is under attack as inefficient and misused through private "rent-seeking" behavior of politicians and civil servants. Downsizing government has been accomplished by restricting government budgets, resulting in cuts that are often disproportionately absorbed by the social sectors. Thus, the model of state responsibility for universal access (Health for All) in primary health care promulgated at Alma Ata in 1978 has been virtually abandoned. Equity-enhancing universal access to basic care has been replaced by so-called health sector reform, promulgated by budget-strapped governments under pressure from international financial institutions such as the World Bank and International Monetary Fund (Gershman and Irwin 2000).

Health sector reform as pursued by these institutions is rather narrowly conceived—priority-setting, privatization, and decentralization. Prioritization has mostly been supply driven rather than demand or consumer driven. Although necessary in any resource-constrained situation, priority-setting or rationing has focused on technologies against specific diseases. Affordable access to appropriate services and technologies tailored to diverse local circumstances has not been equally embraced by reform policies. Some have argued that a mixture of efficiency driven by the private sector and equity protected by the public sector can provide an acceptable blend (World Bank 1993). Yet there is little empirical evidence for such optimism. Indeed, early experiments on the imposition of user fees in public systems to enhance efficiency and cost recovery have neither realized the presumed benefit nor enhanced equity of access (Dahlgren 1994). Private payments for health care naturally place fiscal barriers on universal access by the poor (Stocker et al. 1999). Finally, administrative decentralization has been pursued in an effort to enhance client responsiveness, administrative efficiency, and improved service access. The danger is rapid decentralization of responsibility without the corresponding devolution of authority and requisite human, institutional, and financial resources needed to provide affordable, accessible, and equitable basic health services.

Harnessing Science and Technology

Imbedded in the scientific revolution of globalization are the seeds of health inequity. Because human health is knowledge based, the manner in which knowledge is produced and harnessed to address health problems has powerful distributive effects. The main equity concern in relation to biomedical sciences is the tendency to ignore the diseases suffered by the majority of human beings and to concentrate instead on commercially profitable products. These types of knowledge are particularly evident for "orphan diseases" and the "digital divide," as outlined below.

As we move to decipher the human genome, the potential of biotechnology to transform health is increasingly appreciated. For some diseases, research breakthroughs could result in effective prevention or treatment—against diseases such as Alzheimer's or hypertension—based on an expanding pool of basic knowledge and the research and development capabilities of the pharmaceutical industry. For many diseases that afflict the poor, however, the priority assigned by large pharmaceutical companies not surprisingly is low. Called "market failures," comparatively neglected by the research and development efforts of private industry is the development of technologies against some of the major killers in low-income countries like malaria, tuberculosis, and HIV/AIDS (Pablos-Mendez et al. 1999). The inequity is compounded by the World Trade Organization trade-related intellectual property (TRIPs) agreement that permits patenting of genomic resources on a global basis. Many low-income countries fear loss of control over indigenous genetic materials through intellectual property regimes. Still poorly recognized are the equity implications of "iatrogenesis," illness or death due to abuse or misuse of health technologies. As scientific frontiers are advanced, the inequitable impact of biased or selective research and development by commercial enterprises is likely to exacerbate or even worsen health inequities.

A second source of inequity in the new sciences is the hypothesized growing digital divide in health. Information is recognized as a key component for generating healthful individual behavior as well as healthy cultural norms. The information revolution may empower many, but even more are excluded due to inaccessibility. Digital access depends on basic literacy, primary education, sufficient income to access digital systems, basic electronic infrastructure, and an enabling social environment. The lack of universal literacy and primary education around the world automatically translates into informational inequities. Inequitable information and knowledge access operates at all levels, with inequity compounded at each higher level. Informational exclusion at the individual level would be worsened if systems at the community or national levels are similarly deprived because both the demand for and delivery of information determine equitable access.

Toward a Democratization of Health

Simon Szreter (1997), a public health historian, analyzed health dynamics of the industrial revolution in Britain during the first half of the nineteenth century. He concluded that times of rapid economic change are not necessarily good for health, especially of the poor. There were first of all winners and losers in economic competition. Great disruptions of human ecology, socially and environmentally, occurred. Rapid change also triggered ideological ferment in the cultural negotiations over new values and norms. Many established institutions became obsolete, while new configurations emerged.

Are we entering another round of health change associated with social, economic, and technological transformation? The answer, we believe, is yes. Like a century ago, fresh social responses will be required, this time on a global scale. Several chapters in this book offer the theoretical rationale and practical suggestions for the advancement of more equitable health policies and programs. They involve developing shared equity goals and targets, tracking and monitoring progress, developing new analytical tools, and fashioning equity-enhancing social policies.

Yet for global health, the new millenium does not even begin on a level health playing field. Foege (1998) has characterized health progress in the twentieth century as "spectacular achievement, spectacular inequities." The forces of globalization left unattended could worsen these inequities in the social determinants of health, unequal access to health care, and the imbalanced deployment of health knowledge. As informed by history, the promotion of health equity will require public action on a global scale to articulate its value and to mobilize political commitment to its achievement (Yach and Bettcher 1998a,b). To be effective, the global social response must harness the power of globalization to flip, like the oriental martial art jujitsu, globalizing forces toward equitable outcomes. Because health advances in the twentieth century have been "knowledge based" and "socially driven," mobilization of social action for health equity should focus on the equity dimensions of new knowledge and technologies, new institutional arrangements, and new values and norms.

The more equitable production and dissemination of health knowledge first of all will depend on an educated and informed public. Achieving universal primary education so that all people are able to become agents of their own health is fundamental. So too will be the harnessing of new sciences to solve health problems not adequately addressed by market incentives. Public investment will be required in research and development of new technologies especially against "orphan diseases" neglected by the commercial sector. Broad and effective utilization of new informational and communications technologies can help with the global dissemination of health information, including enhancing the transparency and connectivity of local, national, and global health institutions.

To drive forward social policies for global health equity, strong institutions at the community, national, and global levels are received. Manual Castells (1998) has characterized our globalizing world as a "network society," where people with similar interests can be connected at the global level in real time to pursue shared interests. This connectivity can be employed to build alliances, coalitions, and partnerships among government, business, and civil society. Currently in vogue is the creation of "private–public partnerships," which seek to accomplish specific global health tasks. Recent examples are coordinated actions by diverse global actors networked together for tobacco control, access to essential drugs, research and development of vaccines against malaria and drugs for tuberculosis, and more equitable health policies.

Globalization, above all, requires a renewed focus on the role of global institutions (Bryant and Harrison 1996). The recent revitalization of the WHO offers new hope for global health governance, especially if it can move beyond its historical role as a monolithic world health operating agency. Rather, it must strengthen its recognized normative role for supporting equity-oriented health policies, operating as the "world conscience" of health (Godlee 1997; Lee 1998).

To assume this new role, the WHO must arrest the decline of financial support to U.N. agencies by member governments while it cooperates with, but does not become subservient to, the health activities of multilateral financial institutions. The WHO must cultivate an appropriate place for the consideration of health equity concerns within a range of other institutions, including the World Trade Organization and the International Labor Organization. In global health, we should not accept as a unique authority that of a few nations that claim it is their right to decide for the whole world; nor should we accept financial institutional claims that all human activities become subservient to monetary interests (Buse and Gwin 1998). Leadership by the WHO could help expand the socially shared space for the equity actions by many other actors from private business, academia, and nongovernmental civil society organizations (Evans et al. 2000).

With this positive outlook, we must pave the way toward a universal health democracy in which all people are informed, their voices are heard, and they are able to participate in decisions affecting their own health. The democratization of health will require strong political will, for no longer is it acceptable in a modern age to tolerate unnecessary illness and death in a world with abundant knowledge and resources to prevent such suffering. Good health is the cornerstone of economic progress, a multiplier of a society's human resources, and, indeed, the primary objective of development. Ultimately, we must strengthen the moral or ethical basis of global health equity. Can we promote the emergence of a commonly shared global value for fairness in health?

Health is a basic human right, and, as such, equity in health should have pride of place. Human values such as universality, social solidarity, and social justice provide effective moral bases for global health equity. We must move toward the democratization of health built on both altruism and self-interest to empower global citizens with the basic health knowledge, the voice and participation in health decision making, and the norms and institutions that are able to advance the ideal and the praxis of the indivisibility of global health.

References

Berlinguer G. 1992. Public health then and now: the interchange of disease and health between the old and new worlds. *American Journal of Public Health* 82:1407–1413.

Berlinguer G. 1996. *Volnej Garrafa: la merce finale. Saggio sulla compravendita di parti del corpo umano.* Milano: Baldini c Castoldi.

Berlinguer G. 1999. Globalization and global health. *International Journal of Health Services* 29(3):579–595.

Bryant J.H., Harrison P.F. 1996. *Global Health in Transition: A Synthesis: Perspectives from International Organizations.* Institute of Medicine. Washington, DC: National Academy Press.

Buse K., Gwin C. 1998. The World Bank and global cooperation in health: the case of Bangladesh. *Lancet* 351:665–669.

Castells M. 1998. *The Information Age: Economy, Society and Culture. Vol I, The Rise of the Network Society; Vol II, The Power of Identity.* Berkeley: Blackwell Publishers, Ltd.

Chen L.C. 1998. Globalization: Health Equity or Social Exclusion? Keynote address at the Conference of the International Health Policy Association, Perugia, Italy, September 23, 1998.

Chen L.C., Evans T.G., Cash R.A. 1999. Health as a global public good. In: Kaul I., Grunberg I., Stern M (eds), *Global Public Goods: International Cooperation in the 21st Century.* UNDP. New York: Oxford University Press, pp. 284–304.

Committee on International Science, Engineering, and Technology. 1995. *Global Microbial Threats in the 1990s.* Report of the NSTC Committee on International Science, Engineering, and Technology (CISET) Working Group on Emerging and Re-emerging Infectious Diseases. Washington, DC: National Science and Technology Council.

Dahlgren G. 1994. The political economy of health financing strategies in Kenya. In: Chen L.C., Kleinman A., Ware N.C. (eds), *Health and Social Change in International Perspective.* Boston: Harvard University Press, pp. 453–470.

Desjarlais R., Eisenberg L., Good B., Kleinman A. 1995. *World Mental Health: Problems and Priorities in Low Income Countries.* New York: Oxford University Press.

Diamond J. 1999. *Guns, Germs, and Steel: The Fates of Human Societies.* New York: W.W. Norton & Co.

Evans T.G., Wirth M.E., Chen L.C. 2000. Philanthropy and global health equity in the 21st century. In: Koop C.E., Pearson C.E., Schwarz M.R. (eds), *Global Health in the 21st Century.* New York: Jossey-Bass, pp. 430–439.

Farmer P. 1999. *Infections and Inequalities: The Modern Plagues.* Berkeley: University of California Press.

Foege W.H. 1998. Global public health: targeting inequities. *Journal of the American Medical Association* 279(24):1931–1932.

Gershman J., Irwin A. 2000. Getting a grip on the global economy. In: Kim J.Y., Millen J.V., Irwin A., Gershman J., et al. (eds), *Dying for Growth.* Monroe, ME: Common Courage Press, pp. 11–43.

Godlee F. 1997. WHO reform and global health. *British Medical Journal* 314:1359–1360.

Heise L., Pitanguy J., Germain A. 1994. *Violence Against Women: The Hidden Health Burden.* Washington, DC: The World Bank.

Insitute of Medicine. 1997. *America's Vital Interest in Global Health.* Washington, DC: National Academy Press.

Jamison D., Frenk J., Kaul I. 1998. International collective action in health: objectives, functions and rational. *Lancet* 351(9101):514–517.

Jonas H. 1990 [1985]. *The Principle of Responsibility.* Chicago: University of Chicago. Translated from the German, *Das Prinzip verantwortung.* Frankfurt: Suhrkamp.

Kawachi I., Kennedy B., Lochner K., Prothrow-Smith D. 1997. Social capital, income inequality and mortality. *American Journal of Public Health* 87:1491–1498.

Kumari R. 1989. *Brides Are Not for Burning: Dowry Victims in India.* New Delhi: Radiant Publishers.

Lederberg J. 1997. Infectious Disease as an Evolutionary Paradigm. *Emerging Infectious Disease* 3(4):417–423.

Lee K. 1998. World health: shaping the future of global health cooperation: where can we go from here? *Lancet* 351:899–902.

Lucky R.W. 1998. Moore's Law Redux. *IEEE Spectrum* 35(9):17.

McMichael A., Haines A. 1997. Global climate change: the potential effects on health. *British Medical Journal* 315:805–809.

McNeill W. 1976. *Plagues and Peoples.* Garden City, NY: Anchor Books.

Murray C.J.L., Lopez A. 1996. *The Global Burden of Disease: A Comprehensive Assessment of Mortality and Disability from Diseases, Injuries, and Risk Factors in 1990 and Projected to 2020.* Geneva: World Health Organization.

Pablos-Mendez A., Chacko S., Evans T.G. 1999. Market failures and orphan diseases. *Development* 42(4):79–83.

Patel V., Araya R., de Lima M., Ludermil A., Todd C. 1999. Women, poverty and common mental disorders in four restructuring societies. *Social Science and Medicine* 49(11):1461–1471.

Schoettle E., Grant K. 1998. *Globalization: Implications for the Rockefeller Foundation.* New York: Rockefeller Foundation.

Sen A. 1999. Global justice: Beyond international equity. In: Kaul I., Gunberg I., Stern M.A. (eds), *International Cooperation in the 21st Century.* United Nations Development Program. New York: Oxford University Press.

Stocker K., Waitzkin H., Iriart C. 1999. The exportation of managed care to Latin America. *New England Journal of Medicine* 340(14):1131–1136.

Streeten P. 1998. Unpublished commentary presented at a meeting, Globalization and Human Development, May 25–29 1998, Bellagio Study and Conference Center, Italy.

Szreter S. 1997. Economic growth, disruption, deprivation, disease and death: on the importance of the politics of public health for development. *Population and Development Review* 23:693–728.

Toynbee A. 1992. *Change and Habit: The Challenge of Our Time (Global Thinkers)*. Oxford: Oxford University Press.

Walt G. 1998. Globalization of international health. *Lancet* 351:434–437.

Whitehead M., Diderichsen F. 1997. International evidence on inequalities in health. In: Drever F., Whitehead M. (eds), *Health Inequalities: Decennial Supplement*. Office for National Statistics. Series DS No. 15. London: The Stationery Office.

Wilkinson R. 1996. *Unhealthy Societies: From Inequality to Well-Being*. London: Routledge.

World Bank. 1993. *World Development Report 1993*. Washington, DC: World Bank.

World Health Organization. 1997. *Violence Against Women*. Geneva: World Health Organization.

Wriston W.B. 1992. *The Twilight of Sovereignty: How the Information Revolution is Transforming our World*. New York: Scribner.

Yach D., Bettcher D. 1998a. The globalization of public health, I: threats and opportunities. *American Journal of Public Health* 88(5):735–738.

Yach D., Bettcher D. 1998b. The globalization of public health, II: the convergence of self-interest and altruism. *American Journal of Public Health* 88(5):738–741.

Zacher M.W. 1999. Global epidemiological surveillance. In: Kaul I., Grunberg I., Stern M. (eds), *Global Public Goods: International Cooperation in the 21st century*, UNDP. New York: Oxford University Press, pp. 284–305.

ASSESSING AND ANALYZING THE HEALTH DIVIDE

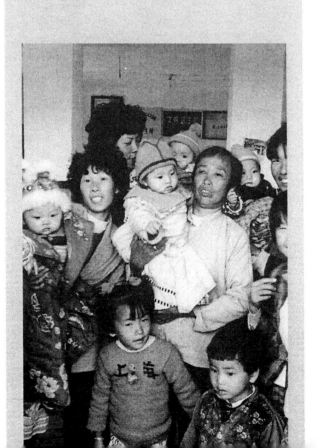

Highlighting injustice—mapping the extent and nature of inequalities in health—is the central theme of this section. Without reliable data on disparities in health, policy makers and populations are less equipped to demand change and monitor progress. We see this as what is perhaps the first injustice—an inability to provide basic statistics that reflect the health status of the entire population. Both effectively and metaphorically, this implies that people do not count.

Simple indicators are often sufficient to focus policy attention on disparities and spur action. To disentangle the root causes of inequities in health, however, more complex measures and techniques are also needed. The next chapter provides a comprehensive approach to the measurement of inequity. It outlines five basic considerations in the choice of health measure, highlighting the ways that assumptions can affect the magnitude and assessment of a given health disparity. A range of measures—new and old, simple and complex—for assessing intergroup and interindividual inequalities in health are reviewed. Amartya Sen then tackles some of the fundamental issues underlying the conception and measurement of equity in health. He raises the following questions, among others: How does the "internal" versus the "external" perspective of a person's health affect assessments of equity? What is the relevance of *health* in health care? How and in what form should we measure health achievement? What criteria do we use to rank health states in order to assess relative inequalities?

The six in-depth country analyses that follow take a wide range of approaches to assessing and analyzing the health divide. The Chinese study, examines whether economic growth has yielded improved health status for all. The authors find that while health for the population as a whole has improved, there is evidence of growing gender and geographic (urban/rural) differentials in health in the context of China's economic integration into the global economy.

The unparalleled health gains and economic progress in Japan in the twentieth century are examined in the context of the cultural ethos of equal outcomes. Historic commitments to gender equity in education and to the health of mothers are deemed important determinants of Japan's rapid health improvement. The analysis reveals significant inequalities in health according to average wealth, income distribution, education levels, television ownership, and occupation grouping.

The chapter on the social burden of ill health in the United States describes the separate and joint effects of household income, race/ethnicity, and gender on health outcomes. The authors argue that sound health equity analysis requires not just an exclusive focus on those at highest risk, but an assessment of the full impact of disparities in health across the social gradient.

In Chile, recent macroeconomic reforms have led to overall improvements in economic and social indicators, but widening socioeconomic gaps in income and health. The authors describe gender, educational, and cause-specific differentials in adult life expectancy at an individual and an ecological level. They argue that the adverse health effects of worsening income inequality may have been offset by the pro-health effects of increased educational attainment.

The Russian mortality crisis is tackled from different angles, elaborating on the temporal, socioeconomic, and spatial variations in gender-specific mortality indices of the Russian population over the last 30 years. Of particular concern is the wide gender gap in mortality in Russia—why do men fare so much worse given that both sexes are exposed to the same general political, social, or economic forces? The chapter takes a close look at the gender gap in mortality, comparing how men and women fare relative to one another within Russia, as well as to the rest of the world, disaggregating the gap into cause-specific components.

Finally, the chapter on Tanzania provides a refreshing qualitative health equity analysis of a specific age group—adolescents. The authors uncover layers of inequities with regard to the policy neglect of adolescents as a group, the bias in the existing policies toward those in school, and the wholesale neglect of male adolescents in programming and policy. The chapter brings to the fore issues such as the underlying instability in the lives and livelihoods of refugees, child laborers, and other marginalized youth. The scope of this final study links this second section of the book, assessing the health divide, to the third section on root causes of inequities in health.

C H A P T E R

5

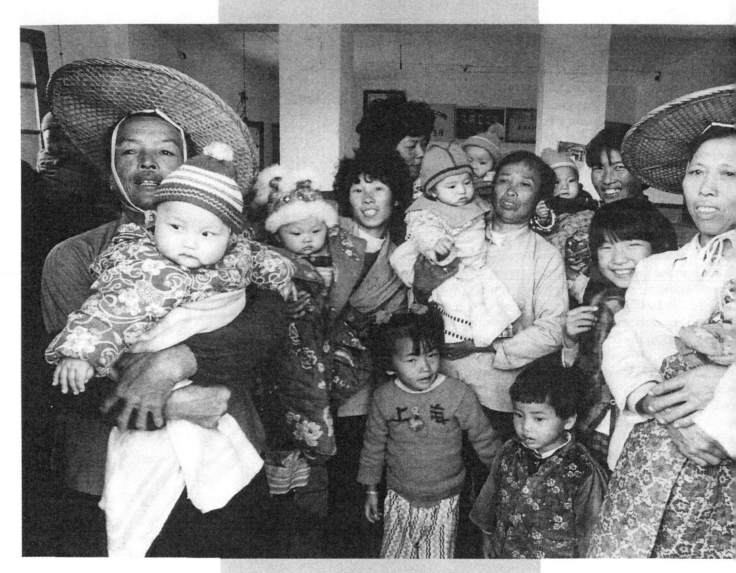

Mothers and children of Putian, Fujian, China.
Source: Sean Sprague/Panos.

Measuring Disparities in Health: Methods and Indicators

SUDHIR ANAND, FINN DIDERICHSEN, TIMOTHY EVANS, VLADIMIR M. SHKOLNIKOV, AND MEG WIRTH

Although part of the variation in health status between individuals is biological in origin, disparities in health between nations and between social groups within nations are largely determined by the way we organize society—locally and globally—along economic, social, and political lines. Moreover, these disparities in health are striking reflections of the powerful stratifying forces that differentiate life opportunities within and between countries. With increasing evidence of significant social stratification in health status, an emerging literature is raising a set of basic issues. These include the need for an accurate quantification of inequalities in health and their trends over time; an assessment of their significance relative to the overall level of health; and an awareness of their causes and consequences. A critical prerequisite to making progress along these lines of inquiry is the availability of reliable and valid measures of health distribution.

The first *Health For All* goal of the World Health Organization (WHO) European Regional Office in 1985 targeted a 25% reduction in inequities in health both within and between countries by improving the level of health of disadvantaged groups and nations (World Health Organization 1991). The absence of a set of health equity indicators has hampered efforts to monitor and evaluate progress toward these ends. In part,

this reflects the traditional focus on aggregate health outcomes, but it is also indicative of the significant challenges in measuring health distribution. These include practical issues on the one hand—such as linking social and health data—and complex issues on the other—such as deciding what norm against which to identify inequities.

This chapter explores critical issues related to the measurement of health equity. Although the distinction between health variations, inequalities, and inequities is important (see chapter 3), our intent here is primarily to focus on issues related to the measurement of health distribution as opposed to the definition of equity. Bringing together principles from such fields as economics, sociology, demography, and epidemiology, a new literature on the measurement of inequalities in health is emerging (Wagstaff et al. 1991; Mackenbach and Kunst 1997; Manor et al. 1997; Anand and Sen 1996; Anand 1998, 1999; Lindholm and Rosén 1998; Gwatkin 1999; Gakidou et al. 1999; Anand and Nanthikesan 2000, 2001).

Drawing on these contributions, we identify five major theoretical and technical considerations underpinning the measurement of health inequalities. This is followed by a critical review of current measures and a presentation of some new measures. The measures are

Figure 1 Two main families of measures of
health equity

Intergroup differentials	
Two groups	**More than two groups**
• Rate ratio	• Slope index
• Rate difference	of inequality
• Low to High ratio	• Concentration
• Shortfall	index
	• Index of
	dissimilarity

Interindividual differentials
• Gini coefficient
• Relative mean deviation
• Atkinson index

grouped into two main families (see Fig. 1): descriptors of variations between individuals and indicators of health inequalities across social groups. Other than describing interindividual or intergroup health inequalities, measures serving purposes such as assessing public health impact and attributing cause are also reviewed (see Fig. 2). The critical issue of measures assessing the effectiveness of interventions is dealt with more extensively in Chapter 21 (health equity impact assessment).

Basic Considerations in Measures of Inequalities in Health Status

In the construction of any measure of health equity, there are at least five issues that must be addressed: (1) the measure of health status and/or health consequence; (2) the population grouping across which health differentials/inequities are described/assessed; (3) the reference group or norm against which differences are measured; (4) the tradeoffs between absolute versus relative measures; and (5) the weights attached

to the (ill) health of individuals/groups at various points along the (ill) health distribution. Below each of these issues is considered.

Health Status Measure

Health is a complex concept with multiple dimensions across each of which it is possible to describe inequalities (see Box 1). It is widely acknowledged that around national averages in health status measures, much inequality may be concealed. In India, for example, the national infant mortality rate is 80 per 1000, while in Orissa state it is 124 per 1000 and in a district of Orissa state it is 164 per 1000 (Drèze and Sen 1995). Less commonly described are inequalities in other dimensions of health such as perceptions of ill health and care-seeking behaviors. An illustration of inequity in care-seeking behavior and access to care is evident in Peru, where 88.4% of women in the lowest income quintile give birth in their homes compared with 5.3% of women in the top income quintile who do so. Furthermore, populations may be stratified according to the socioeconomic consequences of illness. For example, in poor rural areas of China, one-third of the population had to borrow money or sell assets to pay for health care (Hsiao and Liu 1996). It is also conceivable that across some dimensions of health status two groups appear equal but in other dimensions they do not.

The nature and degree of "measurability" embodied in the health indicator across the dimensions outlined earlier will determine the expression of health inequality. In some cases the measures are dichotomous, signaling, for example, the presence or absence of a disease. In other cases the measures reflect a range of ordinal health states as in self-reported health, varying from poor to fair to excellent health. Measures may also be continuous and cardinal such as levels of blood pressure or serum cholesterol level. These basic characteristics of measures—dichotomous/continuous, ordinal/cardinal—determine the mechanics for describing health inequalities and hence cannot be overlooked (Manor et al. 1997; see also chapter 6).

An individual's social position and the social context in which he or she lives heavily influence the self-

Figure 2 Four uses for measures of health equity

Describing differences	**Calculating the public health impact**	**Attributing causality**	**Assessing interventions**
All indicators for measuring differences between groups and between individuals (see Fig. 1)	• Population attributable fraction • Attributable life lost	• Explained fraction • Synergy index • Component analysis	• Change in descriptive measures over time • Health equity impact assessment

perception of disability, symptoms, and suffering. In industrialized countries, poor people report greater illness and also have higher mortality rates than rich people (Idler and Benyamini 1997; Kunst et al. 1995; Kaplan et al. 1996). On the other hand, in developing countries, it is frequently observed that the poor report less ill health than the rich even though the poor have higher mortality rates (Sen 1994; Chen and Murray 1992). For example, the incidence of self-reported morbidity is much higher in the Indian state of Kerala than in Bihar despite higher education levels and greater longevity in Kerala (Sen 1999). Comparison of economic groups within Ghana yield clear patterns of self-reported morbidity increasing with income (Murray et al. 1992).

The question therefore arises as to why the poor in developing countries report less illness even though they are more likely to die prematurely. Some might suggest dismissing the finding on the basis that self-reported health is an inappropriate measure of health status. Measures based on self-assessed health reflect richer (or more educated) persons' greater likelihood to have access to health services, receive diagnoses, and thus report illness; they do not reflect truly poorer health (Sen 1994). When more "objective" criteria of suffering or disability are used, steeper gradients are evident with the poorer groups displaying worse health status (see chapter 7, Table 4; Blaxter 1989; Blank and

Diderichsen 1996). The salutary lesson from these observations is that our understanding of the nature of inequalities in health depends in part on the measure used for health.

In other work, Wagstaff and colleagues (1991) observed that inequalities from mortality in England and Wales in 1981 were more pronounced if measured by years of potential life lost than if measured by death rates. Similarly, Macintyre (1998) suggests that the measures of "years of potential life lost" and "mortality amenable to medical intervention" produce steeper social class gradients than do standardized mortality rates. More recently, Humphries and van Doorslaer (2000) found that in Canada the Concentration Index using self-assessed health consistently shows greater socioeconomic inequality than does the Concentration Index for the Health Utilities Index. These observations underscore the sensitivity of estimations and assessments of health inequality to the chosen measure of health.

Summary measures of health that integrate mortality and morbidity are increasingly used by public health and medical decision makers (Institute of Medicine 1998). Examples of such measures include Disability-Free Life Expectancy (Robine et al. 1993), Quality-Adjusted Life Years (Weinstein and Stason 1976), and Disability-Adjusted Life Years (Murray and Lopez 1996). Their importance for the analysis of health in-

---

BOX 1: DIMENSIONS OF HEALTH STATUS THAT MAY EXHIBIT DIFFERENCES

Risk
In Zimbabwe in the poorest income quintile, 71.8% of females but 86.5% of males have knowledge about the sexual transmission of disease (Pande and Gwatkin 1999).

Perception
Central and Eastern European men report 25% greater ill health than do Western European men (Carlson 1998).

Care-Seeking Behavior
In Peru 88.4% of women in the lowest income quintile give birth in their homes compared with only 5.3% of women in the top income quintile (Pande and Gwatkin 1999).

Diagnosis
Significant differences have been identified between Xhosa-speaking blacks and English-speaking whites in South Africa in the presentation of schizophrenia, but not in its core symptoms (Ensink et al. 1998)

Treatment
In the United States whites are three times as likely to receive a cardiac procedure as are blacks (Daumit et al. 1999)

Incidence of Disease, Disability, and Death
In Namibia the odds of dying before age five years are 37% lower among children of European descent than among children of other ethnic groups (Brockerhoff and Hewitt 1998).

In India the national infant mortality rate is 80 per 1000 live births, but in Orissa state the rate is 124, and in the Ganjam district of Orissa it is 164 (Drèze and Sen 1995).

Socioeconomic Consequences
In poor rural areas of China 25% of people seeking health care had to borrow money to pay for it, and 6% had to sell assets to do so (Hsiao and Liu 1996).

equality is well illustrated from a study in Canada where the gap in life expectancy between the richest 20% and the poorest 20% in the community varied from 6.3 years for overall life expectancy to 14.3 years for disability-free life expectancy (Wilkins and Adams 1983). In the construction of these measures, values are implicitly incorporated that have significant equity implications. They are notable for their assumptions about optimal health profiles by age and sex and weights that differentially value life across age groups, points in time, and states of health (Bleichrodt 1997). For one such measure, the Disability-Adjusted Life Year, the equity implications of its (implicit) assumptions have been examined in detail (Anand and Hanson 1997, 1998). There are also concerns about whether the attempt to provide cardinal rankings of individual health are appropriate for every measure—an issue raised in this volume (see chapter 6) as well as elsewhere (Deaton 1999).

Choice of Population Groupings Across Which Comparisons Are Made

Having selected an appropriate health measure, the next issue concerns the population grouping across which the distribution of health is described. Some argue, for example, that there is a "pure" distribution of health equivalent to the idea of a distribution of income across individuals (Le Grand and Rabin 1986; Anand 1998; Deaton 1999; Gakidou et al. 1999). These so-called interindividual descriptions of health distribution represent an emerging family of measures, discussed later. More typically, inequalities in health have been described according to population groupings such as age, sex, race/ethnicity, education, income, and geographic area of residence. Although some of these groups are relatively easily defined and measured, grouping by other variables—including wealth, race/ethnicity, social capital, and cohesion—poses measurement challenges. Furthermore, there are nontrivial data requirements associated with linking these indicators to health status data (Kunst and Mackenbach 1995; Krieger et al. 1997).

For some social groupings, there are clear hierarchical orderings, for example, by income or education level. For others, such as gender, race, occupation, or region, there may be no obvious ordering. For example, there is no clear social hierarchy between the occupational categories of farm laborers and assembly line workers. In such cases, an association can be made with an underlying, or implicit, social stratification through, for example, a broader description of occupations such as manual and nonmanual (i.e., blue and white collar). Similarly, geographical areas may be described by characteristics that can be ranked. In the Mexican case study (chapter 19), 713 counties were ranked according to a composite measure of socioeconomic disadvantage called the *marginality index*.

The evidence of striking health inequalities across these counties in Mexico, the near health equality across 47 prefectures in Japan (see chapter 8), and the urban/rural health divides in China (see chapter 7) illustrate the multiple approaches to geographical grouping. Although there are several important considerations in choosing a geographical grouping, not least whether the groups constitute administrative or policy making jurisdictions, there is the question of whether certain groupings are more or less likely to reveal health inequalities. Other things equal, the smaller the unit of grouping, the larger the observed inequality. It is not surprising, therefore, that in both Mexico and the United States health inequalities are more accentuated when described across a smaller geographical division—the county—than a larger geographic division—the state (see chapter 19; Murray et al. 1998).

Although a chosen indicator, such as ethnic origin or level of income, may be an important marker of social injustice, its association with health does not necessarily imply anything about the direction of causation. Poor health could lead to low income just as low income could lead to poorer health. Indeed, even the association of a social variable such as ethnicity with health may be due to each of them being causally related to a third factor such as income or education. For example, health differences between blacks and whites in the United States are a marker of class disparities underlying the racial disparity; attributing causality entirely to race may miss an important part of the explanation of the health differences (Navarro 1991). The association between health and income, or between health (inequality) and income inequality, may be disturbing, but it reflects a complex web of pathways linking health and social structure that is far from well understood.

Just as the indicator of health status affects the extent of measured inequalities, so too does the choice of social stratifier, or population grouping (Manor et al. 1997; Macintyre 1998). If comparisons are required over time or across countries, care must be taken to ensure that the underlying definition of social grouping is the same (Kunst 1997; Bartley et al. 1996). Furthermore, the social hierarchy implied by different groupings such as occupation may vary across societies, may change with economic transformation, and may not appropriately reflect women's work. The interpretation of health distributions—measured by an indicator such as occupation—may therefore be different across societies and over time.

Identifying a Reference Group or "Norm"

Integral to describing any inequality or inequity in health is the identification of a reference group or "norm" against which differences are measured. For instance, in a study of ethnic mortality differentials in Nigeria, a privileged ethnic group is used as a benchmark against which the mortality profile of other ethnic groups is compared (Brockerhoff and Hewett 1998). The choice of reference group can affect the magnitude of inequality observed, and the rationale for its selection should be considered explicitly. There are a variety of approaches to identifying a reference group. One approach selects a minimum, or basic, standard below which health performance is judged to be inequitable and above which it is judged to be equitable even though there may be inequality above the threshold. Examples might include achieving 90% childhood immunization coverage, an infant mortality rate (IMR) less than 20 per 1000, or a life expectancy at birth of more than 75 years. In the construction of the Human Development Index and the Gender-related Development Index in the United Nations Development Programme's *Human Development Report 1995*, specific minimum standards for men and women were set across countries (Anand and Sen 1996).

A second approach sets the reference group value at the mean of all groups. This is the case with a measure such as the *index of dissimilarity*, which identifies the amount of health that would theoretically have to be "redistributed" across population groups in order for all groups to have the same mean health, expressed as a fraction of average health (Mackenbach and Kunst 1997). (This index is the same as the relative mean deviation defined in Appendix A.) A problem with identifying the mean as a reference group is the assumption that groups above the mean would need to lower their health status to the mean to achieve greater equality. Even if health cannot be easily redistributed, one can improve the health of the worse-off without having to take it from the better-off. Note, however, that these measures do not place any special weight on the health of the worst-off: The health of the worst-off could deteriorate while relative inequality could improve.

Other measures define inequality with respect to the group with the highest or maximum health status. These measures identify the quanta of health improvement that would have to be gained by other groups in order to reach the health status of the best-off group. The standard may be identified in terms of the highest observed health status (e.g., Japanese life expectancy) or according to some idea of what is biologically maximal (e.g., a life span of 120 years). In South Africa, for example, the magnitude of socioeconomic inequalities in health among black and colored populations is highly sensitive to the choice of reference group (see chapter 14, Table 10). For gender groups, biological differences in the life expectancy of men and women suggest the need for gender-specific maxima. Anand and Sen (1996), recognizing that females have superior survival at all ages relative to males, set different male and female life expectancy norms and assess equity through the respective "shortfalls" from these norms. This approach is the basis of the equity assessment of male and female child mortality rates in Bangladesh (see chapter 16, Figs. 1 and 2 and Table 3).

Both the presence and absence, as well as the magnitude, of inequalities is significantly affected by the reference point used in each measure. The arguments in favor of one reference point or another will involve diverse ethical and biological considerations. For example, various reference points have been suggested for life expectancy at birth for men and women, with the gaps ranging from 2.5 years (Murray and Lopez 1996) to 5 years (Anand and Sen 1996).

Absolute Versus Relative Measures

Another dimension of health inequality measures is whether they are based on relative or absolute differences. Figures 3 and 4 illustrate how our understanding of the magnitude of inequalities is influenced by relative versus absolute measures. In Figure 3, based on a relative measure of inequality in IMR, Vietnam appears to have greater within-country socioeconomic inequality than Mozambique. In contrast, based on an absolute measure (Fig. 4), the level of inequality in Mozambique is greater than in Vietnam. A similar relative versus absolute consideration arose when Sweden was identified as one of the countries with the largest relative occupational inequality in health compared with other European countries (Mackenbach et al. 1997). When absolute levels are compared, however, Sweden ranked among European countries with the lowest level of occupational inequality (Vågerö and Eriksson 1997).

As another example, Table 1 shows time trend data in heart disease mortality among men in England and Wales over the period 1976 to 1992 (Drever and Whitehead 1997). In relative terms, the excess coronary heart disease (CHD) mortality between the low-

Figure 3 Relative inequality in infant mortality rate in Mozambique and Vietnam, 1997

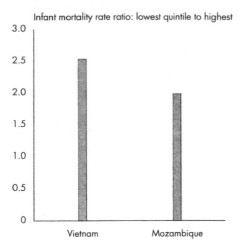

Source: Data from 1997 Demographic and Health Surveys; Pande and Gwatkin 1999.

Figure 4 Absolute inequality in infant mortality rate in Vietnam and Mozambique, 1997

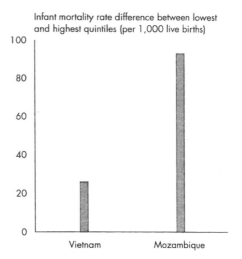

Source: Data from 1997 Demographic and Health Surveys; Pande and Gwatkin 1999.

est and highest social classes increased from 48% to 66% between 1976–1981 and 1986–1992. Thus, the conclusion drawn in Britain is that social inequalities in health have increased over the period (Acheson et al. 1998). In absolute terms, however, the mortality gap between the lowest and highest social classes decreased from 117 to 106 per 100,000. This reflects a larger absolute improvement in CHD mortality in the lowest compared with the highest social classes (an improvement of 97 compared with 86 per 100,000). It could therefore be argued that equity has improved because the absolute mortality gap has decreased. As mentioned earlier, the issue of relative and absolute measures is important, both for intercountry and time-trend comparisons. In general, as the reference group level of ill-

ness/mortality reaches very low levels, relative measures of inequality are likely to show an increase. Conversely, as the reference group level of (ill) health increases, relative measures of inequality are likely to decrease.

Valuing Health Differently Along the Distribution

Assuming that it is possible to identify where changes in the distribution take place, that is, at the lower tail or near the mean, the normative issue arises about how changes in one part of the distribution should be valued relative to changes in another part of the distribu-

Table 1 Mortality from coronary heart disease among men age 35–64 by social class in England and Wales, selected years, 1976–92

(age-standardized rate per 100,000)

	1976–81	1986–92
Social classes		
Highest	246	160
Lowest	363	266
Rate ratio (lowest to highest classes)	1.48	1.66
Rate difference (lowest minus highest classes)	117	106

Source: Adapted from Drever and Whitehead 1997.

tion. It might be argued, for example, that improvements in health among the least healthy should be weighted more than improvements in health among the healthiest. One measure, the Atkinson index (see later), incorporates an "aversion to inequality" parameter, which captures a society's preferences for changes in distribution along its length (Anand 1998). More recently, the WHO (Gakidou et al. 1999) introduced a similar concept as a parameter (called "alpha") that differentially values changes in health at certain points in the distribution.

The Spectrum of Health Inequality Measures

The *Black Report* (Black et al. 1980) indicated increasing (relative) inequalities in mortality in England and Wales from the 1950s to the 1970s. This finding was disputed, in part, by analysis using a different measure indicating improvements in health inequality over the same period (Le Grand and Rabin 1986). These apparently contradictory results reflect the fact that the measures provide information on quite different questions. The *Black Report* measured social class inequalities in health, whereas Le Grand and Rabin's measure described individual variation in longevity without concern for social grouping. There are two fundamental approaches to measuring inequalities in health: (*1*) health differences between population groups and (*2*) health distribution across individuals (see Box 2). The first approach—intergroup disparities—is by far the most common in the literature (and throughout the cases in this volume) and draws on the fields of demography, epidemiology, and sociology. The second approach—interindividual variations—draws largely

on the economic literature related to measures of income distribution. Below we summarize a variety of measures dealing with both of these approaches.

Measures of Intergroup Disparities in Health

Simple range measures

Much of the literature on socioeconomic inequalities in health employs simple "range" measures, *rate ratios* (RR) or *rate differences* (RD), to describe inequalities between groups. These measures compare the range in rates of illness/mortality between the least healthy and the healthiest groups or between the lowest and the highest socioeconomic groups. Selection of the groups for comparison must balance the need to demonstrate the magnitude of the health inequality with the imperative of including sufficiently large population groups to avoid comparisons that are not statistically significant (Mackenbach and Kunst 1997). To calculate the RR or RD may thus require the merging of groups that might suppress some inequalities. While the RR is unitless, independent of average level and scale, the RD depends on both average level and scale. Both are calculated with one group selected as the reference group, and both are insensitive to changes in group size.

A conceptually similar approach is apparent in some measures of socioeconomic inequalities in health distribution. If we rank individuals according to their income, then for each decile or quintile of individuals thus ranked we can estimate their (ill) health status. Comparing the poorest with the richest quintile, for example, we could then make statements of the kind that the infant mortality rate (IMR) of the lowest quintile is 2.5 times higher than that of the highest quintile. The ratio of the health status of the lowest income quintile to the highest income quintile, a variation on the

---

BOX 2: MEASURES USED BY CASE STUDIES IN THIS VOLUME

Rate ratio:	China, Chile, Russia, South Africa	**Years of potential life lost:**	Chile, Mexico, United States
Rate difference:	China, Chile, Russia, South Africa	**Gini coefficient:**	Japan
Shortfall:	Bangladesh, China	**Population-attributable risk:**	Chile, China, United States
Index of dissimilarity:	Chile		
Slope index of inequality:	China, Chile, Mexico, United States	**Explained fraction:**	United Kingdom/Sweden
		Odds ratio:	United Kingdom/Sweden
Relative index of inequality:	Mexico	**Synergy index:**	United Kingdom/Sweden
Concentration index:	China, Mexico	**Arriaga (component) method:**	Chile, Russia

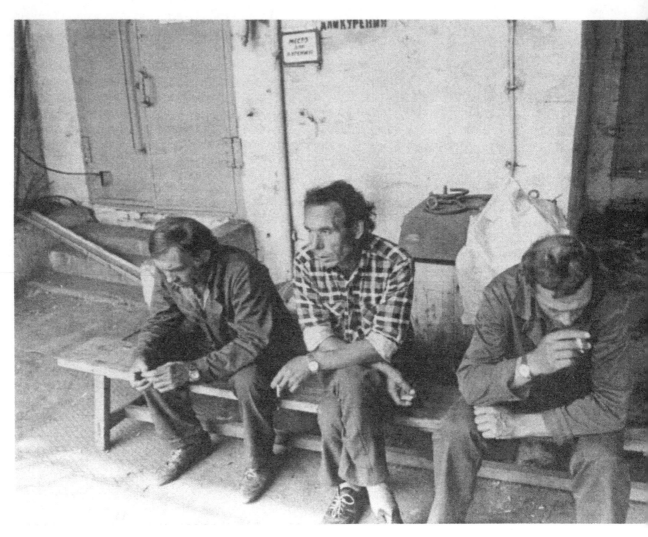

Three unemployed Soviet workers. V.V. Nemtsev, V.A. Vasilyev, V.I. Ryshalo in a shipyard, 1992.
Source: Copyright S. Smolsky; N. Adamovich/Sovfoto/Eastfoto/PictureQuest.

RR called the *low to high ratio*, has been estimated within countries (Pande and Gwatkin 1999). Importantly, this measure does not take into account the health status of the middle three quintiles. Some authors have suggested that this is a drawback (Wagstaff et al. 1991), while others claim that in practice these measures yield estimates of health inequality that are comparable with those based on the complete social-class gradient (Manor et al. 1997). Yet the low to high ratio does have the merit of being a readily interpretable and usable measure of the relative gap in (ill) health between the poor and the rich.

Another simple range measure emerges from the work of Sudhir Anand and Amartya Sen (Sen 1992; Anand and Sen 1996). They identify concepts of equality in health based on comparing *shortfalls* in achievement from some maximum or norm. In the assessment of gender equity of health outcomes, shortfalls in longevity for males and females from their respective biological maxima are compared. These measures invoke the identification of norms for optimal health achievement. As seen in the Bangladesh country-case study (see chapter 16), the differential norms for male and female child mortality rates permitted the identification of persistent gender inequality at a time when direct comparison of male and female rates would have indicated near equality.

Measures based on the entire health distribution

In contrast to measures of health disparity between the two ends of the social hierarchy, there are also measures that express the inequality in health across the full spectrum of socioeconomic status. Such measures recognize the common observation that inequalities in

Figure 5 A histogram illustrating the calculation of the slope index of inequality

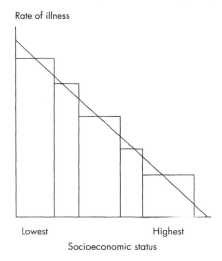

Note: The slope index of inequality takes into account the relative size of the population in each socioeconomic group, indicated by the width of the corresponding bar. The index is calculated as the slope of the weighted least squares regression of group illness rates against the population ranked according to its position in the social hierarchy.

health status exhibit a stepwise gradient across *all* socioeconomic strata. One such measure, which takes account of everyone's level of health according to social position, is the *slope index of inequality* (SII). It is based on a histogram where each bar indicates a group ranked by socioeconomic status, with the width of the bar indicating its population size and the height indicating its level of (ill) health (Fig. 5). The SII is

---

BOX 3: THE CONCENTRATION INDEX

We illustrate the measurement of socioeconomic inequalities in health by use of income as the ranking variable for individuals and groups. If we rank individuals according to their income (e.g., the per capita income of the household to which they belong), then for each decile or quintile of individuals so ranked we can estimate their health (or ill health) status. Comparing the richest with the poorest quintile, for example, we could then make statements of the kind that the infant mortality rate (IMR) of the lowest quintile is 2.5 times higher than that of the highest quintile in India in 1992–1993 (Gwatkin et al. 1999). This measure is akin to the relative index of inequality (RII)—where the calculation of the "slope" does not take into account the health

status of the middle three quintiles. Yet it does provide a readily interpretable and usable measure of the relative gap in ill health between the poor and the rich. The slope index of inequality (SII) for the five quintile groups is a simple extension of this idea, where the "slope" is estimated— through regression—by using information on the health status of all the quintiles.

The concentration index, which is supposed to measure "income-related inequalities in health," is based on precisely this idea applied at the level of the individual rather than the group (see Anand 1999). If we rank n individuals in a population in ascending order of income, with individual 1 labeled as the poorest person and individual n the richest person, and we let h_i be the health status of individual i for i = 1,2, . . . ,n, then the concentration index (CI) can be expressed as the slope of the ordinary least squares regression between h_i and i up to a multiplicative constant. More precisely, it can be shown that

$$CI = 2 \; cov \; (i, h_i)/(n\mu)$$

where $\mu = (1/n) \; \Sigma h_i$ is the average health status of the population (Anand 1983: 315–316). Because the ordinary least squares slope SII in this case is simply cov (i, h_i)/var(i), we have the result that CI and SII are related as follows (Anand 1999):

$$SII = cov \; (i, h_i)/var(i)$$

or

$$SII \; var(i) = cov \; (i, h_i) = CI \; (n\mu)/2$$

so that

$$CI = SII \; [2var(i)/(n\mu)].$$

Therefore, the concentration index CI and SII differ only by a multiplicative constant, which depends on the average health status of the population μ and on its size n (note that var[i] is simply a function of n).

As expressed earlier, the concentration index, CI, measures the covariance between the income ranks of individuals and their health (or ill health) status. This covariance is normalized so that the index always lies between -1 and $+1$, just like any statistical correlation coefficient. It is not a conventional measure of inequality of either the univariate income distribution or the univariate health distribution (such measures vary from 0 when there is perfect equality to $+1$ when there is perfect inequality). Indeed, the income distribution can worsen significantly with no effect on the concentration index as long as the relative ranks of individuals remain the same. For example, the incomes of individuals in the lowest quintile can be reduced by a given absolute amount and the incomes of individuals in the highest quintile increased by the same absolute amount with no change in the concentration index. Similarly, the univariate health distribution can worsen significantly with no effect on the concentration index as long as the covariance between the income ranks and health status of individuals remains the same. The concentration index only captures the correlation between the income ranks of individuals and their health status and is thus akin—subject to a normalization—to the slope index of inequality SII (for details see Anand 1999).

calculated as the slope of the weighted least squares regression of group (ill) health status against the rank ordering of the groups in the social hierarchy. The estimated slope can be interpreted as the absolute difference in (ill) health between successive groups in the social hierarchy while taking into account the (ill) health status of *all* groups (Mackenbach and Kunst 1997: 761). Thus, the larger the absolute value of SII, the greater the inequality. A variant of this measure, the *relative index of inequality* (RII), is calculated by taking the ratio of the (ill) health status only between the bottom and top social groups (cf. the low to high ratio discussed earlier).

The advantage of these measures (SII and RII) is that they do not require the choice of a reference group, and they take into account both the socioeconomic position of groups and their relative size. The SII measure has together with the RD measure the advantage that it is expressed in the same units (e.g., rate) as the health outcome. It should be emphasized that SII requires the groups to be ranked hierarchically according to socioeconomic status. Some have argued, however, that the measure is not easily accessible to policy makers (Mackenbach and Kunst 1997).

Another measure which relates social hierarchy to health is the *concentration index* (CI) (Wagstaff et al.

1991). It turns out to carry exactly the same information as the SII (see Box 3). The CI is defined in terms of the concentration curve which expresses the cumulative proportion of ill health suffered by each cumulative proportion of the population ranked by socioeconomic status (see Fig. 6). Values of the CI lie between "-1" (the poorest suffer all of the ill health) to "$+1$" (the richest suffer all of the ill health), with a value of "0" indicating no correlation between ill health and socioeconomic status (see chapter 7, for an example). The CI is a relative measure in the sense that it is independent of the absolute levels of both (ill) health and income. The CI has the limitation that the actual health gradient across socioeconomic groups, and the corresponding concentration curve, may have a very different shape for two populations and still yield the same correlation coefficient or CI value. Like the SII, the CI may not be readily accessible to policy makers.

Measures of Interindividual Health Distribution

There is a large literature in economics on the measurement of inequality (Atkinson 1970; Sen 1973; Anand 1983; Foster and Sen 1997). Most of this is concerned with measuring inequality in the distribution of

Figure 6 An illness concentration curve

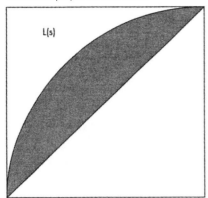

Cumulative proportion of ill health

L(s)

Cumulative proportion of population
ranked by socioeconomic status

Notes: The concentration curve L(s) plots the cumulative proportion of
the population ranked by socioeconomic status, (beginning with the
lowest) against the cumulative proportion of ill health. If L(s) lies
above the diagonal, inequalities in ill health favor the more
advantaged members of society. The farther L(s) lies away from
the diagonal, the greater the inequality.

The ill health concentration index is twice the area between L(s) and
the diagonal. This index has a value of zero when L(s) coincides with
the diagonal and is negative (positive) when L(s) lies above (below)
the diagonal.

Source: van Doorslaer et al. 1997, pp. 96–97.

income (or consumption, wealth, and so on) among
households or individuals. The data sources for such
information include household income and expenditure
surveys, population censuses, and demographic surveys. Inequality measurement is undertaken for a variety of welfare-economic purposes, including international and intertemporal comparison.

We believe that the economic approach to measuring inequality can be applied to individual variations in
the quantity and quality of life. For example, when data
at the individual level become available for measures
that combine mortality and morbidity, such as QALYs
(quality-adjusted life years), we could estimate inequality in quality-adjusted length-of-life in a society.
Though this goal remains distant in most countries due
to insufficient data, the measurement principles discussed here are applicable to measures that combine
the quality and quantity of life. What we have at present is information on the age-at-death of individuals,
collected through vital statistics registers and other
sources. Indeed, this is also the information base for
the age-specific mortality rates used in the construction
of period life-tables.

Thus we could take the cross-section data on those
who die in a given year and, with their age-at-death,
measure inequality in the quantity of life (Le Grand
1989). The problem with this approach, however, is
one very familiar to demographers: the estimates will
be a function of the age structure of the population.
With given mortality rates at different ages, the numbers dying in each age group will depend on the size
of the group, which is determined by previous birth (as
well as death and migration) rates in the society. A
young population will experience many infant and child
deaths, whereas an old population will witness many
elderly deaths. The distribution of age-at-death of individuals will thus be influenced by factors other than
mortality risks in the society. Just as demographers do
not measure average longevity in a population by taking the mean of *this* age-at-death distribution, but
rather measure life expectancy by passing a synthetic
cohort through a life-table, we use the same construct
to measure inequality in length-of-life (for details, see
Anand 1998).

We illustrate the measurement of inequality in
longevity by use of complete life-tables for Russian
males for 1990 and 1995 (Table 2). Three different
types of mean are estimated from the frequency distribution for length-of-life of the cohort (denoted as the
random variable X): the arithmetic mean $X_e(0)$ (which
is simply life expectancy at birth, or e_0); the geometric
mean $X_e(1)$; and the harmonic mean $X_e(2)$. All three
means are "$(1-\epsilon)$ averages" of the length-of-life distribution for different values of ϵ: $\epsilon = 0$ generates the
arithmetic mean; $\epsilon = 1$ generates the geometric mean;
$\epsilon = 2$ generates the harmonic mean (see Anand and Sen
1996). The geometric and harmonic mean life can be
interpreted as indicators that combine average life expectancy $X_e(0)$ with inequality around this average as
measured by the Atkinson index $I(\epsilon)$ for $\epsilon = 1$ and $\epsilon =$
2, respectively. More generally, $X_e(\epsilon)$ may be defined
as the "equally distributed equivalent life" corresponding to the inequality aversion parameter ϵ. Penalizing
inequality around $X_e(0)$, $X_e(\epsilon)$ is that length-of-life
which if enjoyed equally by everyone (perfect equality)
would be judged to be as valuable socially (given the
magnitude of ϵ) as the actual length-of-life distribution
(Atkinson 1970).

For Russian males between 1990 and 1995 there is
a dramatic decrease in life expectancy $X_e(0)$ from 63.8
to 58.43 years, that is, by some 5.4 years or 8.4% (see
Table 2). A different measure of central tendency—the
median life $Q(50)$—falls from 67.02 to 60.52 years for
males between 1990 and 1995. For Russian females
(not shown in Table 2), the corresponding decreases
in life expectancy are less sharp: Life expectancy de-

Table 2 Length-of-life distribution measures for Russian males, 1990 and 1995

Measures	1990	1995
Basic measures of central tendency and dispersion		
Arithmetic mean (life expectancy at birth)	63.80	58.43
Geometric mean	54.14	49.01
Harmonic mean	4.26	4.13
Median	67.02	60.52
Standard deviation	19.39	19.73
Coefficient of variation (= σ / Xe [0])	0.304	0.338
Relative mean deviation	0.232	0.266
Inequality measures		
Gini coefficient	0.163	0.187
Atkinson index		
Inequality aversion parameter 1.0	0.151	0.161
Inequality aversion parameter 1.5	0.581	0.579
Inequality aversion parameter 2.0	0.933	0.929

Note: For the definition of these measures see Appendix A.
Source: Anand 1998.

creases from 74.33 to 71.73 years and median life from 77.7 to 75.62 years. The changes in life expectancy between 1990 and 1995 lead to an increase in the female–male gap from 10.53 years to 13.3 years, which is an historic (and international) high (see also chapter 11).

From the distribution of length-of-life, we can also calculate statistics relating to dispersion around the mean. For Russian males between 1990 and 1995, the standard deviation σ (or square root of the variance) rises from 19.39 to 19.73 years. Together with the fact that arithmetic mean life $X_e(0)$ falls, this leads to an increase in the coefficient of variation $C(=\sigma/X_e[0])$. Another statistical measure of dispersion, the relative mean deviation (sometimes called the "Robin Hood Index"), shows an increase from 0.232 to 0.266.

As in the case of an income distribution (Anand 1983), we can construct a Lorenz curve for the length-of-life distribution. This plots the share of total life-years lived by the shortest lived (100p)% of the population, as p ranges from 0 to 1. The *Gini coefficient* G is defined as the ratio of the area between the Lorenz curve and the diagonal of perfect equality to the area below the diagonal (an equivalent mathematical definition is given in Appendix A). For Russian males there is a significant increase in G from 0.163 to 0.187 (and

for females from 0.114 to 0.130). Note, however, that these Gini coefficients for length-of-life are much lower than those for income (approximately 0.45 in Russia). See Anand (1998) for a discussion of the use of positive and normative inequality measures in comparing inequality *across* spaces—in particular, health and income.

Other measures of inequality implicitly weight different parts of the length-of-life distribution differently (for estimates, see Anand and Nanthikesan 2000). The *Atkinson indices* I(ϵ) explicitly incorporate such weighting through the parameter ϵ, which expresses a society's ethical (or political) aversion to inequality (see Appendix A). From a minimum value of $\epsilon = 0$, where there is no aversion to inequality, increasing values of ϵ attach relatively greater weight to years lived at earlier ages. This is reflected in the decrease in "equally distributed equivalent life" $X_e(\epsilon)$ in Table 2 with the progression from arithmetic to geometric to harmonic mean life.

The values of the inequality aversion parameter ϵ in Table 2 are chosen arbitrarily ($1 \leq \epsilon \leq 2$) and span a range of interesting results. When the inequality aversion parameter ϵ is equal to 1, the numerical value of inequality expressed by the Atkinson index is similar in magnitude to the Gini coefficient and increases from

1990 to 1995. When ϵ increases to 1.5 (2), the magnitude of the Atkinson index in 1990 increases sharply from 0.151 to 0.581 (0.933). Surprisingly, however, at these higher values of 1.5 or 2 of the inequality aversion parameter ϵ, the Atkinson index actually *decreases* between 1990 and 1995, indicating a reduction in inequality. This reflects the fact that in Russia during 1990 to 1995, although infant mortality deteriorated slightly, adult mortality worsened markedly. This led to a small increase in the share of total life-years lived by the youngest age groups (the shortest lived 2% of the population). Because higher values of the inequality aversion parameter have the effect of disproportionately valuing additional (share of) years lived at younger relative to older ages, at values of $\epsilon = 1.5$ or more an improvement in the Atkinson index is observed.

In the above example, the highest value chosen for the inequality aversion parameter is $\epsilon = 2$. Empirical studies among health care politicians in Sweden have, however, come up with values for the parameter as high as 6 (Lindholm and Rosén 1999). The latter estimates are based on a survey asking politicians to choose among intervention programs with different outcomes in terms of efficiency and equity.

The attraction of interindividual measures of health distribution is that they avoid the issues associated with choice of population grouping, and hence facilitate more reliable international and intertemporal comparisons. These measures do not address (socioeconomic) group inequalities in health directly, but could be developed to provide estimates of the contribution of group inequalities to overall interindividual inequality. As with other measures, they may be elusive to policy makers in their current form.

Measures Assessing Impact and Cause

Measures of public health impact

From a policy perspective it is helpful to assess the extent to which health inequalities hinder maximal overall health performance. The *population attributable fraction* (AF_p) (or population attributable risk) is a measure that attempts to answer this question. In particular, it measures the proportional reduction in the overall rate of illness that would occur if all groups had the same rate of illness as the reference group (see Box 4). The reference group selected in AF_p is the group with the best health status or lowest rate of illness—and not necessarily the group with the highest socioeconomic status. Unlike rate ratios or rate differences, the AF_p can be calculated across multiple groups and is sensitive to the population sizes of these groups.

The AF_p may also be calculated in absolute terms. For example, in Chile (see chapter 10) it was found that adult male life expectancy would increase by 8.65 years if all adult males had the health status of the highest education group. When the AF_p is applied to mortality, it is often termed the *population attributable life lost* (PALL) measure (see chapter 9).

BOX 4: CALCULATING THE PUBLIC HEALTH IMPACT

If we have a population in which a certain proportion p belongs to the *exposed* and therefore more-ill group and the other is the reference group, we can calculate a rate ratio (RR) between the two. The attributable fraction can then be calculated as

$$AF_p = (p[RR - 1]) / (p[RR - 1] + 1)$$

Often we will have to control for confounders such as age, and we can then calculate a standardized mortality (or morbidity) rate (SMR). The SMR is the ratio between the observed mortality rate in the exposed group and the rate that would be expected if the age-specific risks in the reference group were applied to the age structure of the exposed group. In that case,

$$AF_p = p_c (SMR - 1) / SMR$$

where p_c is the proportion *among the cases* of ill health that belong to the exposed group. Although this is a simple way of calculating the attributable fraction, the SMR has important limitations as it can only be compared with the reference group and not the SMR of other groups that are based on different age distributions.

The calculation of AF can be done even in situations in which there is more than one exposed group:

$$AF_p = \Sigma \ p_i \ AF_{pi}$$

An absolute measure of the reduction in the overall rate of illness is obtained by multiplying the proportionate reduction in the overall rate of illness by the overall rate of illness.

Explained fractions and the synergy index

It is important to distinguish (*1*) the association between socioeconomic status and health and (*2*) the causal pathways that link social position to disease outcome (see also chapter 2 on the social basis of disparities in health). If occupation, for example, is associated with certain exposures, such as job strain or pesticides, these exposures may be thought of as *mediating causes* of ill health. In explaining inequalities in health, it will be useful to quantify and compare the role played by each exposure. The explained fraction (XF), a measure based on the odds ratio, can be calculated to estimate the proportion of excess risk explained by mediating risk factors (Lynch et al. 1996; Hallqvist et al. 1998; see also Box 5). The explained fraction compares the odds ratio before and after controlling for the mediating factor(s). If the odds ratio were calculated before and after controlling for the presence of pesticides, we would be able to estimate the effect of pesticides as a mediating risk factor in explaining the morbidity or mortality differences between groups. The Anglo-Swedish study in this volume applies this technique when analyzing potential pathways in the causation of social inequalities in health.

Disaggregating social inequalities in life expectancy by age and disease group

Although intergroup disparities in life expectancy can be calculated easily, it is not obvious how these can be linked to intergroup differentials in mortality rates at different ages and from different causes. The difficulty lies in life expectancy being a nonlinear function of mortality rates at different ages (for details, see Chiàng 1984; Namboodiri and Suchindran 1987) and in the selection of population weights for age group–specific life expectancies. Nevertheless, procedures are available that allow us to quantify the contribution of intergroup differences in mortality rates to differences in life expectancy (see Appendix B).

As an example, we consider the racial differentials in mortality among men in the United States. U.S. mortality statistics by cause are available by 5-year age groups for the three major ethnic groups—white, black, and "other." According to the 1990 census, the percentages of these groups in the male population were 84.2%, 11.9%, and 3.9%, respectively. Life-tables for these racial groups yield the following estimates of life expectancy at birth in 1990: 71.9 years for all men, 72.7 years for white men, 64.6 for black men, and 78.1 years for "other" men. The three groups show a remarkable range of mortality patterns. The life expectancy of "other" men is higher than that of men in Japan or Iceland, which have the world's highest levels for a national population. The life expectancy of white men is close to the West European average, whereas the life expectancy of black men is close to the low levels of life expectancy found in countries of Eastern Europe. What factors underlie these vast intracountry ethnic disparities in survival?

BOX 5: CALCULATING THE EXPLAINED FRACTION AND SYNERGY INDEX

If the odds ratio after adjustment for confounders but before the potential mediating cause is entered into the adjustment model is OR′ and the same odds ratio after introduction of the potential mediating cause to the model is OR″, then the explained fraction (a proportion) can be calculated as

$$XF = ([OR' - 1] - [OR'' - 1])/(OR' - 1)$$

The effect of such a cause might not, however, be the same across different social positions. Population groups are more or less susceptible to a cause of disease depending on the constellation of causes to which they are exposed. This implies that exposures that are evenly distributed across social positions still might play a role in explaining the inequality (Hallqvist et al. 1998) as the effect (in terms of rate difference or odds ratio) might be different across social positions or contexts.

When one cause modifies the effect of the other, they might interact in the sense that they are part of the same pathway. Such an interaction is important information for policy makers as the effect of one cause will be reduced if exposure to the other is reduced.

To test if two contributing causes (A and B) are part of the same pathway, a measure of interaction can be calculated. If the odds ratio for those exposed to both is OR_{AB} and those exposed to only one of them is OR_A or OR_B, a *synergy index* (SI) can be calculated as

$$SI = (OR_{AB} - 1)/([OR_A - 1] + [OR_B - 1])$$

Thus, the synergy index expresses the odds among the doubly exposed compared with the added effect of the two exposures considered separately (Rothman and Greenland 1998; Lundberg et al. 1996).

Table 3 Decomposition of the difference in life expectancy at birth between white and black males by age and cause of death in the United States, 1990

(years)

Age (years)	Infectious diseases	Cancers	Cardiovascular diseases	Respiratory diseases	Digestive diseases	Other diseases	Injuries and violence	All causes
0	0.02	0.00	0.02	0.03	0.01	0.66	0.03	0.78
1–4	0.01	0.00	0.01	0.01	0.00	0.03	0.05	0.10
5–14	0.01	0.00	0.00	0.01	0.00	0.01	0.05	0.08
15–29	0.10	0.01	0.04	0.02	0.01	0.07	0.72	0.97
30–44	0.44	0.10	0.29	0.09	0.11	0.26	0.48	1.76
45–59	0.18	0.55	0.77	0.12	0.15	0.33	0.17	2.27
60–74	0.07	0.64	0.73	0.08	0.06	0.27	0.07	1.92
75 and over	0.04	0.21	0.01	−0.08	0.00	0.12	0.00	0.29
All ages	0.88	1.50	1.88	0.28	0.33	1.75	1.56	8.18

Source: Shkulnikov 1998.

To shed some light on the reasons for such gaps in life expectancy, we can disaggregate the interethnic differences by age and cause of death using "component analysis" (Andreev 1982; Arriaga 1984; Pressat 1985). This method allows us to attribute the overall difference in life expectancy between two population groups by age and cause (see Appendix B). Applying the method, we can estimate the contribution of different causes of death to the observed racial differences in life expectancy at birth in the United States. Between the two largest racial groups, white and black Americans, there is a difference in life expectancy of 8.2 years in 1990 (see Table 3). Almost one-half of this difference arises from mortality differences in the middle age groups (between the ages of 30 and 60). Among major causes of death, cardiovascular diseases, injuries from accidents and violence, and neoplasms (cancers) are the greatest contributors to the overall difference. Excess cardiovascular mortality of black males makes the largest contribution between the ages of 45 and 75 years, while accidents and violence are most important among young adults aged 15 to 44 years. Infectious diseases play a significant role between the ages of 30 and 44 years, perhaps reflecting the disproportionate concentration of deaths from human immunodeficiency virus among young African Americans (Feldman and Fulwood 1999; Lai et al. 1997).

Such a "component analysis" is important from a policy perspective. The pinpointing of age groups, racial groups, and causes of death may facilitate a more efficient use of scarce resources for reducing inequalities. Both the Chilean and the Russian case studies in this volume use component analysis to examine the cause-

and age-specific contributions to the gap in life expectancy between education groups (see chapters 10 and 11).

Discussion

This chapter has attempted to review a set of fundamental issues in health equity measurement as well as some actual measures—old and new. A prerequisite to using any of these measures is the availability of data. Unfortunately, in many countries, especially those likely to have the poorest health, the required data are lacking. In such situations, innovative methods of data collection and analysis, including qualitative and rapid assessment techniques, will be needed to understand the nature of the health distribution. Even when data are relatively abundant, however, equity analysis can be hampered by the absence of *joint* information on health and socioeconomic variables.

Assumptions are explicitly or implicitly made in each of five areas of measurement: choice of health measure; choice of stratification variable to describe socioeconomic inequalities; choice of reference group or norm; choice of absolute or relative measure; and choice of valuation of health along different points of the distribution. These assumptions can affect the magnitude and assessment of a given health inequality. Efforts to measure inequality should attempt to provide the rationale for choice in these areas. It would seem prudent to demonstrate the (in)sensitivity of the measures to alternative assumptions. In the end, however, these choices should not seen as purely mechanical or mutually exclusive. For instance, choosing one health measure should not obviate the need for examining other measures that reflect complementary dimensions of health. The complexities inherent in the nature of health and its distribution argue for a plurality of measurement approaches.

Sophisticated adjustments to, or refinements of, measures are not always required to identify inequalities. Simple indicators may prove adequate to the task. For example, large differences in life expectancy between groups—social, gender, or other—are likely to be sufficient evidence of inequality to mobilize policy makers. In general, however, policy must be buttressed by valid indicators that describe inequalities, assess causes, and monitor the progress of interventions—which will often call for refined measurement. Whether it is a simple or complex undertaking, measurement must lie at the heart of any effort to understand and redress inequalities in health.

References

Acheson D., Barker D., Chambers J., Graham H., Marmot M., Whitehead M. 1998. *The Report of the Independent Inquiry into Inequalities in Health.* London: The Stationery Office.

Anand S. 1983. *Inequality and Poverty in Malaysia: Measurement and Decomposition.* New York: Oxford University Press.

Anand S. 1998. Measuring Inequality in Longevity. Paper presented at the GHEI Workshop on Measuring Inequalities in Health, St. Catherine's College, Oxford, October 27–28.

Anand S. 1999. Inter-individual and inter-group inequalities in health. Mimeograph. St. Catherine's College, Oxford.

Anand S., Hanson K. 1997. Disability-adjusted life years: a critical review. *Journal of Health Economics* 16(6):685–702.

Anand S., Hanson K. 1998. DALYs: efficiency versus equity. *World Development* 26(2):307–310.

Anand S., Nanthikesan S. 2000. A compilation of length-of-life distribution measures for complete life tables. Working Paper Series, Vol. 10 No. 7, Harvard Center for Population and Development Studies, Cambridge, MA, June.

Anand S., Nanthikesan S. 2001. The evolution of inequality in length-of-life: France 1806–1987, Working Paper Series, Vol. 11, No. 3, Harvard Center for Population and Development Studies, Cambridge, MA, February.

Anand S., Sen A. 1996. Gender inequality in human development: theories and measurement. In: UNDP, *Background Papers: Human Development Report 1995*, pp 1–20. New York: United Nations Development Programme.

Andreev E. 1982. Metod komponent v analize prodoljitelnosty zjizni [The method of components in the analysis of length of life]. *Vestnik Statistiki* 9:42–47.

Arriaga E. 1984. Measuring and explaining the change in life expectancies. *Demography* 21:83–96.

Atkinson A.B. 1970. On the measurement of inequality. *Journal of Economic Theory* 2:244–263.

Bartley M., Carpenter L., Dunnell K., Fitzpatrick R. 1996. Measuring inequalities in health: an analysis of mortality patterns using two social classifications. *Sociology of Health and Illness* 18:455–475.

Black D., Morris J.N., Smith C., Townsend P. 1980. Inequalities in health (The Black Report). In: Townsend, P., Whitehead, M., Davidson, N. (eds), *Inequalities in Health: The Black Report and The Health Divide.* 2nd ed. London: Penguin.

Blank N., Diderichsen F. 1996. Social inequalities in the experience of illness in Sweden: a "double suffering." *Scandinavian Journal of Social Medicine* 24:81–89.

Blaxter M. 1989. A comparison of measures of inequality in morbidity. In: Fox J. (ed), *Health Inequalities in European countries*, pp. 199–230. Aldershot: Gower.

Bleichrodt H. 1997. Health utility indices and equity considerations. *Journal of Health Economics* 16:65–91.

Brockerhoff M., Hewett P. 1998. Ethnicity and Child Mortality in Sub-Saharan Africa. Policy Research Division Working Paper No. 107. New York: The Population Council.

Carlson P. 1998. Self-perceived health in East and West Europe: another European health divide. *Social Science and Medicine* 46(10):1355–1366.

Chen L., Murray C. 1992. Understanding morbidity change. *Population and Development Review* 18(3):481–503, 593, 595.

Chiang C.L. 1984. *The Life Table and Its Applications.* Malabar, FL: R.E. Krieger Publishing Co.

Daumit G.L., Hermann J.A., Coresh J., Powe N.R. 1999. Use of cardiovascular procedures among black persons and white persons: a 7–year nationwide study in patients with renal disease. *Annals of Internal Medicine.* 130(3):173–182.

Deaton A. 1999. Inequalities in income and inequalities in health. Working Paper 7141. http://www/nber.org/papers/w7141. National Bureau of Economic Research, Cambridge, MA, May.

Drever F., Whitehead M. (eds). 1997. *Health Inequalities. Decennial Supplement.* Series DS No. 15. London: The Stationery Office.

Drèze J., Sen A. 1995. *India: Economic Development and Social Opportunity.* Delhi: Oxford University Press.

Ersink K., Robertson B., Ben-Arie O., Hodson P., Tredoux C. 1998. Expression of schizophrenia in black Xhosa-speaking and white English-speaking South Africans. *African Medical Journal* 88:883–887.

Feldman R.H., Fulwood R. 1999. The three leading causes of death in African Americans: barriers to reducing excess disparity and to improving health behaviors. *Journal of Health Care for the Poor and Underserved* 10(1):45–71.

Foster J.E., Sen A. 1997. On economic inequality: after a quarter century. Annex to expanded edition of Sen A. 1973. *On Economic Inequality.* Oxford: Clarendon Press.

Gakidou E.E., Murray C.J.L., Frenk J. 1999. *A Framework for Measuring Health Inequality.* Global Program on Evidence for Health Policy Discussion Paper No. 5, October 1999. Geneva: World Health Organization.

Gwatkin D. 1999. Information on poor–rich differences with respect to health, nutrition and population. World Bank internal mimeo.

Gwatkin D., Guillot M., Heuveline P. 1999. The burden of disease among the global poor. *Lancet* 354:586–589.

Hallqvist J., Diderichsen F., Theorell T., Ahlbom A. 1998. Is the effect of job strain due to interaction between high psychological demand and low decision latitude? *Social Science and Medicine* 46:1405–1415.

Hsiao W.C., Liu Y. 1996. Economic reform and health—lessons from China [editorial]. *New England Journal of Medicine* 335(6):430–432.

Humphries K.H., van Doorslaer E. 2000. Income-related health inequality in Canada. *Social Science and Medicine* 50:663–671.

Idler E., Benyamini Y. 1997. Self-rated health and mortality: a review of twenty-seven community studies. *Journal of Health and Social Behavior* 38:21–37.

Institute of Medicine. 1998. *Summarizing Population Health: Directions for the Development and Application of Population Metrics.* Field M.J., Gold M.R. (eds). Washington, DC: National Academy Press.

Kaplan G.A., Pamuk E., Lynch J.W., Cohen R.D., Balfour J.S. 1996. Inequality in income and mortality in the United States: analysis of mortality and potential pathway. *British Medical Journal* 312:999–1003.

Krieger N., Williams D.R., and Mosse N.E. 1997. Measuring social class in US public health research: concepts, methodologies and guidelines. *Annual Review of Public Health.* 18:341–378.

Kunst A.K. 1997. Cross-National Comparisons of Socio-Economic Differences in Mortality. Dissertation, Erasmus University, Rotterdam.

Kunst A.K., Geurts J.J.M, van den Berg J. 1995. International variation of socioeconomic inequalities in self-reported health. *Journal of Epidemiology and Community Health* 49:117–123.

Kunst A.K., Mackenbach M.P. 1995. *Measuring Socio-Economic Inequalities in Health.* Regional Office for Europe. Copenhagen: World Health Organization.

Lai D., Tsai S.P., Hardy R.J. 1997. Impact of HIV/AIDS on life expectancy in the United States. *AIDS* 11(2):203–207.

Le Grand J. 1989. An international comparison of distributions of ages-at-death. In: Fox J. (ed), *Health Inequalities in European Countries.* Aldershot: Gower Press.

Le Grand J., Rabin M. 1986. Trends in British health inequality: 1931–83. In: Culyer A.J., Jonsson B. (eds), *Public and Private Health Services.* Oxford: Blackwell.

Lindholm L., Rosén M. 1998. On the measurement of the nation's equity adjusted health. *Health Economics* 7:621–628.

Lundberg M., Fredlund P., Hallqvist J., Dederichsen F. 1996. A SAS program calculating three measures of interaction with confidence intervals. *Epidemiology* 7:655–656.

Lynch J.W., Kaplan G.A., Cohen R.D., Tuomilehto J., Salonen J.T. 1996. Do cardiovascular risk factors explain the relationship between socioeconomic status, risk of all-cause mortality, cardiovascular mortality and acute myocardial infarction? *American Journal of Epidemiology* 144(10):934–942.

Macintyre S. 1998. Social inequalities and health in the contemporary world comparative overview. In: Strickland S.S., Shetty P.S. (eds), *Human Biology and Social Inequality.* 39th Symposium Volume of the Society for the Study of Human Biology. Cambridge: Cambridge University Press, pp. 22–33.

Mackenbach J.P., Kunst A.E. 1997. Measuring the magnitude of socioeconomic inequalities in health. *Social Science and Medicine* 44:757–771.

Mackenbach J.P., Kunst A.K., Cavelaars A.E., Groenhof F., Geurts J.J. 1997. Socioeconomic inequalities in morbidity and mortality in western Europe. The EU Working Group on Socioeconomic Inequalities in Health. *Lancet* 349:1655–1659.

Manor O., Matthews S., Power C. 1997. Comparing measures of health inequality. *Social Science and Medicine* 45(5):761–771.

Murray C.J.L., Lopez A. 1996. *The Global Burden of Disease: A Comprehensive Assessment of Mortality and Disability from Diseases, Injuries, and Risk Factors in 1990 and Projected to 2020.* Geneva: World Health Organization.

Murray C.J.L., Michaud C.M., McKenna M.T., Marks J.S. 1998. *U.S. Patterns of Mortality by County and Race: 1965–1994.* Cambridge: Harvard Center for Population and Development Studies.

Murray C.J.L., Yang G., Qiao X. 1992. Adult mortality: levels, patterns and causes. In: Feachem R.G.S., et al. (eds), *The Health of Adults in the Developing World.* Oxford: Oxford University Press, pp. 23–111.

Namboodiri K., Suchindran C.M. 1987. *Life Table Techniques and Their Applications.* Orlando: Academic Press.

Navarro V. 1991. Race or class or race and class: growing mortality differentials in the United States. *International Journal of Health Services* 21(2):229–235.

Pande R., Gwatkin D. 1999. Country-Level Information on Poor–Rich Differences with Respect to Health, Nutrition and Population. Provisional Data. Washington, DC: World Bank.

Pressat R. 1985. Contribution des écarts de mortalité par âge à la différences des vies moyennes. *Population* 4–5:766–770.

Robine J.M., Mather C.D., Bone M.R. (eds) 1993. Calculation of Health Expectancies: Harmonization, Consensus Achieved and Future Perspectives: 6th REVES International Workshop. Colloque INSERM, Vol. 226. Paris: Editions INSERM.

Rothman K., Greenland S. 1998. *Modern Epidemiology*, 2nd ed. New York: Lipincott.

Sen A. 1973. *On Economic Inequality.* Oxford: Clarendon Press.

Sen A. 1992. *Inequality Reexamined.* Cambridge, MA: Harvard University Press and Oxford: Clarendon Press.

Sen, A. 1994. Objectivity and position: assessment of health and well-being. In: Chen L.C., Kleinman A., Ware N.C. (eds), *Health and Social Change in International Perspective.* Cambridge, MA: Harvard University Press.

Sen A. 1999. *Development as Freedom.* New York: Alfred A. Knopf.

Shkolnikov V.M. 1998. Class-Based Measurement of Inequalities in Length of Life. Paper presented at the Workshop on Measuring Inequalities in Health, St. Catherine's College, Oxford, October 27–28.

Vågerö D., Eriksson R. 1997. Socioeconomic inequalities in morbidity and mortality in western Europe. Correspondence. *Lancet* 350:516.

van Doorslaer E., Wagstaff A., Bleichrodt H., Calonge S., Gerdtham Ulf-G, Gerfin M., Geurts J., Gross L., Häkkinen U., Leu R., O'Donnell O., Propper C., Puffer F., Rodriguez M., Sundberg G., Winkelhake O. 1997. Socioeconomic inequalities in health: some international comparisons. *Journal of Health Economics* 16(1): 93–112.

Wagstaff A., Paci P., van Doorslaer E. 1991. On the measurement of inequalities in health. *Social Science and Medicine* 33:545–577.

Weinstein M.C., Stason W.B. 1976. *Hypertension: A Policy Perspective.* Cambridge, MA: Harvard University Press.

Wilkins R., Adams O.B. 1983. Health expectancy in Canada, late 1970s: demographic, regional, and social dimensions. *American Journal of Public Health* 73(9):1073–1080.

World Health Organization. 1991. *Updating of the European Health for All Targets.* Regional Office for Europe (document EUR/RC41/Inf.Doc./1 Rev.1). Copenhagen: WHO.

APPENDIX A. FORMULAE FOR LENGTH-OF-LIFE DISTRIBUTION MEASURES

We generate a frequency distribution for length-of-life (denoted as the random variable X) by passing a synthetic cohort of individuals through the age-specific probabilities of dying given in a complete life-table (viz., the probability of dying at age x conditional on having survived to age (x − 1). This shows the fraction f_i of individuals from the cohort who live to age x_i, where x_i is the midpoint (usually) of age interval i (except for the first age interval) in the complete life-table, that is, for i = 1,2, . . . ,100.

Hence,

$$\sum_i f_i = 1$$

From this distribution of length-of-life, we can calculate many statistics relating to both the central tendency (mean) and the dispersion around it. We provide here the formulae for the length-of-life distribution measures used in the text (for details, see Anand 1998; Anand and Nanthikesan 2000).

Equally distributed equivalent life $X_e(\epsilon)$ corresponding to the inequality aversion parameter $\epsilon \geq 0$ is defined as

$$X_e(\epsilon) = \begin{cases} \left(\sum_i f_i x_i^{1-\epsilon}\right)^{1/(1-\epsilon)} & \text{for } \epsilon \geq 0, \epsilon \neq 1 \\ \\ \exp\left(\sum_i f_i \log x_i\right) & \text{for } \epsilon = 1 \end{cases}$$

For $\epsilon = 0$, this expression reduces to the arithmetic mean life $X_e(0)$, or life expectancy e_o:

$$X_e(0) = \sum_i f_i x_i$$

For $\epsilon = 1$, we get the geometric mean life $X_e(1)$:

$$X_e(1) = \exp\left(\sum_i f_i \log x_i\right)$$

For $\epsilon = 2$, we get the harmonic mean life $X_e(2)$:

$$X_e(2) = \left(\sum_i f_i x_i^{-1}\right)^{-1}$$

The median is defined as the 50th quantile, or Q(50), with the length-of-life of half the individuals in the cohort below it and of half above it.

The standard deviation σ is defined as the square root of the variance of length-of-life, that is,

$$\sigma = \left[\sum_i f_i(x_i - X_e(0))^2\right]^{1/2}$$

Other statistical indices of dispersion include the coefficient of variation and the relative mean deviation:

$$\text{Coefficient of variation } C = \sigma/X_e(0)$$

$$\text{Relative mean deviation } M = \sum_i f_i|x_i - X_e(0)|/X_e(0)$$

The formulae for the other inequality measures used are given in the following expressions:

$$\text{Gini coefficient } G = \sum_i \sum_j f_i f_j |x_i - x_j|/2X_e(0)$$

The Atkinson index $I(\epsilon)$ for inequality aversion parameter ϵ is defined as

$$I(\epsilon) = 1 - [X_e(\epsilon)/X_e(0)]$$

Hence, for $\epsilon = 1.0$, 1.5, and 2.0, we have the following expressions for the corresponding Atkinson indices:

$$I(1.0) = 1 - [X_e(1.0)/X_e(0)]$$

$$I(1.5) = 1 - [X_e(1.5)/X_e(0)]$$

$$I(2.0) = 1 - [X_e(2.0)/X_e(0)]$$

APPENDIX B. DECOMPOSITION AND WEIGHTING OF THE LIFE EXPECTANCY

Decomposition of a Difference in Life Expectancies

The method of so-called component analysis allows a difference between two life expectancies to be split into contributions of elementary differences in age-specific mortality rates:

$$e_x^2 - e_x^1 = \sum_{y \in [x,W]} \epsilon_y$$

$$\epsilon_y = \frac{1}{2l_x^2}[l_y^2(e_y^2 - e_y^1) - l_{y+1}^2(e_{y+1}^2 - e_{y+1}^1)]$$
$$- \frac{1}{2l_x^1}[l_y^1(e_y^1 - e_y^2) - l_{y+1}^1(e_{y+1}^1 - e_{y+1}^2)]$$

where 1 and 2 are the two population groups to be compared, x and y are ages, W is the oldest age group (usually 85+, 95+, or 100+), and ϵ_y is the component of the overall difference induced by age y.

If cause-specific data are available, a further decomposition according to causes of death (j) can be performed as follows (Andreev 1982):

$$\epsilon_y = \sum_j \epsilon_{y,j}$$

$$\epsilon_{y,j} = \frac{M_{y,j}^1 - M_{y,j}^2}{M_y^1 - M_y^2} \cdot \epsilon_y$$

where $M_{y,j}^1$ is a central death rate in population group 1, age group y and cause of death j; and M_y^1 is a central death rate in population group 1, age y for all causes combined.

Weights of Population Group in the Life-Table Cohort

Developing weights by which life expectancies of different population groups can be weighted together to an average can be done by the following method. In general, to obtain the appropriate weights for group-specific life expectancies, one should solve the system of two equations:

$$e_x l_x = \sum_i l_x^i e_x^i$$

$$l_x = \sum_i l_x^i$$

where i denotes population strata and x is age. Variables e_x^i are known, and the weights (or fractions) l_x^i/l_x are unknown. If there are only two population groups (n = 2) the above system of equations has only one simple solution:

$$l_x^1 = \frac{l_x(e_x - e_x^2)}{e_x^1 - e_x^2}$$

$$l_x^2 = l_x - l_x^1$$

There are, however, multiple solutions if $n > 2$. It seems reasonable to choose the weights characterized by a minimum distance from the proportions of groups in the overall population. It can be shown that the weights l_x^i/l_x can be derived as the first n elements of the vector $\mathbf{z}$ having dimensions $(n + 2)*1$. This vector can be yielded from

$$\mathbf{z} = \mathbf{A}^{-1} \cdot \mathbf{b}$$

where $\mathbf{A}$ is a matrix $(n + 2)*(n + 2)$ and $\mathbf{b}$ is a vector $(n + 2)*1$:

$$\mathbf{A} = \begin{bmatrix} 2 & 0 & 0 & .. & .. & .. & 0 & 1 & e_x^1 \\ 0 & 2 & 0 & .. & .. & .. & 0 & 1 & e_x^2 \\ 0 & 0 & 2 & .. & .. & .. & 0 & 1 & e_x^3 \\ .. & .. & .. & .. & .. & .. & .. & .. \\ .. & .. & .. & .. & .. & 2 & 0 & .. & .. \\ 0 & 0 & 0 & .. & .. & 0 & 2 & 1 & e_x^n \\ 1 & 1 & 1 & .. & .. & .. & 1 & 0 & 0 \\ e_x^1 & e_x^2 & e_x^3 & .. & .. & .. & e_x^n & 0 & 0 \end{bmatrix},$$

$$\mathbf{b} = \begin{bmatrix} 2(P_{x+}^1/P_{x+}) \\ 2(P_{x+}^2/P_{x+}) \\ 2(P_{x+}^3/P_{x+}) \\ .. \\ .. \\ 2(P_{x+}^n/P_{x+}) \\ 1 \\ e_x \end{bmatrix}$$

where P_{x+}^i/P_{x+} is a proportion of stratum i in overall population aged x and over. The obtained weights l_x^i/l_x characterize the sensitivity of the overall life expectancy to the life expectancies in specific population groups.

In the case of the racial differentials in life expectancy within the U.S. male population, the weights can be estimated as follows:

$$\mathbf{A} = \begin{bmatrix} 2 & 0 & 0 & 1 & 72.7483 \\ 0 & 2 & 0 & 1 & 64.5717 \\ 0 & 0 & 2 & 1 & 78.1041 \\ 1 & 1 & 1 & 0 & 0 \\ 72.7483 & 64.5717 & 78.1041 & 0 & 0 \end{bmatrix}$$

$$\mathbf{b} = \begin{bmatrix} 2*0.8413 \\ 2*0.1190 \\ 2*0.0387 \\ 1 \\ 71.8752 \end{bmatrix}$$

The resulting vector $\mathbf{z}$ is a product of inverse matrix $\mathbf{A}^{-1}$ and vector $\mathbf{b}$:

$$\mathbf{z} = \begin{bmatrix} 0.8413 \\ 0.1273 \\ 0.0314 \\ -0.1660 \\ 0.0023 \end{bmatrix}$$

Thus, the weights are 0.841, 0.127, and 0.031 for white, black, and "other race" men.

These weights are slightly different from the population shares of racial groups given in vector $\mathbf{b}$ (see above).

CHAPTER
6

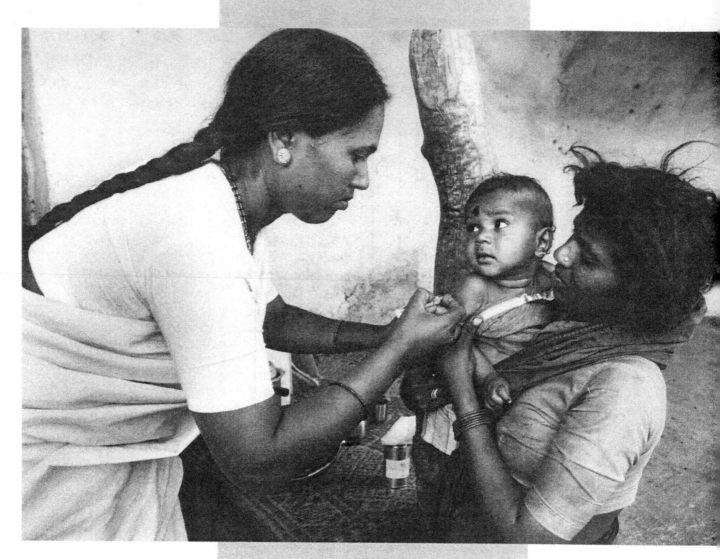

Tribal family receiving vaccination.
Andhra Pradesh, India.
Source: Liba Taylor/Panos.

Health Equity:
Perspectives, Measurability, and Criteria

AMARTYA SEN

In a famous essay, Frank Ramsey, the mathematical philosopher and economist, asked the question: "Is there anything to discuss?" He came to the conclusion that there was not much to discuss because many of our debates deal with only apparent—not real—disagreements. He proposed an analogy with an imagined dispute. Someone says, "I went to Grantchester this afternoon," and the other responds, "No, I didn't!" What looks like a disagreement may be nothing of the sort, but merely disparate statements regarding different events that are—wrongly—taken to be the same event (such as your and my going to Grantchester, respectively).

Ramsey is certainly right about many apparent debates that masquerade as real disputes. I am afraid, however, that there are genuine disputes as well. This is especially so in the subject that I have been asked to address. Analysis of equity in health inevitably depends on many contentious issues, which can be resolved in very different ways that are thoroughly open to discussion, disputation, and scrutiny.

Difficulties in the conceptualization of equity in health care can arise, I would argue, from any of the following distinct components of that exercise:

1. Selection of *informational bases of health assessment* (particularly the choice between "external" and "internal" perspectives in evaluating the state of health)
2. Choice of an appropriate *concept of individual advantage* (dealing particularly with the distinction between judging advantage by the extent of health *care* as opposed to judging it by the *achievement* of good health or the *freedom to achieve* good health)
3. Presumption regarding the extent of *measurability of health status* (particularly the choice between *cardinal* and *ordinal* measurement, the use of *complete* or *partial orderings*, and so forth)
4. Determination of an acceptable *criterion* of equity (along with choice of relative emphases on *conglomerative or aggregative efficiency* and *distributive equity*)

In a short chapter like this, I do not have the opportunity of addressing these questions in an adequate way. I shall concentrate mainly on answering the first question and then supplement that analysis by briefer observations on the other issues. The questions themselves have importance of their own in indicating the need for appropriate scrutiny in understanding the demands of health equity. Even when the answers to these different questions call for more investigation, it may be useful to have an unclouded view of what the pivotal issues are that underlie the exercise of assessing health equity (and that of seeing their implications for public policy).

Informational Basis in Assessing Health

Ideas of good health and ill health are themselves open to some disputation. What kind of information should we use to judge the goodness or badness of health?

A crucial distinction concerns the difference between the "internal" and the "external" views of illness and health. Medical anthropologists provide interesting and important investigations of health and illness in an "internal" perspective: not as observed by a doctor or an outside expert, but by the patient himself or herself. In contrast, medical statistics are often—per force—detached from *self-perception* and rely on *externally observed medical findings* (such as diagnosed ailments of particular types). The allocation of resources is often influenced powerfully by this choice of focus.

This raises an important question about the informational basis of judgements of good and bad health. Should we go by self-perception of bad health (what the patient herself thinks), or should we concentrate, instead, on professional assessment of illness and indifferent health? This also raises a question about the relevance and usefulness of indirect indicators (such as mortality rates and life expectancy).

Practitioners of medical anthropology have been particularly active in recent years to show the relevance of the internal perspective—well illustrated, for example, by the major contributions of Arthur Kleinman and his colleagues (Kleinman 1980, 1986, 1988, 1995; Kleinman et al. 1997). These works are illuminating and insightful especially in bringing out the importance of *suffering* and *jeopardy* as central features of illness. No mechanically observed medical statistics can provide an adequate understanding of these aspects of poor health. Pain, as Wittgenstein had noted, is inescapably a matter of self-perception. If you *feel* pain, you do *have* pain, and if you *do not feel* pain, then no external observer can sensibly reject the view that you *do not have* pain. In dealing with this aspect of illness, the empirical material on which health planners, economic allocators, and cost–benefit analysts frequently rely may, thus, be fundamentally deficient. There is a need to draw on the rich discernment provided by the difficult but deeply rewarding anthropological understanding of these matters. These insights and comprehension are important, and the analysis of health equity as well as the deter-

mination of priorities of health care can be enriched by taking fuller note of them.

The question that does arise, however, is this: Because of the relevance of the internal perspective, can we conclude that the external perspective is redundant? I would argue that we cannot, because internal perception has its own limitations. This is obvious enough when we consider the understanding of complicated illnesses, of which many patients may have very limited knowledge, particularly in assessing their seriousness and reaching the associated prognosis. Also, if a disease is endemic to a region, a patient with no knowledge of other places and other experiences (and no awareness of the possibility of preventing or curing the ailment) may easily take the suffering to be a part of the "human condition" rather than seeing it as avoidable—and in need of preventive or curative intervention. It is, thus, extremely important not to reject or ignore the external views merely on the ground of the relevance of the internal view. Indeed, both perspectives are important, and it is a question of taking a broad enough approach to have an informationally adequate framework.

Positionality and Situation in Health Diagnosis

To recognize the abiding importance of external diagnosis does not, in any way, undermine the far-reaching relevance of the internal view, which medical anthropologists have done so much to illuminate and emphasize in recent years. I am not advocating a return to exclusive reliance on "expert judgement," ignoring the ideas and feelings of the person most directly involved, to wit, the patient. When the external and the internal views diverge, however, there are important cases in which the external view has a cogency and reach that may not be similarly manifest in the internal view.

The internal view of the patient is not only *informed* by knowledge to which others do not have access, but it is also *limited* by the social experience of the person in interpreting what is happening and why. A person reared in a community with a great many diseases may tend to take certain symptoms as "normal" when they are clinically preventable and remediable. Also, a person with little access to medical care and little education about medical matters can take certain bodily conditions as inescapable, even when they are thoroughly amenable to effective medical treatment. Thus the internal view, while informationally rich in one respect, is also informationally limited in very serious ways (even though the informational limitation comes here from a different direction compared with the restrictions that apply to the external view).

The dependence on contingent social experience can be a very significant limitation in the epistemology of the internal view and has a direct bearing on the domain and reach of mainstream anthropological approaches. Let me illustrate the issue with an example. Consider the different states of India, which have very diverse medical conditions, mortality rates, educational achievements, and so on. The state of Kerala has the highest level of longevity (a life expectancy much above 70 years for men and 76 years for women) compared with the Indian averages of 59 or 60 years, respectively. It so happens, however, that Kerala also has incomparably the highest rate of reported morbidity. Even when we make *age-specific* comparisons, Kerala has remarkably higher rates of reported illnesses than any other Indian state so that the difference is not just a reflection of the higher age pattern of the Kerala population. At the other end, the low-longevity states in India such as Bihar (with life expectancy well below that of the Indian average) also have much lower rates of reported morbidity.

Do we, then, accept self-perceived assessment of health as a criterion of good and bad health and declare the state of Bihar to be blessed with much higher achievement of health than Kerala? Or do we go by the evidence of mortality rates (*lowest* in Kerala among all states), confirmed also by the professional analyses of medical practitioners (also *lowest* in Kerala), to take exactly the opposite view based on self-diagnosed morbidity (*highest* in Kerala) (Sen 1985, 1993, 1999)?

There is a need also to address the *explanatory* question as to why this dichotomy arises. It does seem odd that a population—that of Kerala—in which self-perceived illness and disease are so rampant should be exactly the population that lives the longest and avoids preventable epidemics and pestilence most successfully. The picture cannot be disentangled by simply ignoring self-perceptions, as some medical practitioners seem inclined to do (to the irritation, entirely justified, of those informed by anthropological analysis). In fact, instead of ignoring self-perceptions, we have to see why they arise and what they tell us about the continued prevalence of avoidable morbidity and mortality. For example, it can be sensibly argued that the population of Kerala with its very high literacy rate and with the most extensive public health facilities in the country is in a much better position to diagnose and perceive particular illnesses and do something about them than the populations of other states in India.

Indeed, seeking medical attention is not only a reflection of the *awareness* of a health condition, it is also a way of *achieving remedy*. Most people go to the doctor to get medical help rather than to influence medical statistics. The illiterate and medically ill-served population of Bihar may have little perception of illness. While that is no indication that there is little illness to perceive, it is frequently symptomatic of the fact that little remedying is being attempted. There is no real mystery here once the "positional" conditions are woven into the interpretation of medical statistics (Sen 1992, 1993, 1994).

This way of understanding and explaining the dissonance between the perceived morbidity rates and observed mortality rates fits well into what is found in a further comparison of reported morbidity rates—that between Kerala and India, on the one hand, and the United States, on the other. Such comparisons can be found in a work by Lincoln Chen and Christopher Murray (1992). It emerges from disease-by-disease comparison that while Kerala has much higher reported morbidity rates for most illnesses than the rest of India, the United States has *even higher* rates for the same illnesses. Thus, if we insist on going by self-reported morbidity, we would have to conclude that the United States is the least healthy in this comparison, followed by Kerala, with the rest of India enjoying the highest level of health (led by the states most backward in health care and education, such as Bihar and Uttar Pradesh).

The approach for which I have tried to argue invokes the idea of "positional objectivity," seeing the perception of reality in terms of the observers' "position" in relation to the things being observed (Sen 1993). It is crucially important to socially "situate" the statistics of self-perception of illness, taking note of the connection between self-perception, on the one hand, and levels of education and public health facilities, on the other. In analyzing equity in the allocation of health care, it would be, in this analysis, a great mistake to take low perception of morbidity as positive evidence of good health status.

A more credible picture can be constructed through *combining* diagnostic investigations of medical practitioners with the statistics of mortality and causes of death, supplemented by social analysis in trying to make sense of reported perceptions of morbidity. While attaching adequate importance to the privileged information of self-perception of the patient, we also have to recognize the limits of actual social experience related to health care, education, and other social parameters. An adequate grasp of positionality and situational differences of different groups of people is crucial for making sense of the diverse observations involved—covering external assessment as well as self-perception and mortality information as well as morbidity data.

The Relevance of Health in Health Care

If the foregoing analysis is right, then when investigating health status we have to make use both of "internal" and "external" perspectives. When the two perspectives happen to coincide (as they may, in many comparisons), the conflict may not be observed, but in general a health equity analyst cannot expect to escape the need to deal with both sets of information. The chosen priorities must be lucid and open to public scrutiny.

There is perhaps a more basic—at least a *prior*—question here, which relates to the second item in the previous listing of issues. How relevant is health achievement when judging the equity of health policy? Can the exercise not be done entirely on the basis of equity in providing health services and health care? If health care is open to all, in contrast with the situation in, for example, the United States (where, it appears, more than 40 million people do not manage to get any medical insurance), should we not decide that the need for health equity has been adequately served? Equality in the delivery of health care may be easier to assess than equality in health achievement, and is it not right that health equity should be concerned only with the former, not the latter?

If we are attracted by justice in the process rather than by the results achieved, and if we take a fairly proximate view of what constitutes a "process," then this claim may indeed have some plausibility. Neither of the conditional premises is, however, easy to justify. Can we judge the fairness of a process of delivering, for example, kidney dialysis by noting that everyone gets the same amount of time on a dialysis machine no matter what exactly one's kidney needs? If, on the other hand, we evaluate the equity of the process of health care delivery by relating it to human diversity and differential needs, can we ignore the connection with likely *results* (e.g., on the functioning of the kidney, in the example considered)? It is hard to justify the view that fairness or equity in *health care* can be dissociated from the actual results—the health outcome—achieved through the respective processes or from the *freedoms* enjoyed by the individuals involved

to achieve particular results using the processes under examination.

Indeed, it is easy to see that if we are concerned with the real freedom that people enjoy, or with the actual well-being that individuals have, then the assessment of health equity cannot adequately be pursued in terms of mere quantification of health *care*. In judging the value of health care, we have to examine what it does to the lives of the people involved, not just the magnitude—or extent—of the care they receive. This involves, inescapably, the need to judge individual advantage in terms of the health conditions they achieve or the opportunity of good health that they enjoy. That, in turn, requires that the analysis of health equity has to be linked with comparisons of quality of life, or of capabilities, or of some other way of looking at comparative opportunities of leading good lives and achieving what one has reason to value. Also note must be taken of the fact that health care is only one way of achieving good health (or the freedom to achieve good health), and other policies, related to economic and social conditions, can also influence the health status of the population. Equity of health care delivery has to be integrated with other ways of improving health, in particular, and the quality of life and substantive freedoms, in general (Sen 1992; Nussbaum and Sen 1993; Roemer 1996; Ruger 1998).

Measurability of Health Achievement

We cannot, thus, escape the need to assess good and bad health, but how—and in what form—do we measure health achievement? This is the third issue outlined earlier. Should we insist only on getting a *ranking* of health status, without any kind of a "cardinal" measurement of it? Must this ranking be presumed to be complete?

I have discussed elsewhere the technical issues involved in such measurability problems (Sen 1970, 1973). Let me recollect, very briefly, some of the main alternative formulations of measurability. Perhaps the most elementary kind of measurement is one that takes the form of a "partial ordering," whereby some of the alternatives can be ranked vis-à-vis each other, but not all pairs of alternatives can be so ranked. We may decide that x is definitely better (or involves better health) than y, and also better than z, and yet we may not be able to rank y against z. More demandingly, we can have a complete ordering whereby every pair of alternatives can be ranked vis-à-vis each other. This ordering property can be translated in most cases into a numerical ordering, with a higher numerical valuation standing for superiority. This is called *ordinal measurement*. The next step beyond this is cardinal measurement. While ordinality requires that comparisons be confined to what is more and what is less (differences in health status without specification of the *size* of differences), cardinal measurement permits comparison of differences (and of differences of differences, and so on). A further extension of measurement would permit the comparison not only of differences (and differences of differences, and so on) but also of *ratios*. This is called *ratio scale measurement*. There are various other types of measurement as well and also different extents of partial measurement, such as partial cardinality (Sen 1970, 1982, 1997; Basu 1980).

In studying equity or inequality, economists tend to concentrate on variables like income, which admit ratio scale measurement, going even beyond cardinality. It is difficult, however, to expect that this will work for the condition of health. "I am twice as well in health this year as I was in the last" is not a statement that is likely to make a great deal of sense (even though it is easy enough to understand the ordinal comparison: "I am in better health this year than I was last year"). In fact, in most cases, even cardinal measurability may be somewhat problematic, because *differences* in values may be hard to measure and compare (Sen 1982). Neither the internal perspective of the sense of being well, nor the external evaluation of the state of a person's health, would typically allow such measurement. Quite often, an ordering or ordinal measurement may be as far as we can go. If cardinality is to be used, it may be at most partial so that some differences may be ranked without there being any guarantee that all differences can be similarly ranked.

Criteria and Measurability

Because the standard measures of inequality used in economics (such as the Gini coefficient, the coefficient of variation, standard deviation of logarithms, and so forth) all require *more* than ordinal measurement (in fact, typically need ratio scale measurement), there is unlikely to be any kind of immediate translation of measures of *income inequality* into corresponding measures of health inequality. Thus the vast and rather definitive literature on "economic inequality" cannot be easily translated into a corresponding understanding of health inequality.

I would like to emphasize here that even with ordinal information, it is possible to make some kinds of substantive judgements of equity. Indeed, John Rawls's famous theory of justice only uses ordinal comparison (Rawls 1971, 1993; see also Sen 1970 and Daniels 1975, 1985). That approach tends to concentrate on making the worst-off groups as well-off as possible (in Rawls' *Difference Principle*), and this task does not demand more than ordinal measurement.

We can, in fact, go well beyond the Rawlsian criteria as well, on the basis of ordinal information. Indeed, even *difference comparisons* of some types can be made on the basis of ordinal logic alone. The concept of "ordinal intensity" characterized in the literature on social choice theory can be useful here. For example, if we rank four states in the decreasing order of w, x, y, z, then we can say that the difference between w and z is larger than that between x and y. Thus the mere ordering of these four alternatives also tells us something about the differences as well (Sen 1982).

This may not look like much, but it turns out that comparisons of ordinal intensity may often be adequate for quite sophisticated judgments on health equity. Consider, for example, the important critique by Sudhir Anand and Kara Hansen of the use of DALY (disability-adjusted life years) as aggregate evaluative statistics (Anand and Hansen 1997, 1998). The neglect of equity considerations in this way of assessing health achievement of a group is, however, a major limitation (see also Foster and Sen 1997). Among these grounds of criticism is Anand and Hansen's crucial point that if DALY were to be minimized for a nation as a whole, then priority would be systematically given to catering to the interests of people who were able bodied over those who were already afflicted with disability. Saving an able-bodied person gives more credit in reducing "good years" lost—central to the DALY approach—than saving a person already with some disability. This entails, however, that a person who is disadvantaged already—with some disability—would be disadvantaged further through relative neglect in public policy if policy priorities were to be based on DALY (with the consequent preference for serving the interests of the able bodied). Also, this would make the health inequality greater than in the absence of intervention. Although cardinal comparisons can be used to make such judgements, the conclusions do not *require* cardinal comparison; ordinal intensity comparisons would suffice (Foster and Sen 1997).

This issue is important especially because many measures of health—based on either internal or external perspectives—may face difficulties in cardinalization (not to mention ratio scale quantification). Better or worse health may not have the measurement possibilities that income or physical output may have, which have tended to be the informational ingredients of equity judgments in welfare economics. Recent progress in the measurement of economic inequality is to a great extent due to the constructive leadership of A. B. Atkinson (1983).

In fact, given the conflict of criteria (not least the conflict between "external" and "internal" perspectives, discussed earlier in this essay), we may often fall short even of a complete ordering. If we take the common elements, the "intersections" of different orderings (based, for example, on external and internal perspectives respectively), we get a partial ordering, with articulate comparison of alternatives in some pairs, but not in others. For these cases too, the idea of "ordinal intensity" can work and may be actually used in many practical comparisons. The possible usefulness of this approach demands greater investigation and scrutiny.

Health equity, like all other kinds of equity, cannot escape the need to examine inequalities in the relevant variable, in this case health condition (and, correspondingly, the freedom to achieve good health condition). For this a partial ordering is the most elementary requirement, and the more complete that partial ordering is, the more extensive will be the possible reach of such investigation. To see whether inequality is greater in one case than in another, we can go some substantial distance through the use of ordinal intensity. We must not overlook what we can do even with the minimal extents of measurability that we are likely to find in the field of health assessment. To go beyond that would require various hybrid measures that do not overpresume the extent of measurability that health variables may have, but at the same time try to stretch the available information as far as it will go with the analytical techniques that are available to us. For example, combining the purely aggregative framework of DALY (or quality-adjusted life year, QALY) with adjustment for inequality in health conditions is likely to be a very fruitful exercise.

This may indeed provide a reasonable way of approaching the fourth question—establishing an acceptable criterion of health equity. In general, the criteria that we might wish to use when assessing health equity would depend, among other things, on what we could do with the plausible extents of measurability. To frame it the other way, the information we seek (on the basis of direct observation or based on some combination of observation and interpretation) has to respond to the informational *need* of the criteria proposed for use, without going beyond the limits of feasibility (Sen 1970, 1973, 1992). For example, even without any explicit use of criteria of equity, just the assessment of aggregate health achievement (e.g., for a community) would have need for interpersonal comparability with cardinal measurability of some kind so that positive differences in one direction can be contrasted with negative differences in the other. It is not quite clear to what extent this can be sensibly done. Even though arbitrary assumptions can be used to get numbers that look concrete (as many rough and ready "aggregate" figures do), they may not bear much critical scrutiny on the extent of measurability that has been implicitly invoked. This is a major neglect in the contemporary literature on health equity.

Ultimately, the possibility of using particular criteria of health equity is limited by (*1*) the analytical requirements of measurability demanded respectively by each specific criterion and (*2*) the extent of actual measurability that is consistent with the nature of the available and usable information. In this overall exercise, the different questions identified earlier are closely linked with each other. Any research agenda that attempts to carry forward what has already been achieved must take adequate note of these interdependences. Much remains to be done.

References

Anand S., Hansen K. 1997. Disability-adjusted life years: a critical review. *Journal of Health Economics* 16(6):685–702.

Anand S., Hansen K. 1998. DALYs: efficiency versus equity. *World Development* 26(2):307–310.

Atkinson A.B. 1983. *Social Justice and Public Policy*. Cambridge, MA: MIT Press.

Basu K. 1980. *Revealed Preference of the Government*. Cambridge: Cambridge University Press.

Chen L., Murray C. 1992. Understanding morbidity change. *Population and Development Review* 18(3):481–503, 593, 595.

Daniels N. (ed.) 1975. *Reading Rawls*. Oxford: Blackwell.

Daniels N. 1985. *Just Health Care*. Cambridge, England: Cambridge University Press.

Foster J., Sen A. 1997. *On Economic Inequality* after a quarter century. In: Sen A. (ed), *On Economic Inequality*. Oxford: Clarendon Press, pp. 109–149.

Kleinman A. 1980. *Patients and Healers in the Context of Culture*. Berkeley: University of California Press.

Kleinman A. 1986. *Social Origins of Disease and Distress*. New Haven, CT: Yale University Press.

Kleinman A. 1988. *The Illness Narrative: Suffering, Healing and the Human Condition*. New York: Basic Books.

Kleinman A. 1995. *Writing at the Margin: Discourse Between Anthropology and Medicine*. Berkeley: University of California Press.

Kleinman A., Das V., Lock M. (eds). 1997. *Social Suffering*. Berkeley: University of California Press.

Nussbaum M., Sen A. (eds). 1993. *The Quality of Life*. Oxford: Clarendon Press.

Rawls J. 1971. *A Theory of Justice*. Cambridge, MA: Harvard University Press.

Rawls J. 1993. *Political Liberalism*. New York: Columbia University Press.

Roemer J. 1996. *Theories of Distributive Justice*. Cambridge, MA: Harvard University Press.

Ruger J.P. 1998. Aristotelian Justice and Health Policy: Capability and Incompletely Theorized Agreements. Ph.D. thesis, Harvard University.

Sen A. 1970. *Collective Choice and Social Welfare*. San Francisco: Holden-Day; republished, Amsterdam: North-Holland.

Sen A. 1973. *On Economic Inequality*. Oxford: Clarendon Press. Extended edition, 1997.

Sen A. 1982. *Choice, Welfare and Measurement*. Oxford: Blackwell; republished, Cambridge, MA: Harvard University Press, 1997.

Sen A. 1985. *Commodities and Capabilities*. Amsterdam: North-Holland.

Sen A. 1992. *Inequality Reexamined*. Cambridge, MA: Harvard University Press; republished Oxford: Clarendon Press.

Sen A. 1993. Positional objectivity. *Philosophy and Public Affairs* 22:126–146.

Sen A. 1994. Objectivity and position: assessment of health and well-being. In: Chen L., Kleinman A., Ware N. (eds), *Health and Social Change: An International Perspective*. Cambridge, MA: Harvard University Press.

Sen A. 1997. *On Economic Inequality*, 2nd ed. Oxford: Clarendon Press.

Sen A. 1999. *Development as Freedom*. New York: Knopf; republished, Oxford: Oxford University Press.

CHAPTER
7

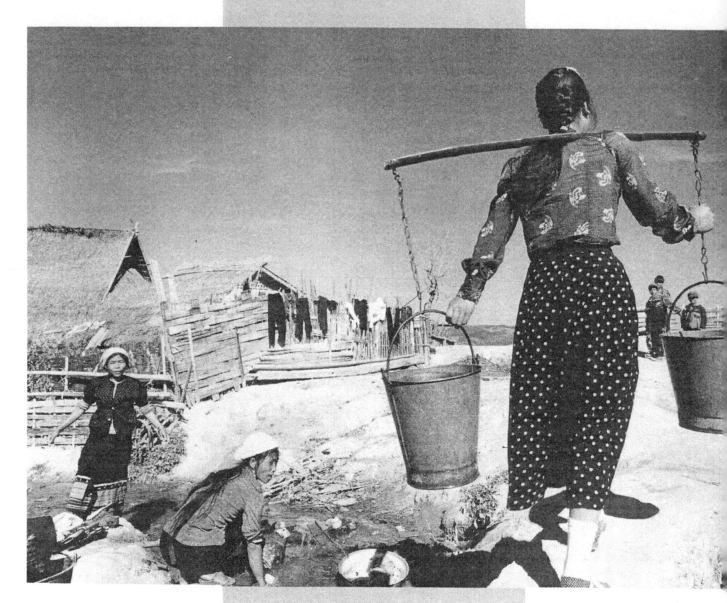

Girls fetching water. "Wa" minority village.
Cangyan Yunnan, S.W. China, 1995.
Source: Rhodri Jones/Panos.

China: Increasing Health Gaps in a Transitional Economy

YUANLI LIU, KEQIN RAO, TIMOTHY EVANS, YUDE CHEN,
AND WILLIAM C. HSIAO

China's outstanding health achievements before the 1980s and her rapid economic growth over the past decade are well documented (Sidel 1972; Newell 1975; World Health Organization and UNICEF 1975; Sidel and Sidel 1982; Ye et al. 1982, Hartland-Thunberg 1989; World Bank 1997b). Less well known, however, is the impact of the transition from a socialist to a market economy on overall health development and equity in health and health care. Since the initiation of the economic reform process 20 years ago, China's real output has increased 9% annually, nearly quadrupling the size of the economy (Tseng et al. 1994). Productivity gains have permitted substantial improvements in real income and notable progress in reducing poverty (World Bank 1996). As is shown in Table 1, China's economy in 1995 in terms of total gross domestic product (GDP) was four times its size in 1980, when China had just begun its economic reforms.

Yet rapid economic growth does not necessarily guarantee a desirable distribution of resource gains. Rather, in China, as in most transitional economies, reforms have spawned an increasing income gap between different subpopulations (United Nations Development Programme 1997). In 1980, the difference in annual per capita income between the rural residents and their urban counterparts was 243 yuan (equivalent to about U.S. $30). By 1995 the income differential increased to 650 yuan (approximately U.S. $75). In 1981, China was a relatively egalitarian society as indicated by relatively low levels of income inequality (a Gini coefficient of 0.29). By 1995, however, the rise in income inequality was the most rapidly accelerating ever (a Gini coefficient of 0.39) (World Bank 1997a). This evidence, along with concerns about the relative neglect of peripheral economic areas (rural and geographically remote) and their populations has led to a specific focus on interregional gaps in socioeconomic status in China's tenth 5-year plan (2001 to 2006) (Xing Hua She 1999).

It is less clear what the implications of economic reform have been for the health status of the Chinese population. Life expectancy has increased steadily from about 68 years at birth in 1980 to approximately 71 years in 1995 (see Table 1). The infant mortality rate (IMR) has declined gradually over the same period from 41 per 1000 live births in 1980 to around 35 per 1000 in 1995 (see Table 1). According to the 1999 *World Health Report*, China's health performance has slipped considerably in the last 20 years. In 1972 China's infant mortality rate was 67% lower than predicted based on level of income, whereas in 1992 its

China

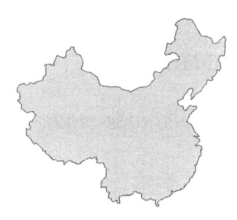

Total population (millions), 1997	1,244.2
Human development index, 1999	0.701
Human development index rank, 1999	98
Infant mortality rate (per 1,000 live births), 1997	38
Real GDP per capita (PPP$), 1997	3,130
Public spending on health as percentage of GDP, 1995	—

— Not available.
Source: UNDP 1999. [Human Development Report]

infant mortality rate was only 33% lower than predicted (World Health Organization 1999). The incidence of infectious diseases has decreased dramatically from 2080 per 100,000 in 1980 to 176 per 100,000 in

1995 (see Table 1). In the context of decreasing fertility rates and an aging population, an epidemiological transition has also been witnessed. While infectious diseases have been successfully brought under control, chronic and degenerative diseases have become the major cause of disease burden, especially in urban areas. Over the 8-year period from 1985 to 1993 there has been an increase in noncommunicable diseases as a percentage of total deaths as well as a substantial rise in the morbidity rate for chronic disease (Liu et al. 1998). China's experience may help to answer a question of great importance to other countries with developing and transitional economies: Does economic reform and growth necessarily improve health status for all (Hsiao and Liu 1996)?

There is a growing concern that populationwide aggregate statistics are masking significant inequality in the health status of subpopulations differentiated by geographic location, gender, and level of socioeconomic development. For example, in 1994 the coastal province of Zhejiang had a maternal death rate of 23.74 per 100,000, whereas that of the inland province Qinghai was 215.37 per 100,000 (Huang and Liu 1995). Data obtained in 1988 indicate that deaths from all major causes among residents in rural areas were 10% to 100% higher for specific age groups than those of urban residents (Ministry of Health 1988). The IMR is also consistently greater in rural than in urban areas, and there is evidence that the gap has been growing during economic transition (Huang and Liu 1995; Wang 1996). Even among rural communities the IMR

Table 1 Socioeconomic and health indicators in China, selected years, 1980–95

Indicator	1980	1985	1990	1995
Income				
GDP (billions of yuan)	443	700	893	1,636
Urban per capita income (yuan)	430	535	668	1,093
Rural per capita income (yuan)	187	311	330	443
Health				
Life expectancy at birth (years)	68	69	70	71[a]
Infant mortality rate (per 1,000 live births)	41	40	38	35[b]
Deaths from infectious disease (per 100,000)	3.07	0.97	0.80	0.62
Incidence of infectious disease (per 100,000)	2,080	875	292	176
Doctors (per 1,000)	1	1	2	2
Hospital beds (per 1,000)	2	2	2	2

a. Estimated using data from the 1993 National Sample Survey of Cancer Mortality.
b. Estimated using data from Huang and Liu 1995.
Source: Ministry of Health 1998; Huang and Liu 1995.

has been found to vary substantially—from 29.3 to 72 per 1000 live births in 1990 (Ministry of Health 1994). A recent study of 30 of China's poorest counties found that the average IMR increased from about 50 per 1000 live births in the late 1970s to 72 per 1000 live births in the late 1980s (Liu et al. 1996). Nutrition statistics also indicate a relative deterioration in the health status of rural populations. Surveys in nine provinces in 1987 and 1992 showed that the percentage of stunted children in rural areas had actually increased (World Bank 1992). Furthermore, in one of the most comprehensive studies to date, Shen et al. (1996) find that data on growth of Chinese children (measured as height for age) indicate increasing disparities between urban and rural areas despite aggregate improvement overall. Reflecting these trends in child health, life expectancy in rural areas is lower than in urban areas for all age groups. More worrisome still is evidence that suggests increasing rural/urban differentiation in the life expectancy across age and gender groups during the period 1981 to 1994 (Huang and Liu 1995).

These descriptive statistics indicate that health inequalities between different population groups may be a serious and growing problem in China and thus warrant research and policy attention. To this end, the primary consideration guiding the equity focus of this case study is its relevance to policy. Political attention and action may not be effectively generated by studies that consider dimensions of socioeconomic inequalities for which there are no realistic policy options. For example, even though income inequality is found by an increasing body of literature to be strongly correlated with community health (Wilkinson 1992a, 1996), policies for the reduction of income inequality are lacking or politically infeasible. Indeed, one of the motivations underlying the movement of former socialist countries toward a market economy is the belief that increasing income inequality is a necessary incentive to and natural consequence of economic development. Given our concern for policy relevance, this study considers two major dimensions of health equity in China: gender inequality and interregional inequality in health.

Gender equality is a prominent policy issue in China that has been addressed in successive governments since the founding of the People's Republic of China in 1949. Indeed, China has been proud of her record in gender equality in labor participation, education, and health care. For example, concerted efforts have been made to promote women to senior government positions. The specific policy of training female health workers to staff village health posts at the grassroots level is intended to enhance women's labor participation in the health sector and increase health care uti-

lization by women (United Nations Development Program 1997). These positive policy initiatives, however, must be balanced with a persistent patrilineal system that places greater value on the male child and discriminates against the female. This strong preference for sons may have been exacerbated by the "one child per family" policy. Given this historical legacy, a question arises: Have the economic reforms led to the emergence of greater gender inequality? If so, it may signal an inadequacy of current policies toward gender equality in health.

The second major issue addressed in this chapter concerns trends in interregional inequality in health since the onset of reforms. As China has opened its doors to the outside world, the coastal regions have been poised to seize opportunities presented by their proximity to world markets, access to better infrastructure, and an educated labor force. The coastal regions have benefited through the increased autonomy and tax base arising from the decentralization of China's fiscal system as well as the central government's policies to stimulate foreign investment. As a result, interprovincial inequality has risen. According to a World Bank (1997a) estimate, interprovincial inequality accounted for one-fourth of total inequality in income in 1995 and explained one-third of the increase since 1985. Given this context, is there a similar pattern of interregional inequality in health? This chapter explores recent trends in gender and regional inequality in health with a specific interest in the impact of economic transition and identification of actionable policy to rectify inequities judged intolerable.

Following a description of the methods and data, the main findings on gender and regional inequalities in health are presented. Of academic and policy interest is not only the magnitude but also the major determinants of the health inequalities. We employ regression analysis to study possible determinants of population health, using data from 62 counties, representative of China's rural population of 800 million. The chapter concludes with a summary of major findings, possible policy implications, and issues for future research.

Data, Methods, and Measures

This study takes advantage of extensive data on health and health care in China, such as those in the 1981 and 1990 censuses. The study primarily relies, however, on the 1993 National Health Services Survey (Ministry of Health 1994). With a stratified multistage sample design, this survey was carried out on a nationally representative sample of 90 cities and counties. In each sampled city and county, in-depth interview surveys were conducted on about 600 households. Over 200,000 individuals provided information on self-reported health status, health care, and socioeconomic status through household interviews. The 1993 National Health Services Survey also provided information about area characteristics such as population size and rural/urban composition, which facilitated interregional analysis.

Measuring Gender Inequality in Health

Gender inequality is measured with respect to three major questions. First, do Chinese women enjoy an "adequate" level of female advantage in life expectancy? We address this question by comparing China's female advantage in life expectancy (the difference between female and male life expectancy) to that of Japan. Urban and rural differences in female advantage are indicated by comparing the female advantage in rural China with that in urban China, using the latter as a reference point to measure "shortfall."

The second question pertains to the problem of "missing women" (Sen 1990). This phenomenon relates to practices that favor boys' survival over girls' survival, such as cessation of childbearing when the desired number of sons is reached, sex-selective abortion or infanticide, and female neglect during early childhood. Under conditions of relatively equal treatment for both sexes, 105 to 106 males are born for every 100 females to compensate for the greater biological vulnerability of males (Hull 1990; Johansson and Nygren 1991; Zeng et al. 1993). By comparing sex differences in the mortality rates of boys and girls under 5 years of age in developing countries with the West model life-tables and by comparing the recorded sex ratio at birth to a "normal" ratio of 106, one can calculate the total number of "missing girls," namely, the number of excess deaths in those aged 0 to 4 years and the number of excess abortions (Anand and Sen 1995).

The third question we ask is what particular health problems (other than reproductive health problems) do women suffer more frequently than men? To address this question, male and female prevalence rates of self-reported injuries and psychosis from the 1993 National Health Survey and suicide incidence are compared.

Measuring Interregional Inequalities in Health

To examine interregional inequalities in health status, indices of mortality and morbidity are derived. Four morbidity indicators are constructed from the 1993 Household Health Survey. The "two week morbidity rate" is based on the question: Have you been ill or injured in the past 2 weeks? The answer to this question indicates self-perceived health status. "Chronic diseases" is based on the question: In the last 6 months, did you have any chronic illnesses diagnosed by health professionals? Here, a clinical diagnosis is required, meaning that the "manifestation" of the chronic diseases in our data is conditional on the patient's having seen a doctor. "Health limitations" are reflected in the answer to the question: In the last 6 months, did you have any functional limitations due to illness or injury? If yes, the respondent is asked to specify what kind of limitations are experienced (a seven item multiple choice list is presented, ranging from walking difficulties to urine control). Finally, each household member is asked whether he or she is disabled ("disability") based on China's legal definition (Ministry of Health 1994).

Area-based income measures are used to derive a socioeconomic ranking of regions. This scheme served as part of the sampling framework for the 1993 survey. Based mainly on per capita income of the region, China's 2400 cities and counties were grouped into seven areas. The urban sample was categorized into big cities (Big City), medium cities (Med City), and small cities (Sm City), while rural counties were classified according to level of wealth, with "Cnty 1" representing the richest and "Cnty 4" representing the poorest areas.

Measuring Socioeconomic Inequalities in Health

A number of summary indicators are used to express the size of health inequalities by income group. Using 1993 National Health Services Survey data, we ranked individuals by their income and divided them into income deciles. The following indicators of health inequality between income groups were then derived: (1) the rate difference (between the lowest and highest income decile), (2) the rate ratio (of the lowest vs. highest income decile), and (3) the population attributable risk, which is the reduction in overall morbidity rates that would occur in the hypothetical case that all persons would experience the rate of the highest income decile group (Kunst and Mackenbach 1994). An illness concentration index "C_{ill}" (Wagstaff et al. 1991) provides a summary of the distribution of health across the entire socioeconomic spectrum. The "C_{ill}" ranges from -1 (when only the most disadvantaged person is ill) to $+1$ (when only the least disadvantaged person is ill) and takes a value of zero when all individuals have the same morbidity irrespective of their socioeconomic position.

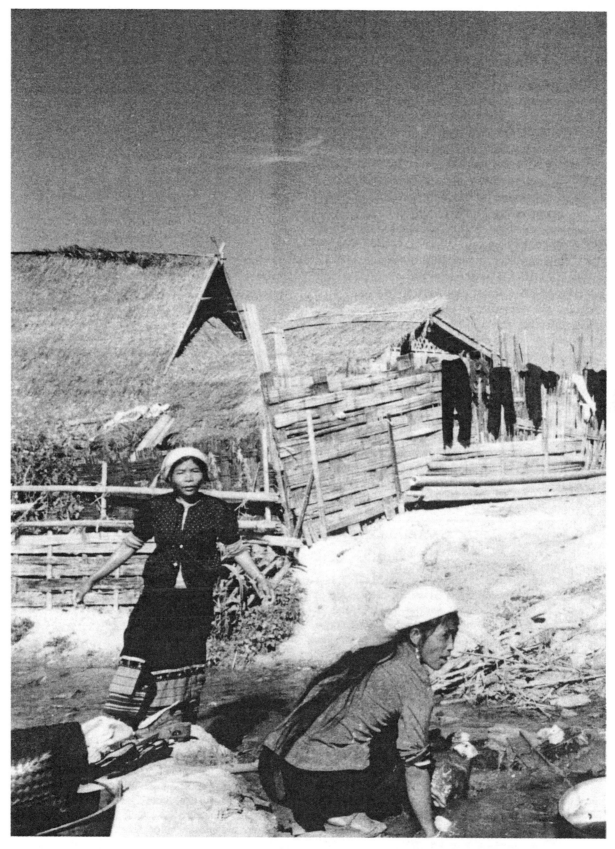

Girls fetching water. "Wa" minority village. Cangyan Yunnan, S.W. China, 1995.
Source: Rhodri Jones/Panos.

Developing an Ecological Model of County Level Health

We also assess the relative importance of different factors associated with interregional inequalities in health through an ecological analysis of 62 counties in China (see Table 5). Although selection of an ecological unit of analysis has many risks and uncertainties (Norcliffe 1982; Jerrett et al. 1998; Wilkinson 1996; Fiscella and Franks 1997), the county is chosen here because it is a relatively autonomous political and geographical unit and of increasing importance in the context of economic reforms based on decentralization (United Nations Development Programme 1997). Within this geographical unit, strong social, cultural and economic ties are likely to exist. Counties vary in population size with an average population of about 400,000.

To explain the variation in life expectancy at birth and infant mortality rate across different counties, we include a set of independent variables, following a model proposed by Evans and Stoddart (1994). In this model, the determinants of health are categorized into two major interrelated groups: socioeconomic environment and biophysical environment (see Box 1). These broad categories, in turn, condition an individual's behavioral and biological responses to external stimuli. Within this broad framework, we have attempted to select variables that might act as proxies for these fundamental social causes (Link and Phelan 1996) such as income inequality (Wilkinson 1996) and environmental quality (Patrick and Wickizer 1995). We have also incorporated variables to control for county differences in lifestyle, health care, and water supply. Data for the illiteracy rate and for the two dependent variables, life expectancy and infant mortality rate, are from the 1990 census. The rest of the independent variables are constructed from the 1993 National Health Services Survey data set.

Results

Gender Inequality in Health

As shown in Figure 1, Chinese women have experienced a consistently greater life expectancy than men over the period 1972 through 1992, a gap that appears to be constant over time. This reflects a gradual and parallel improvement in life expectancy at birth of about 5 years for both sexes. Although these trends appear to be consistent with global patterns and expectations of female advantage over males in life expectancy, if Japan is used as a benchmark female gains in life expectancy in China are not as dramatic. The shortfall in life expectancy compared with that in Japan is larger for females than for males. Relative to the female/male gap in life expectancy in Japan, Chinese females are experiencing lower gains in life expectancy compared to males. Turning to the disaggregation by

---

BOX 1: VARIABLES USED IN THE ECOLOGICAL MODEL

Geographic and Demographic Variables
Geographic characteristics pertain to a community's biological and physical environment. Given the association of remote mountainous areas with serious poverty and ill health (Liu et al. 1998), in regression analyses we include a dichotomous variable (mountain region), which takes the value of 1 if the county is a mountainous region.

As our dependent variables are not standardized by age, we used two control variables—the percentage of total population who are under 15 years of age and the percentage who are 60 years and over.

Socioeconomic Variables
Per capita GDP is included as a measure of the overall economic status of the county. Although most of China's rural counties are predominantly engaged in agriculture, some counties have a sizable industrial base in the economy. The percentage of the population engaged in full-time farming captures this difference. Educational levels are represented by the illiteracy rate. Lifestyle variables include regular tobacco use and alcohol consumption among adults. Income inequality is represented by the widely used Gini coefficient. For each county, we ranked families by per capita income (adjusted for family size) to calculate the county-level Gini coefficients.

Sanitation and Health Care Variables
Sanitation conditions are obviously important for population health, and we have included the proportion of the county population with access to tap water. Health care availability is represented by the number of doctors per 1000 residents, and lack of health care access is assessed by using the percentage of villages with no health post as a proxy (percent of villages without primary health care). Health care coverage for special groups in the population is measured by the proportion of children under age 6 years enrolled in prepaid health care for children programs, which provides routine physical check ups for growth monitoring purposes and immunization services. Actual health resource inputs are measured by per capita total health care expenditures. (See Table 5 for results.)

Figure 1 Life expectancy and infant mortality rate by sex in China, selected years, 1972–92

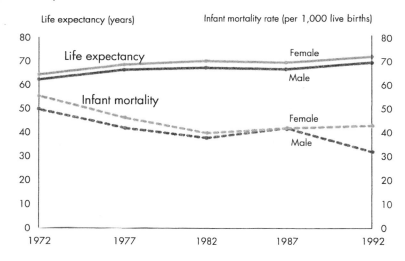

Source: Huang and Liu 1995.

urban versus rural residence, female advantage over males in longevity is much lower in the rural areas in both 1981 and 1991 (Fig. 2). In fact, the urban/rural gap in female advantage is increasing. In other words, rural Chinese women have not enjoyed the same level of advantage in life expectancy over men as their urban counterparts.

Unlike trends in life expectancy, the infant mortality rate (IMR) over the period 1972 through 1992 indicates an initial survival disadvantage for males that diminishes until the mid-1980s and thereafter becomes a survival advantage compared with females (see Fig. 1). Notably, there has been a steady increase in infant mortality among females since its low point in 1982. These figures do not, however, reflect the increasingly documented phenomenon of sex-selective abortion (Mason 1995; Das Gupta and Li 1997). Das Gupta (1998) has estimated that for every 1000 female births in China, between 61 and 94 girl children are "missing" as manifested in a markedly skewed sex ratio at birth. The 1994 National Population Sample Survey revealed a sex ratio of 116.3 males to 100 females, which is substantially higher than the biologically expected ratio at birth of 106 males to 100 females.

In addition to gender inequality in child survival, there are emerging insights from gender comparisons of nonfatal health outcomes. Of particular concern is the remarkably high disability rate among girls in the age group of 0 to 4 years. The female morbidity rate tends to be higher than that of males for all age groups except for children under 10 years of age. In almost all

the regions sampled, especially in rural areas, female children between 0 and 9 years of age arc reported to have lower morbidity than male children.

Consistent with gender distributions reported elsewhere in the world, men are more prone than women to suffer certain causes of ill health such as injury and poisoning, while for other conditions, such as psychosis, women appear to be at greater risk (Fig. 3). In contrast, whereas in most countries men's suicide rates

Figure 2 Female advantage in life expectancy in urban and rural China, 1981 and 1991

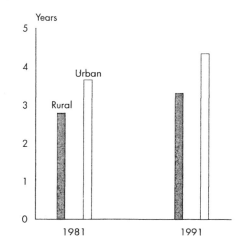

Source: Huang and Liu 1995.

Figure 3 Prevalence of selected health conditions by sex in China, 1993

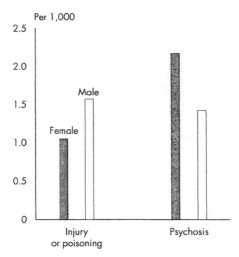

Source: Ministry of Health 1994.

are considerably higher than women's, in China this pattern is reversed. Deaths from suicide among women in 1989 were about 30% higher than among their male counterparts (see Table 2).

Interregional Inequalities in Health

As shown in Table 3, a clear socioeconomic gradient in life expectancy and IMR is present. For example, while big cities with the highest average income enjoy the highest life expectancy of 74.5 years, the poorest counties (rural Cnty 4) have a life expectancy as low as 64.5 years. Similarly, moving from big cities to small cities and rural regions with lower income, we observe a sharp increase in IMR and mortality from infectious diseases.

Table 3 also includes age-standardized morbidity rates. For the prevalence of "disability" there is a similar socioeconomic gradient as found for mortality statistics, while other morbidity indicators such as the "2 week morbidity rate," "chronic diseases," and "health limitations" do not display the same pattern. In fact, people living in big cities seem to report more chronic diseases and physical limitations than do their counterparts in smaller cities and rural regions.

Socioeconomic Inequalities in Health

Table 4 presents age-standardized morbidity rates by income decile (lowest vs. highest decile), simple indices of health inequalities (rate ratio, rate difference, and population attributable risk), and the illness concentration index (C_{ill}) for each of the four health indicators. Because income source and relative purchasing power are very different for urban and rural populations, we rank them separately and only present the inequality statistics for rural population groups. All of the four morbidity measures reflect an unequal socioeconomic distribution, that is, the concentration indices have a negative sign, indicating that lower income groups bear a disproportionate share of the morbidity

Table 2 Suicide rate by sex in selected economies, various years
(per 100,000)

Economy	Year	Total	Male	Female	Rate ratio
Hungary	1990	38.2	61.4	18.8	3.3
Sri Lanka	1986	33.2	46.9	18.9	2.5
USSR	1990	21.1	34.4	9.1	3.8
China	1989	17.1	14.7	19.6	0.8
Japan	1991	16.1	20.6	11.8	1.7
Australia	1988	13.3	21.0	5.6	3.8
Singapore	1990	13.1	14.7	11.5	1.3
Hong Kong	1989	10.5	11.8	9.1	1.3
India	1988	8.1	9.1	6.9	1.3
Korea, Rep. of	1987	7.9	11.5	4.4	2.6
Thailand	1985	5.8	7.1	4.5	1.6
Mexico	1990	2.3	3.9	0.7	5.6

Source: Desjarlais et al. 1994

Table 3 Socioeconomic and health indicators in cities by size and rural counties by income level, in China, 1993

Indicator	Urban[a]			Rural[a]			
	Big-city	Med-city	Sm-city	Cnty 1	Cnty 2	Cnty 3	Cnty 4
GDP per capita (yuan)	5,002	4,070	3,040	2,523	1,305	939	664
Income per capita (yuan)	2,291	1,947	1,158	927	677	561	441
Population in agriculture (percent)	n.a.	n.a.	n.a.	81.0	89.0	91.5	95.2
Rate of illiteracy and semi-illiteracy (percent)	9.6	14.8	14.2	26.4	26.8	28.1	50.7
Life expectancy (years)	74.5	71.3	70.0	71.0	69.0	68.3	64.5
Infant mortality rate (per 1,000 live births)	15.8	17.1	30.1	29.3	34.5	44.2	71.8
Two-week morbidity rate (per 1,000)[b]							
Female	12.6	12.8	9.2	9.1	9.9	9.0	9.7
Male	12.8	12.4	9.9	8.9	10.4	9.9	9.0
Prevalence of chronic disease (per 1,000)[b]							
Female	13.5	13.8	13.2	7.7	7.6	8.8	10.6
Male	13.6	13.3	13.2	7.5	7.9	8.7	11.3
Prevalence of health limitations (per 1,000)[b]	11.1	11.8	8.50	8.1	9.6	10.3	12.1
Prevalence of disability (per 1,000)[b]							
Female	6.4	7.5	8.5	10.6	10.8	11.5	12.5
Male	6.3	7.6	9.5	9.9	10.3	12.3	12.4

n.a. Not applicable.
a. China's 2,400 cities were grouped into seven areas based mainly on per capita income as follows: big city, medium city, and small cities represent the groupings of urban areas; Cnty 1 (richest)–Cnty 4 (poorest) represent the grouping of rural counties.
b. Age standardized: $\Sigma p_i (m_i)/\Sigma p_i (M_i)$, where m_i is the region-specific morbidity rate for age group i; M_i is the population morbidity rate for age group i; and p_i is the number of surveyed people in age group i.
Source: Ministry of Health 1994.

Table 4 Summary statistics of socioeconomic inequalities in health in China, 1993

Indicator[a]	Rate per 1,000		Rate ratio	Rate difference	Population attributable risk (percent)	Illness concentration index
	Bottom income decile	Top income decile				
Two-week morbidity	14.54	11.77	1.24	2.78	8.00	−0.03
Chronic disease	14.89	11.05	1.35	3.84	1.00	−0.05
Health limitations	5.01	2.19	2.29	2.82	25.00	−0.12
Disability	4.59	1.53	3.00	3.06	32.00	−0.18

a. Age-standardized estimates.
Source: Ministry of Health 1994.

burden. The level of socioeconomic inequality is small-est for "2 week morbidity" and greatest for "disability." When the concentration indices of urban and rural pop-ulations are compared, the illness concentration index for the rural population is consistently greater.

Determinants of County Level Health

Table 5 summarizes the regression results of the eco-logical variables associated with variation in life ex-pectancy and infant mortality. The first regression model accounts for approximately 35% of the variance in life expectancy in 1990. Only two variables, GDP per capita and doctors per 1000, display a significant positive relationship with life expectancy. In contrast, the IMR model accounts for a much higher percentage of the variance in IMR. Four variables exert a statisti-cally significant effect on IMR. Although an increase in per capita GDP is negatively correlated with IMR, the coefficient is statistically insignificant. In contrast, increasing income inequality is significantly associated

with an increase in IMR. In addition to income in-equality, higher levels of illiteracy are strongly related to higher IMR.

One significant difference between the life ex-pectancy and IMR models occurs with lifestyle and health care variables. Except for the number of doctors per 1000 residents, these variables have no significant relation to life expectancy, but are significantly associ-ated with IMR. A 10% increase in the number of smok-ers as a percentage of the adult population is associ-ated with an increase of 13 infant deaths per 1000 live births. Importantly, an increase in the percentage of children receiving health care under the prepayment program is associated with a decrease in IMR.

Discussion

Measurement and Methodological Issues

As has been noted elsewhere in this volume (see chap-ter 5) and is illustrated, in this chapter, the magnitude of the inequalities in health depends to a large extent

Table 5 Coefficients from regression analysis of life expectancy and infant mortality rate by county in China, 1993

Explanatory variable	Life expectancy[a]	Infant mortality rate[a]
Intercept	0.0001	0.0001
Mountainous region	–0.2163	0.0055
Percentage of population in agriculture	–0.0729	0.0967
GDP per capita	0.4160**	–0.1143
Gini coefficient	–0.0776	0.3867**
Percentage of population age 15 and under	0.2299	0.0624
Percentage of population age 60 and over	0.1154	–0.0744
Illiteracy rate	–0.1633	0.3495**
Percentage of villages without primary health care	0.0714	0.1336
Water supply (access to tap water)	0.1075	–0.1449
Medical expenditure per capita	–0.1284	0.1113
Doctors per 1,000	0.2708*	–0.0029
Enrollment in prepaid child health program	0.1279	–0.3819**
Regular tobacco use	–0.0864	0.2741*
Regular alcohol consumption	–0.0797	–0.0833
Number of observations	62	62
F probability	0.0010	0.0001
Adjusted R^2	0.3473	0.5202

* Significant at 0.5 percent.
** Significant at 0.1 percent.
Note: Coefficients show the relationship between the explanatory variable and life expectancy.
a. Standardized estimate.
Source: Authors' calculations based on data from Ministry of Health 1994.

on the type of morbidity measure used. Urban residents' higher propensity to report illness than rural residents in China (Ministry of Health 1994), for example, suggests caution in interpretation of the interregional inequalities in morbidity as they may reflect differences in perceptions of health, access to health care, or populations at different stages of epidemiological transition rather than inequalities in health status (Liu et al. 1998). International comparisons are similarly sensitive to outcome measures. Depending on the index used, China's health inequality indices compare either favorably or unfavorably with those reported by some countries that belong to the Organization for Economic Co-operation and Development (van Doorslaer and Wagstaff 1997).

Likewise caution is recommended when interpreting the results of the regression models of intercounty variation in life expectancy and infant mortality. Employing the same set of independent variables, the models selected different variables as significant correlates of the two health outcome measures. We should be careful when generalizing our research results on determinants of "health inequality" because the relative impact of the economic versus health care factors vary depending upon the health outcome used. Life expectancy at birth reflects the survival probabilities of the whole population, while IMR, even when used as a "social barometer," measures the survival probability of a single age group, namely, infants. As implied by our results, health care may not play a significant role in stratifying the general health of the population as reflected in the life expectancy outcomes. Access to care may be a key stratifier, however, of the survival of certain vulnerable population groups, such as infants.

Policy Implications

This initial exploration of China's health experience with economic reform has shed light on the more global question of whether economic reform improves health status for all (Hsiao and Liu 1996). The evidence on growing gender and geographic stratifications in health in the context of reforms suggests quite clearly that, although health continues to improve in China, it has not improved for all. The prohibitive costs of health care in rural areas threaten further disparities between rural and urban populations.

A national survey showed that the percentage of untreated patients in poor counties is higher than in rich counties. In-depth case studies of three poor rural counties revealed the fact that 41% of sick peasants did not seek medical treatment because of financial difficulties. As policy studies indicate that it is price, not a short-age of services, that prevents rural poor from obtaining adequate health care, rural cooperative health care in the form of community health funds and better drug management will be increasingly important priorities (Gu 1999). In this regard, the Government's next 5 year plan, which deals with regional inequalities, is timely and might benefit from including a focus on health in addition to other dimensions of socioeconomic status such as education.

Gender Inequality in Health

With respect to gender inequality, our findings reveal the expected female survival advantage in life expectancy over males. The data also indicate modest improvements in both women's and men's life expectancies since the onset of economic reforms. These improvements, however, are less than expected when compared with levels of health in countries at a similar stage of economic development. According to World Bank statistics (1994), the female advantage in life expectancy in middle-income countries is about 6 years compared with only 3 years in China. Although the female advantage over males in terms of life expectancy appears to be increasing slowly, this reflects a deceleration of improvements in male longevity rather than a "catching up" of female survival relative to international norms. Of further concern, however, is the slower rate of improvement in longevity in rural areas such that there is a growing gap between urban and rural women's advantage in life expectancy.

In contrast to trends in life expectancy, the overall improvement in IMR is more pronounced among boys than girls: In other words, male IMR has moved from an inferior to a superior position relative to girls during the course of economic reforms. Although these data may be subject to sex biases in reporting, data quality has continuously improved since the late 1980s, when China established monitoring sites for surveillance of maternal and child health. The regression analysis for 62 counties suggests that the correlates of lower IMR are greater income equality, higher literacy, and better access to a prepaid health care program for children. Although further analysis is necessary to understand whether these correlates are sex specific, we might hypothesize that boy children would be more likely to benefit from free health care than their female counterparts. Insofar as reforms have exacerbated income inequality, it might also be argued that there is a greater negative impact on girls' lives relative to boys'.

This deterioration in female IMR is highly compatible with the evidence of persistent, if not worsening, social discrimination against females and the phenomenon of "missing girls" (Das Gupta 1998). Son preference is attributed to the economic needs for strong men to work in the fields and for old age support (Xie 1997) as well as the patrilineal imperative to continue the family line. The compromised health status of the Chinese female is further revealed by evidence of unusually high disability rates among girl children as well as by the gender reversal in suicide rates. It is quite likely that the economic upheaval associated with reform in combination with the "one child per family" policy (introduced in the late 1970s) has accentuated the problem of missing girls and, more generally, the ill health sequelae of female disadvantage (Ren 1995).

Interregional Inequalities in Health

With respect to interregional inequalities in health, our findings concur with observations elsewhere of better health in urban than rural areas (Shen et al. 1996). Results also indicate strong socioeconomic gradients from rural poor to urban rich across a variety of health outcomes. Although the direct relationship of these inequalities to economic reforms cannot be ascertained, it appears that geographic areas closer to the engines of economic reform enjoy better health outcomes. This argument is supported by the county level analysis of determinants of life expectancy and IMR (see Table 5). Regression findings indicate higher county GDP, income equality, number of doctors, literacy, and prepaid health programs as important correlates of better health. Economic reforms have undoubtedly accentuated the relative concentration of economic activity, social services, and educated population and therefore contributed to the further stratification of health opportunity between urban areas and the rural periphery.

Monitoring Health Inequalities

Our findings, although tentative, indicate that monitoring gender differentials in health particularly among infants and children is a necessary first step to understanding and responding to the problems of female suicide and missing girls. Similarly, redressing the vast regional inequalities depends on the capacity to monitor health and health inequalities at regular intervals. Although China's first National Health Services Survey in 1993 is a step in the right direction, this study indicates that more accurate information on neonatal and postneonatal survival and mental health would help to illuminate gender inequalities. More generally, if these surveys are to be the basis for monitoring inequalities in health, they must reflect equity priorities or goals

and employ reliable indicators of health inequalities. In this regard, this chapter may help to initiate this process by presenting for the first time measures of health inequality including shortfall equality and concentration indices for use as benchmarks and to evaluate change over time.

Beyond benchmarks, however, this study offers some initial avenues to explore for narrowing gaps in health outcomes between regions or counties and gender. First, the correlates of higher county level infant mortality, such as illiteracy, lack of access to health services, and parental smoking, are not new. The challenge is to develop interventions that will reach these populations and be truly equity enhancing. Perhaps more formidable is the issue of cultural gender bias as expressed by missing girls and anomalous rates of suicide among women. Changing the status of women in society and raising the value of girls to their parents relative to boys are long-term undertakings. Insofar as these inequitable trends appear to be accentuated by reforms, at the macro level, at least, a clearer articulation of these and other equity goals will provide the necessary legitimacy for what will undoubtedly be a long journey toward greater health equity in China.

References

Anand S., Sen A. 1995. *Gender Inequality in Human Development: Theories and Measurement*. New York: United Nations Development Program.

Das Gupta M. 1998. "Missing Girls" in China, South Korea and India: Causes and Policy Implications. Working paper series No. 98-03, Harvard Center for Population and Development Studies.

Das Gupta M., Li S. 1997. Gender Bias and the Marriage Squeeze in China, South Korea and India 1920–1990: The Effects of War, Famine and Fertility Decline. Working Paper Series No. 97-05, Harvard University Center for Population and Development Studies.

Desjarlais R., Eisenberg L., Good B., Kleinman A. 1995. *World Mental Health: Problems and Priorities in the Low-Income Countries*. New York: Oxford University Press.

Evans R.G., Stoddart G.L. 1994. Producing health, consuming health care. In: Evans R.G., et al. (eds), *Why Are Some People Healthy and Others Not?* New York: Aldine de Gruyter.

Fiscella K., Franks P. 1997. Poverty or income inequality as predictor of mortality: longitudinal cohort study. *British Medical Journal* 314:1724–1727.

Gu X. 1996. *Financing of Health Services in Poor Rural China*. Shanghai: Baija Press.

Hartland-Thunberg P. 1989. *A Decade of China's Economic Reform: Challenges for the Future*. Washington, DC: Center for Strategic and International Studies.

Hsiao W.C., Liu Y.L. 1996. Economic reform and health—lessons from China. *New England Journal of Medicine* 335(6):430–432.

Huang Y., Liu Y. 1995. *Mortality Data of the Chinese Population*. Beijing, PRC: The Chinese Population Press.

Hull T.H. 1990. Recent trends in sex ratios at birth in China. *Population and Development Review* 16:63.

Jerrett M., Eyles J., Cole D. 1998. Socioeconomic and environmental covariates of premature mortality in Ontario. *Social Science and Medicine* 47(1):33–49.

Johansson S., Nygren O. 1991. The missing girls of China: a new demographic account. *Population and Development Review* 17:35.

Kunst A.E., Mackenbach J.P. 1994. The size of mortality differences associated with educational level in nine industrialized countries *American Journal of Public Health* 84(6)932–937.

Link B.G., Phelan J.C. 1996. Editorial. Understanding sociodemographic differences in health: the role of fundamental social causes. *American Journal of Public Health.* 86(4):471–172.

Liu Y., Hu S.L., Wei F., Hsiao W.C. 1996. Is community financing necessary and feasible for rural China? *Health Policy* 38(3):155–171.

Liu Y., Rao K., Fei J. 1998. Economic transition and health transition: comparing China and Russia. *Health Policy* 44(2):103–122.

Mason K. 1995. *Is the Situation of Women in Asia Improving or Deteriorating?* Asia-Pacific Research Report No. 6. Honolulu: East-West Center Program on Population.

Ministry of Health. 1988. *Health Statistics in China.* Beijing: Ministry of Health.

Ministry of Health. 1994. *Research on National Health Services—An Analysis Report of the Research on National Health Services—An Analysis Report of the National Health Services Survey in 1993.* Beijing: Ministry of Health.

Ministry of Health. 1998. *China's Health Statistics Yearbook of 1997.* Beijing: Ministry of Health.

Newell K.W. 1975. *Health by the People.* Geneva: World Health Organization.

Norcliffe G.B. 1982. *Inferential Statistics for Geographers: An Introduction.* London: Hutchinson.

Patrick D.L., Wickizer T.M. 1995. Community and health. In: Amick B., Levine S., Tarlov A., Walsh D. (eds), *Society and Health,* pp 46–92. New York: Oxford University Press.

Ren X. 1995. Sex differences in infant and child mortality in three provinces in China. *Social Science and Medicine* 40(9):1259–1269.

Sen A., 1990. More than 100 million women are missing. *New York Review of Books* 37(20):61–66.

Shen T., Habicht J.-P., Chang Y. 1996. Effect of economic reforms on child growth in urban and rural areas of China. *New England Journal of Medicine* 335:400–406.

Sidel V.W. 1972. The barefoot doctors of the People's Republic of China. *New England Journal of Medicine* 286:1292–1299.

Sidel R., Sidel V.W. 1982. *The Health of China: Current Conflicts in Medical and Human Services for One Billion People.* Boston: Beacon Press.

Tseng W., Burton D., Mihaljek D., Khor H.E., Eochhar K. 1994. *Economic Reform in China: A New Phase.* Washington, DC: International Monetary Fund.

United Nations Development Programme (UNDP). 1997. *China: Human Development Report.* Beijing: UNDP.

UNDP. 1999. *Human Development Report 1999.* New York: UNDP.

van Doorslaer E., Wagstaff A. 1997. Income-related inequalities in health: some international comparisons. *Journal of Health Economics* 16:93–112.

Wagstaff A., Paci P., van Doorslaer E. 1991. On the measurement of inequalities in health. *Social Science and Medicine* 33.545–557.

Wang F. 1996. *Summary of the Current Condition of Chinese Women and Children.* Beijing: Ministry of Health.

Wilkinson R.G. 1992a. Income distribution and life expectancy. *British Medical Journal* 304:165–168.

Wilkinson R.G. 1996. *Unhealthy Societies—The Afflictions of Inequality.* London; New York: Routledge.

World Bank. 1992. *China—Strategies for Reducing Poverty in the 1990s.* Washington, DC: World Bank.

World Bank. 1994. *Social Indicators of Development.* Baltimore: Johns Hopkins University Press.

World Bank. 1996. *World Development Report 1996: From Plan to Market.* New York: Oxford University Press.

World Bank. 1997a. *China 2020—Disparities in China, Sharing Rising Incomes.* Washington, DC: World Bank.

World Bank. 1997b. *China: Issues and Options in Health Financing.* Washington, DC: World Bank.

World Health Organization and UNICEF. 1975. *Meeting Basic Health Needs in Developing Countries: Alternative Approaches.* Geneva: World Health Organization.

World Health Organization 1999. *World Health Report 1999.* Geneva: World Health Organization.

Xie Z. 1997. Demand of Childbearing of Chinese Farmers and its Changes in Zhejiang Province, China. Paper presented at the workshop on Son Preference in China, South Korea and India, Harvard University, Cambridge, MA.

Xing Hua She. 1999. *People's Daily.* June 24, 1999.

Ye X.F., Huang D.Y., Hinman A.R., Parker R.L. (eds). 1982. Health services in Shanghai County: introduction to Shanghai County. *American Journal of Public Health* 72:13–18.

Zeng Y., Tu P., Gu B.C., Xu Y. 1993. Causes and implication of the increases in China's reported sex ratio at birth. *Population and Development Review* 19:283.

CHAPTER 8

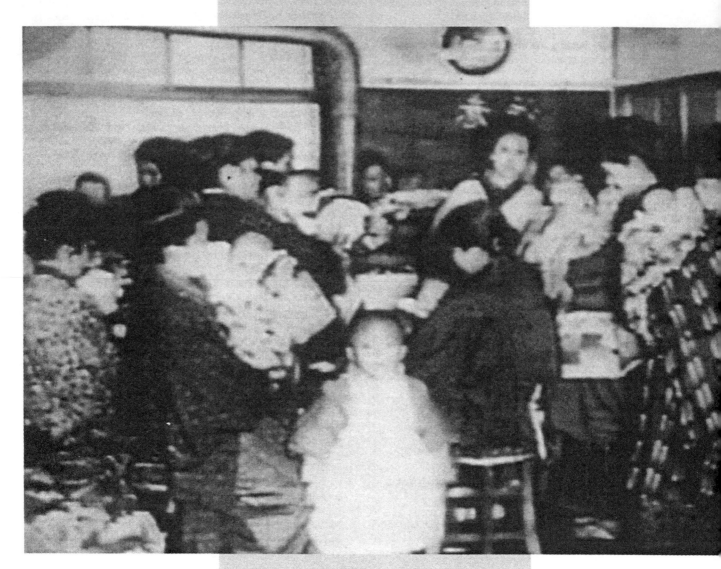

A still frame from a documentary film of a health education campaign in Japan, circa 1920.
Source: Video Pack Japan.

Japan: Historical and Current Dimensions of Health and Health Equity

TOSHIHIKO HASEGAWA

If I summarize the principle for the education of women, it is to train women for ryosai kenbo *[good wives and wise mothers]. . . . [T]he foundation of our national strength and prosperity depends on education. The foundation of education depends on women's education. The stability of the nation depends on women's education.*

—Mori Arinori circa 1900 (Matsui 1996)

Japan has attracted considerable attention as the country with one of the highest life expectancies and the lowest infant mortality rates in the world. That these dramatic health outcomes were achieved over a relatively short period of time makes them all the more extraordinary (see Table 1 and Fig. 1). Although the achievements in health over the last century have been lauded, the main factors explaining the impressive health progress in Japan have not been fully explained (Jannetta 1987; Johansson 1987; Marmot and Davey Smith 1989). Furthermore, the focus on impressive gains in average health indicators may have obscured the issue of inequalities in health within Japan. This chapter has two main objectives: first, to examine the long-term historical antecedents of the unparalleled improvements in the population's health as a whole and, second, to analyze patterns of past, current, and future health inequalities in Japanese society.

Historical Analysis: Social and Health Progress in the Twentieth Century

It is in the context of the Japanese cultural attitude of *yokonarabi*, or "same to the next person," that inequalities and inequities in health must be assessed and understood. This outcome-oriented approach contrasts with the equality-of-opportunity approach that characterizes American egalitarianism (Fukatsu and Nagata 1998). Although it is not clear how this ethic evolved in Japan, there is evidence of the existence of such an attitude before the Edo and Tokugawa eras (1603–1867). Some scholars have proposed that an outcome-oriented egalitarian ethos was deeply embedded in an agrarian rice paddy–based society (Nakane 1967). This ethic also underpinned the Meiji period in which the foundations for the modern Japanese state were laid—a long-term vision that emphasized human development and well being through hygiene campaigns, provision of universal education, and support of the patriarchal family (Miyaji and Lock 1994). In 1946, the New Constitution of Japan enshrined these principles in Article 25, Clause 2, stating that "in all spheres of life, the state shall use its endeavors for the promotion and extension of social welfare and security and of public health." Despite rapid urbanization and economic transformation in the post–World War II period,

Japan

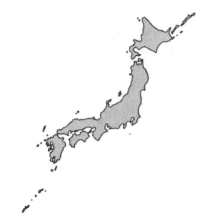

Total population (millions), 1997	126.0
Human development index, 1999	0.924
Human development index rank, 1999	4
Infant mortality rate (per 1,000 live births), 1997	4
Real GDP per capita (PPP$), 1997	24,070
Public spending on health as percentage of GDP, 1995	5.6

Source: UNDP 1999. [Human Development Report]

this cultural ethos remains prevalent in Japan today. More recently, however, the egalitarian image of Japan has been challenged by the emergence of a number of subcultures defined by gender, occupation, and education that are stratified according to economic privilege and social prestige (Sugimoto 1997).

This chapter considers the broader social context, including education and income inequality and its relationship to progress in health, in four distinct historical periods over the last century: pre-1920, 1920–1940, 1950–1970, and 1970–2000 (Murayama et al. 2000). In the first two decades of the twentieth century, Japan's infant mortality rate (IMR) hovered around 150 per 1000, peaking during the 1918–1919 flu epidemic

Table 1 Infant mortality rate in selected OECD countries, 1920 and 1995
(per 1,000 live births)

Country	1920	1995
Japan	166	4
United States	107	8
England and Wales	97	6
Sweden	65	4

Source: Mitchell 1998a, 1998b, 1998c.

at about 180 per 1000 (Fig. 2). Since 1920, Japan has experienced the most rapid decline in IMR among countries that belong to the Organization for Economic Cooperation and Development (OECD), with the fastest decreases occurring between 1945 and 1970 (see Fig. 2). In 1920, infant mortality in Japan was the highest in OECD countries, but by 1995 it had assumed the lowest ranking among this group of countries (see Table 1). At the close of the twentieth century (1995), the Japanese infant mortality rate was 4.26 per 1000.

1890–1920

Although marked by concerns about data quality, the period of 1890–1920 may be characterized by persistently high rates of infant mortality, which reached a peak around 1920 at the time of the influenza pandemic (see Fig. 2). It has been postulated that these average figures hide divergent trends. In urban areas affected by heavy industrialization, poor labor safety standards, and unsanitary living conditions, there were significant increases in infant mortality, while in rural agricultural areas there was modest improvement. This period marks the only time during the twentieth century when infant mortality in rural areas was lower than that in urban areas.

Until the 1870s, primary school attendance rates were low and reflected significant gender bias, with a female to male ratio of 1:4. In the mid-1870s, the first school to train women teachers was established. In 1879, an education order advocating decentralized school policy encouraged the education of girls based on the premise that *ryosai kenbo*, "a good wife and wise mother," was a prerequisite for developing "a rich nation and making strong soldiers" (Ministry of Education 1972; National Institute of Education 1974). In the late 1890s and early 1900s a series of policies led to compulsory, free primary education and increased training and employment of female teachers. As rates of primary school attendance approached 100% around 1900, the gender gap diminished, and the female to male ratio became 1:1 where it has remained ever since (Fig. 3). One could argue that the benefits to health conferred on a family through educated mothers were universally available to the Japanese population by the time this first generation of educated girls began to bear children.

1920–1940

The second historical period reviewed (1920–1940) is characterized by a steady decline in the high IMR, a health improvement that is best understood in the larger social context (see Fig. 2). In the wake of World

Figure 1 Trends in life expectancy at birth in selected countries, 1963–95

Female

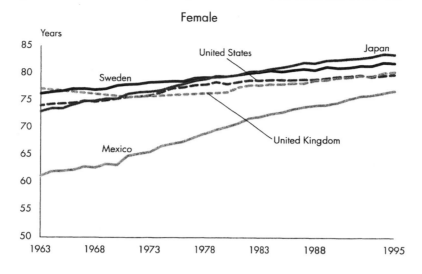

Male

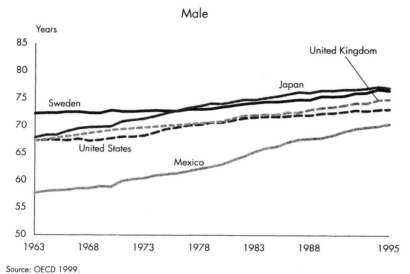

Source: OECD 1999.

Figure 2 Trends in the infant mortality rate in selected OECD countries, 1900–96

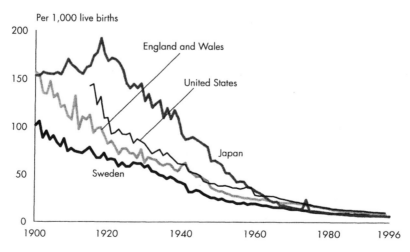

Source: OECD 1999.

Figure 3 Trends in school attendance rate by sex in Japan, 1880–1997

Primary school, 1880–1910

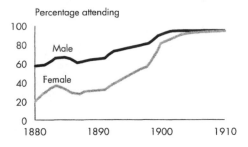

Junior high school, 1910–46

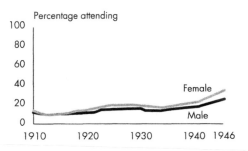

High school, 1951–80

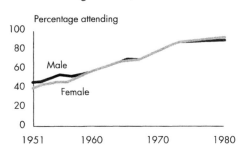

University and junior college, 1964–97

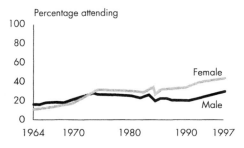

Source: Ministry of Education 1880–97.

War I and the early days of a capitalist system marked by increasing income disparity, food shortages, and "rice riots," a new social era known as "Taisyo Democracy" emerged. During this period feminist, socialist, and labor movements flourished and yielded notable

accomplishments, not the least of which was universal suffrage. Feminists such as Raicyo Hiratsuka, and Kikue Yamakawa brought to the fore issues of chastity, abortion, and the abolition of licensed prostitution. A birth control movement was also initiated, drawing on Margaret Sanger's 1922 visit to Japan and on a broad-based coalition of Malthusians and neo-Malthusians, eugenicists, and women's rights activists (Ishihara 1999).

There was a surge of activity aimed at making medical care more accessible to the poor, and in 1926 Japan established a social insurance system (Shigeki 1986). In the 1920s medical movements for the poor included Jippi Shinryojyo (cost-price clinic activities), Musan Shinryojyo (Proletariat clinic movement), and Syakai-Igaku Kenkyukai (the Society for the Study of Social Medicine). In response to the rice riots of 1918, the government established a National Institute of Nutrition in 1920 (Koseisyo Gojyunenshi Hensyu Iinkai 1988), and municipalities adopted policies aimed at improving nutrition and opened maternal and child health centers in the 1920s (Mouri 1972). From 1900 to the 1930s, the number of midwives trained in modern medicine increased steadily (Fujime 1998; Kondo 1998). In 1933, Aiiku Kai, founded to promote maternal and child health, implemented basic surveys on infant mortality to inform policy and implemented Aiiku-son village demonstration projects to improve infant health (Mouri 1972).

In addition to these important contextual changes favoring health, there is also the likelihood that previous investments in universal access to primary education began to yield their health dividends. The percentage of babies whose mothers were exposed to primary education increased steadily toward 100% before World War II with a concomitant decline in infant mortality. The fact that mothers' exposure to primary school increased dramatically during this period may in itself be an important factor explaining the success and uptake of the progressive social movements. This unique confluence of a cohort of educated women at a time of increased social welfare activism and policy making laid a firm foundation for the rapid advances in health status that occurred across the population.

It is interesting to note, however, that not all trends were necessarily pro-health. Income inequality was very high, equivalent to that in present-day Latin America, and showed an upward tendency until World War II.

1950–1970

Despite the dramatic rate of improvement in health, life expectancy in Japan in the 1960s was still one of the lowest among OECD nations. After World War II, the third period reviewed (1950–1970) is characterized by a steep and steady decline in infant mortality (see Fig. 2). During this time the Ministry of Health and Welfare had an active policy of supporting maternal and child health activities through a health center network that specialized in prevention and succeeded in controlling infectious disease through public health activities. After the constitutional mandate, equality was made a primary objective of the health system, and by 1961 Japan achieved universal and compulsory health insurance.

The gender roles imposed by the state ("good wives and wise mothers") in the Meiji period intensified in post-war Japan when rapid economic development became the major goal of the nation (Miyaji and Lock 1994). Some have argued that this widespread attitude toward women has led to their subordination and hindered their professional development. Critics of the burdens placed on women have noted that the post-war Japanese society has re-created women as education-oriented mothers, welfare agents, and supplementary workers (Matsui 1996). In fact, given the importance of women's social position for health improvement, some researchers have noted that the low IMR in Japan is somewhat at odds with women's subordinate position in society. This paradox may not be so surprising, however, given the *ryosai kenbo* policy in which the social status of Japanese women may be relatively low, but the status of motherhood is high.

Following the war, the high school advancement rates increased dramatically, and female high school attendance surpassed that of males (from less than 50% for boys and 40% for girls to about 95% for girls and 93% for boys by the late 1970s; see Fig. 3). The universality of high school education reflects the momentum from previous investments in primary education as well as the enactment of the Fundamental Law of Education passed in 1947, making primary and junior high school mandatory. This nationwide law led to dramatic declines in the differentials between prefectures in educational attainment beyond primary school. Even high school and junior college attendance rates surpassed those of males in this period (Fig. 3). However, female university attendance was lower than male, perhaps reflecting the persistence of *ryosai kenbo* ideology and the fact that many women ended their education after junior college in order to marry.

In the post-war period, the Japanese economy went through an initial period of restructuring, landowner reform orchestrated by the U.S. army occupying Japan, infrastructure repair, and democratization. Some of these reforms, along with a surplus of labor, led to economic expansion and a general improvement in living conditions. The immediate post-war era saw very low levels of income inequality as the restructuring period appears to have had an equalizing effect (a measure of income iequality, the Gini coefficient, dropped to 0.3 immediately after the war) (Minami 1994, 1996). This situation was short lived, however, as the rapid disappear-ance of surplus labor and increasing wages of skilled workers led to more unequal income distribution.

1970–2000

In the fourth period (1970–2000), the rate of decrease in the IMR slowed considerably, perhaps reflecting the fact that physiological limits of child survival were being approached (see Fig. 2). By the 1980s, however, in the space of two decades, male and female longevity in Japan became one of the highest in the world. After 1960, increases in life expectancy in Japan were mainly due to survival improvements at older ages, most notably with a major decline in stroke mortality. Among females, life expectancy has remained the highest globally since 1980 and has become the world's gold standard for calculating premature mortality.

This period represents the beginning of the expansion of the Japanese economy as GDP per capita increased at near exponential rates through the late 1980s. The economy was driven largely by growth in the technology and service sectors, leading to an increased number of skilled laborers and higher wages. The differentiation between skilled and unskilled labor resulted in increased income inequality, which has persisted through the current recession. Over the last 30 years, income inequality levels in Japan have been very similar to those in the United States—much higher than in Canada although lower than in Brazil, Thailand, or Sri Lanka. In a cross-country analysis of the Gini coefficient among countries that have comparable data, Japan sits in a lower group, but certainly not the lowest (see Fig. 4).

Interprefectural Trends in Inequality in Health

In an attempt to understand whether the gains in population health have been accompanied by improvement in health distribution, I begin with a geographic analysis. The distribution of health may be assessed using a subnational geographic unit. The prefecture, as an administrative area, proved to be a useful and valid unit of analysis in Japan for several reasons. First, the prefecture is the unit that has direct administrative power in the economic, education, and health sectors. Second, the prefecture has specific jurisdiction over health centers, the locus of preventive health care ac-

Figure 4 Trends in income inequality in selected countries, 1960–92

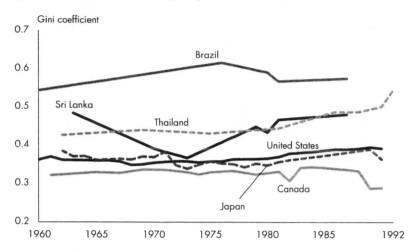

Note: The Gini coefficient is a measure of the degree of inequality. The higher the Gini coefficient the greater the inequality.

Source: Deininger and Squire 1996.

tivity. Finally, the boundaries between prefectures have not changed since the Meiji Restoration, enabling long-term analysis.

The prefectural maps from 1930, 1960, and 1990 reflect the equitable geographic distribution of the dramatic improvement in IMR over the century (see Fig. 5). In 1930, there was an absolute rate difference of 100 infant deaths per 1000 between the best and the worst prefectures. This difference declined to less than 30 per 1000 in 1960 and to less than 3 per 1000 in 1990, a disparity between areas comparable with that in the United Kingdom (Stationery Office 1997). The remarkable improvements in both health and its distribution across prefectures in the last half century are illustrated in Figure 6. At low levels of life expectancy before World War II, there was high inequality in average life expectancy between prefectures (a Gini coefficient of greater than 0.3). After World War II, as life expectancy has steadily improved, interprefectural disparity has dropped to extremely low levels (a Gini coefficient of less than 0.05).

To extend the historical analysis, prefecture-level data from 1930 onward were used to model the correlates of health status at 10 year intervals (see Tables 2 and 3). The regression analysis in Table 2 uses prefectural data on educational level, GPP (gross prefectural product) per capita ("economy"), and the number of midwives and medical doctors to test the explanatory value of these variables in predicting IMRs in prefectures. Income inequality was not included in this model as values for the Gini coefficient do not extend back to 1930,

the first decade included in this IMR analysis. Higher prefectural wealth is associated with lower infant mortality in 1940, 1960, and 1970, whereas in 1930, 1950, 1980, and 1990 there does not appear to be an association. In 1950 and 1980, higher levels of education were correlated with lower IMR. Neither the number of midwives nor medical doctors was correlated with IMR at these seven points in time. Thus, in this model, the "health sector" factors have less association with the IMR in a prefecture than broader social factors such as education and GPP per capita.

A similar prefectural analysis was carried out using a measure of adult health—life expectancy at age 40 years (see Table 3). Data for these models could be gathered only for the period 1965 through 1990 at 5 year intervals. In addition to the economic, health resources, and education variables used previously, several others were added, including economic inequality (prefectural Gini), medical doctors per capita, access to water, television access, and average temperature. Among men, the more prosperous the prefecture in which they lived, the greater the adult life expectancy in 1970 and 1980. In contrast, greater income inequality within prefectures was associated with lower life expectancies in 1970, 1985, and 1990. Television access was associated with better adult male life expectancy in 1965 and 1975, and higher air temperature was associated with better adult male life expectancy in 1965 and 1970. For women, greater income inequality was associated with lower life expectancy at age 40 years in 1965, but not in other years. Of note,

Figure 5 Infant mortality rate by prefecture in Japan, 1930, 1960, and 1990

Per 1,000 live births

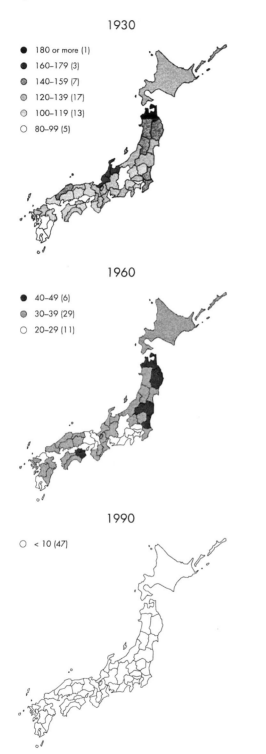

1930

- ● 180 or more (1)
- ● 160–179 (3)
- ◉ 140–159 (7)
- ◉ 120–139 (17)
- ○ 100–119 (13)
- ○ 80–99 (5)

1960

- ● 40–49 (6)
- ◉ 30–39 (29)
- ○ 20–29 (11)

1990

- ○ < 10 (47)

Note: The numbers in parentheses refer to the number of prefectures with the corresponding infant mortality rate. The increase in the number of prefectures between 1960 and 1990 reflects changes in boundaries

Source: Ministry of Health and Welfare, Japan.

education is not associated with adult life expectancy for men in any of the years studied, while for women, education is positively associated with adult longevity in all years except 1965. The proportion of the prefecture residents with access to television also appears to be very strongly correlated with women's longevity in all years except 1965, whereas for men this is true only in the earlier years.

The number of doctors and midwives does not appear to be correlated with life expectancy at age 40 years for men or women in any of the years measured. Until the 1970s, stroke was the main cause of death among adults in Japan. Given the association between colder climates and cerebrovascular disease, I hypothesize that living conditions in colder areas may have been correlated with high mortality due to strokes (Igarashi and Murao 1978). Until the 1970s construction of Japanese homes was quite poor, such that in the winter people were liable to suffer sudden changes of temperature, especially in northern districts (Tohoku and Hokkaido districts). Thus, there is a strong inverse relationship between temperature and death rates before the 1970s. Living conditions were improved over the course of the 1970s, however, with better insulated homes and heating, perhaps explaining the disappearance of the association between temperature and mortality.

Thus, the regression results present fairly different scenarios for adult men and women. For males, economic well being (both absolute and in terms of income inequality) is associated with greater adult life expectancy in 1970 and 1980. For women, however, the variables of access to television and access to education appear to have far greater effect on variation in longevity.

Occupational Distribution of Mortality in Japan

In addition to a geographic analysis of health distribution, this study also considered the distribution of health outcomes across occupational groups. The analysis of prefectural disparities in health shows evidence of precipitous declines in the health gap for both IMR and longevity. To fully explore the pattern of health inequalities in Japan, however, an occupational analysis was undertaken. A significant literature on the nature of the Japanese workplace exists, although research into specific occupational gradients in health is minimal. A comparative study in 1980 (Kagamimori et al. 1988) found that there were steeper gradients in standardized mortality ratios between occupations in Japan than in Great Britain. The study also documented that, as has

Figure 6 Trends in life expectancy at birth and in inequality of life expectancy across prefectures in Japan, 1884–1995

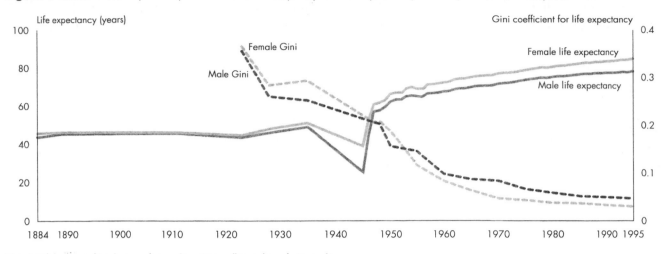

Note: A Gini coefficient of 0 indicates perfect equality, a Gini coefficient of 1 perfect inequality.
Source: Ministry of Health and Welfare, Japan.

been found in other countries, the all-cause occupational mortality rate in Japan was negatively associated with occupational grade, that is, lower occupational grades in Japan such as service and blue collar workers had higher mortality rates. There is also a growing body of literature on psychosocial job stress and its adverse effects on health in Japan that emphasizes, among other things, a greater focus on job stress among women (Kawakami and Haratani 1999). Evidence of occupational stratification complicates the picture of Japan as an egalitarian society.

This section examines a few findings from a larger analysis of occupational gradients in mortality (Hasegawa and Miyao 1998). The occupational analysis is undertaken based on *Jinkou Doutai Touke* (Vital Statistics of Japan), which cover the whole population. From the period 1960 through 1990 there appear to be significant differences in the age-standardized mortality profiles of different occupational groups for men. Commensurate with the overall decline in mortality levels, there is a similar decline for all male occupational groups (see Fig. 7). Closer inspection of the male occupational trends reveals that the declines were not as steep for certain groups. The gap in mortality between the managerial, professional/technical, clerical, and sales workers lessened considerably over the 25 year period examined. Service workers and agriculture, fishery, and forestry workers have, how-

Table 2 Partial correlation coefficients from a stepwise regression analysis of the infant mortality rate in prefectures in Japan, selected years, 1930–90

Explanatory variable	1940	1950	1960	1970	1980
Education level		−0.462**			−0.448**
Economy	−0.406**		−0.647***	−0.745***	
Number of midwives					
Number of doctors					
Adjusted R²	0.146	0.195	0.405	0.545	0.183

Note: Coefficients show the relationship between the explanatory variable and life expectancy. No results are shown for 1930 or 1990, as none of the variables was significant.
** Significant at the 1 percent level.
*** Significant at the 0.1 percent level.
Source: Author's calculations.

Table 3 Partial correlation coefficients from a stepwise regression analysis of life expectancy at age 40, by sex, in prefectures in Japan, selected years, 1965–90

Dependent variable	Explanatory variable	1965	1970	1975	1980	1985	1990
Male life expectancy at age 40	GDP per capita		0.497***		0.390**		
	Number of doctors and midwives						
	Education level						
	Income inequality		−0.240*			−0.366*	−0.344*
	Diffusion rate of televisions[a]	0.277*		0.298*			
	Average temperature	0.562***	0.289**				
	Adjusted R^2	0.335	0.422	0.068	0.133	0.114	0.098
Female life expectancy at age 40	GDP per capita						
	Number of doctors and midwives						
	Education level		0.314*	0.358**	0.316*	0.349**	0.446**
	Income inequality	−0.276*					
	Diffusion rate of televisions[a]		0.282*	0.495***	0.446**	0.400**	0.380**
	Average temperature	0.645***	0.398**				
	Adjusted R^2	0.39	0.419	0.33	0.287	0.266	0.369

* Significant at the 5 percent level.
** Significant at the 1 percent level.
*** Significant at the 0.1 percent level.
Note: Coefficients show the relationship between the explanatory variable and life expectancy.
a. Measures household ownership of televisions.
Source: Author's calculations.

ever, enjoyed less improvement in their health relative to the other occupational groups; in relative terms, the gap between the service/agricultural worker groups and the others is greater in 1990 than in 1960. An analysis of causes of death in these two groups (service and agricultural) compared with the population average reveals that they are at increased risk for all of the major causes of death.

Women show markedly different age-standardized occupational trends over the shorter period of time for

Figure 7 Trends in age-standardized mortality rates for men age 20–59 by occupation in Japan, 1960–90

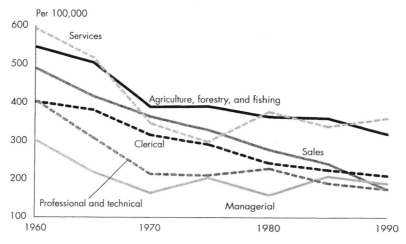

Source: Ministry of Health and Welfare, Japan; author's analysis.

Figure 8 Trends in age-standardized mortality rates for women age 20–59 by occupation in Japan, 1980–90

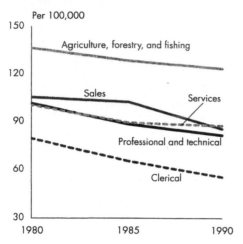

Source: Ministry of Health and Welfare, Japan; author's analysis.

which data were available, 1980 through 1990 (see Fig. 8). As one might expect, female mortality rates are substantially lower than male rates. Like men, those women involved in agriculture appear at significantly higher mortality risk in both 1980 and 1990. In contrast to men, female clerical workers appear to have the lowest mortality rates, lower than even professional/technical workers. A further intriguing finding (preliminary due to small numbers) suggests that "female managers" have the highest mortality rate among all female occupational groups.

Discussion

The four-period historical qualitative analysis reveals a strong social commitment to universal access to education and gender equity in educational attendance as well as pioneering movements socializing public health. In the early phase of the construction of the modern state of Japan, the main focus of the social sector policies was primary education and the securing of health service human resources such as medical doctors and midwives. In the wake of World War II, Japan shifted to an overriding focus on economic development. Although social and economic policies were often instituted for very different ends (such as imperialism or industrialization), it seems that the serendipitous combination and sequencing of these policies has led to ex-

traordinarily favorable health outcomes. The century's early investments in education, nutrition, and public health—with a special focus on women—most certainly allowed Japan to attain its unrivaled population health status and may have fueled its spectacular economic growth. The trends in social inequities in health, however, are less conclusive.

In Japan, over the twentieth century, the interprefectural differences between the lowest and highest IMR areas decreased from 100 to 3 per 1000. An obvious advantage of analysis by this geographic unit is its eventual use as a policy entry point. However, it is likely that smaller geographic or administrative divisions would reveal greater variations in health; a smaller unit of analysis would likely be more sensitive to disadvantaged populations such as ethnic minorities or low-skilled workers and identify wider disparities in health (see chapter 19).

Although prefectural inequalities in health appear modest, the regression analyses from different decades indicate strong associations with socioeconomic differentials. Gross prefectural product (GPP) per capita and levels of primary and secondary educational attainment are strongly associated with differentials in infant mortality. For adult women, education and household ownership of televisions appear to be strongly associated with longevity, while for men increasing GPP per capita and lower inequality in prefectural income distribution are associated with greater longevity at age 40 years. These results are in keeping with the broader literature on social inequalities in health (Wilkinson 1996) and suggest that social stratification in Japan is of some consequence for health and that social inequalities between prefectures explain variation in health achievement.

Also of note are the distinct gender patterns in explaining geographic differentials in life expectancy at age 40 years. Men's survival appears to have stronger links to prefectural income and income distribution, while education and television ownership levels correlate with female survival rates. These findings lend support to the idea of gender-specific determinants of inequality in health. Furthermore, it is possible that there is temporal and health outcome specificity to determinants of inequality in health given the way stratifiers of health outcomes change over time and differ depending on the health outcome measured—IMR or life expectancy at age 40 years.

A remarkable finding in this analysis is that primary education for women has provided profound and long-lasting health dividends. The cohort of women born around 1890—the first to benefit from universal primary education—had a direct impact on the decline in IMR in the 1920s. This education might also be linked to increases in life expectancy in the 1960s and 1970s as evidenced by the strong association between women's education and adult life expectancy. Economic growth could have enhanced this effect, but education seems to have been the basis for these health improvements. A clear policy implication is that the encouragement of female primary education should be a high priority for health achievement. Detractors might qualify this recommendation, noting that although the policy of "good wife, wise mother" may have been beneficial to the health of women and children, other dimensions of women's well being may not have been as well served (Matsui 1996).

While the analysis of prefectures indicates small geographic inequalities in health, the occupational analysis tells another story. Wide differentials in health across occupational groups are revealed for men, with the lower occupational levels suffering higher mortality. Although the overall trends in the occupational gradient for men suggest decreasing inequality over time, mortality rates for male agricultural and service workers continue to lag unacceptably behind. Among women, agricultural workers are similarly disadvantaged relative to other occupational groups. Somewhat surprisingly, however, mortality rates among female professional workers are as high as among service workers and appear higher than among clerical workers. Further analysis, however, suggests that the clerical worker mortality rates may be artificially low given their greater likelihood to exit the formal workforce when ill (Hasegawa and Miyao 1998). Even if the clerical worker rates are underestimated, the finding of the highest death rates among female managers suggests that for women in Japan the classical occupational gradient, found among Japanese men as well as for men and women in other countries, may not adequately capture the complex nature of disadvantage and discrimination experienced by women in the workforce. One hypothesis is that though they are classified under the same occupational category, the actual jobs might be quite different for men and women. In other words, gender norms "allocate" men into certain types of managerial or professional jobs or industries and women into others. Alternatively, this finding might reflect the duress of workplace discrimination or the strain of handling both domestic and career responsibilities. Clearly much more information is required about the nature of work by occupation and gender before making statements about the level and magnitude of occupational inequity in health for Japanese women.

The occupational analysis provides an indication that significant stratification along one axis, for example, occupation, might coexist with high equity in another dimension of the social sphere, for example, access to primary education and health care. Although education and health care are universal and an egalitarian social ethic prevails, stratification in health by occupation remains pronounced in Japan.

The long-standing commitment to egalitarianism in Japan underlies extraordinary gains in health and impressive relative equality in health distribution. This egalitarian ethos, however, may be "selectively" applied to certain carefully circumscribed population groups, thereby excluding ethnic minorities or even women. For example, mortality in minority ethnic groups, particularly among males, is higher than the overall Japanese age-standardized mortality rate; for example, the mortality rate of Korean males living in Japan is 1.7 times that of the average Japanese male. This inequity demands further scrutiny. Demographic changes, such as the rapidly burgeoning elderly population, pose frontier equity challenges such as the intergenerational allocation of resources and the gendered burden of care. A number of disconcerting trends, including increased suicide rates in males and other sociobehavioral patterns related to cigarettes, diet, and alcohol, are likely to stratify health outcomes in the future (Cockerham et al. 2000).

In summary, research over the last several decades has called into question the "classlessness" of Japanese society, pointing to occupational gradients, clear delineations between working and middle classes, biases against ethnic minorities, and gender discrimination (Schultz 1995; Brinton 1989). A social commitment to equity is laudable and has clearly benefited the population as a whole, but the evidence presented here reiterates the fact that social or health systems may still generate inequities, about which society must remain vigilant.

Despite the evidence of social gradients in longevity, overall achievement in health outcomes in Japan are remarkable. Japan's unparalleled attainment in longevity occurred despite significant income inequality because of the early achievement of equality in female primary education. Thus, the role of female primary education—early in a nation's development—may be the single most important lesson for other countries from the Japanese experience.

I thank Dr. Fabienne Peter, Harvard Center for Population and Development, and Dr. Michael Marmot, Department of Epidemiology and Public Health University College London, for their informative comments, which have been reflected in various parts of this study. The study is financially supported by the Rockefeller Foundation under its "Global Health Equity Initiative." This report is based on the results of a collaborative work of team members. They are listed by their affiliations at the time the study was completed in 1999:

Primary investigator: Toshihiko Hasegawa, MD, MPH, National Institute of Health Services Management; General secretariat: Kunichika Matsumoto, PhD candidate of Waseda University; Editorial Adviser: Indermohan S. Narula, MBBS, MPH, MTropMed (Liverpool)

Conceptual studies: Equity, equality, and Japanese culture: Nobuko Fukatsu, PhD candidate of the University of Tokyo; Yu Nagata, PhD candidate of Jochi University. Health transition: Toshihiko Hasegawa, MD, MPH, National Institute of Health Services Management; Nobuko Murayama, MSc, PhD, National Institute of Health Services Management; Hisayoshi Kondo, MD, PhD candidate of Nippon Medical School; Koya Tabata, BS, graduate student of Tokyo Institute of Technology

Cross-sectional comparative study: Occupation: Yoko Hori, MS, PhD candidate, Department of Public Health, Graduate School of Medicine, Nagoya University; Tomoyuki Watanabe, MS, PhD candidate, Department of Public Health, Graduate School of Medicine, Nagoya University; Junichi Mase, PhD, graduate School of Mathematics, Nagoya University; Masaru Miyao, MD, PhD, Graduate School of Mathematics, Nagoya University; Toshihiko Hasegawa, MD, MPH, National Institute of Health Services Management. Ethnicity: Toshihiko Hasegawa, MD, MPH, National Institute of Health Services Management; Akiko Ishihara, BA, Master Degree candidate, Kyoto University; Region: Masahide Kondo, MD, MS, PhD candidate of London School of Hygiene and Tropical Medicine; Toshihiko Hasegawa, MD, MPH, National Institute of Health Services Management

Historical Trend Analysis: Manpower management: Hisayoshi Kondo, MD, PhD candidate of Nippon Medical School. School attendance analysis: Maki Yoshinaka, PhD candidate of Tsukuba National University; Kyoko Okamura, BA, National Institute of Health Services Management; Toshihiko Hasegawa, MD, MPH, National Institute of Health Services Management. Income inequality and regional disparity: Kunichika Matsumoto, PhD candidate of Waseda University; Sumihiko Oohira, PhD, Professor, Shizuoka Prefecture University. Socioeconomic determinants of child mortality: Nobuko Murayama, MSc, PhD, National Institute of Health Services Management

References

Brinton M. 1989. Gender stratification in contemporary urban Japan. *American Sociological Review* 54:549–564.

Cockerham W., Hattori H., Yamori Y. 2000. The social gradient in life expectancy: the contrary case of Okinawa in Japan. *Social Science and Medicine* 51:115–122.

Deininger K., Squire L. 1996. A new data set measuring income inequality. *World Bank Economic Review* 10(3):565–591.

Fujime Y. 1998. *Sei no rekishi gaku*. Tokyo: Fuji Press.

Fukatsu N., Nagata Y. 1998. *Measurement of Equity, Equality and Japanese Culture*. Working paper of National Institute of Health Services Management. Tokyo: National Institute of Health Services Management.

Hasegawa T., Miyao M. 1998. Analysis on Occupation and Gender. Working paper of National Institute of Health Services Management. Tokyo: National Institute of Health Services Management.

Igarashi T., Murao M. 1978. Epidemiological survey of cerebro-cardiovascular diseases and Iwamizawa in Hookaido. *Hokkaido Igaku Zasshi* 53(2):79–115.

Ishihara A. 1999. Yamamoto Senji no sanjiseigen undo [Senji Yamamoto on the birth control movement]. Master's thesis, Graduate School of Kyoto University, Kyoto.

Jannetta A.B. 1987. *Epidemics and Mortality in Early Modern Japan*. Princeton, NJ: Princeton University Press.

Johansson S.R., Mosk C. 1987. Exposure, residence and life expectancy: disease and death during the economic development of Japan, 1900–1960. *Population Studies* 41(2):207–236.

Kagamimori S., Matsubara I., Sokejima S., Skine M., Matsukara T., Nakagawa H., Naruse Y. 1988. The comparative study on occupational mortality, 1980 between Japan and Great Britain. *Industrial Health* 36(3):252–257.

Kawakami N., Haratani T. 1999. Epidemiology of job stress and health in Japan: review of current evidence and future direction. *Industrial Health* 37:174–186.

Kondo H. 1998. Historical Analysis of the Distribution of Medical Doctors' Manpower Management in the Primary Care Delivery System. Working paper of National Institute of Health Services Management. Tokyo: National Institute of Health Services Management.

Koseisyo Gojunenshi Hensyu Iinkai. 1988. *Koseisho Gojunenshi*. Tokyo: Koseimondai Kenkyukai.

Marmot M.G., Smith G.D. 1989. Why are the Japanese living longer? *British Medical Journal* 299:1547–1551.

Minami R. 1994. Senzen nihon no shotoku bunpu. *Keizaikenkyu* 45(3):193–202.

Minami R. 1996. *Nihon no keizai hatten to shotoku bunpu*. Tokyo: Iwanami Press.

Ministry of Education. 1972. *Gakusei hyakunennshi*. Tokyo: Gyosei.

Mitchell B.R. 1998a. *International Historical Statistics: Africa, Asia and Oceania, 1750–1993*. London: Macmillan.

Mitchell B.R. 1998b. *International Historical Statistics: The Americas 1750–1993*. London: Macmillan.

Mitchell B.R. 1998c. *International Historical Statistics: Europe, 1750–1993*. London: Macmillan.

Mouri T. 1972. *Gendai Nippon syoni hokenshi [Contemporary History of Children's Health in Japan]*. Tokyo: Domesu Press.

Murayama N., Matsumoto K., Hasegawa T. 2000. Historical Analysis of the Impact of Socio-economic Factors on the Interregional Inequality of Child Mortality Rate in Japan. Working paper of National Institute of Health Services Management. Tokyo: National Institute of Health Services Management.

Nakane C. 1967. *Tatesyakai No Ningen Kankei*. Tokyo: Kodansha.

National Institute of Education. 1974. *Nihon kindai kyouiku hyakunennshi*. Tokyo: Kyoiku Kenkyu Shinkokai.

Organization for Economic Co-operation and Development. 1999. *Organization for Economic Co-operation and Development Health Data 1998: a Comparative Analysis of 29 Countries*.

Washington, DC: Brookings Institution Press/Inter-American Development Bank.

Schultz T.P. 1995. *Aging, Immigration and Women in the Labor Force: Japan Compared to Other OECD Countries.* Center Discussion Paper No. 743. New Haven, CT: Economic Growth Center, Yale University.

Shigeki N. 1986. [The Role of Medical Technology in the Mortality Decline of Modern Japan]. *Journal of Public Health* 33:529–533, 605–616.

Stationery Office. 1997. *Regional Trends 1997.* No. 32. London: The Stationery Office.

Sugimoto Y. 1997. *An Introduction to Japanese Society.* Cambridge, MA: Cambridge University Press.

United Nations Development Programme (UNDP). 1999. *Human Development Report 1999.* New York: UNDP.

Wilkinson R. 1996. *Unhealthy Societies: The Afflictions of Inequality.* London: Routledge.

CHAPTER
9

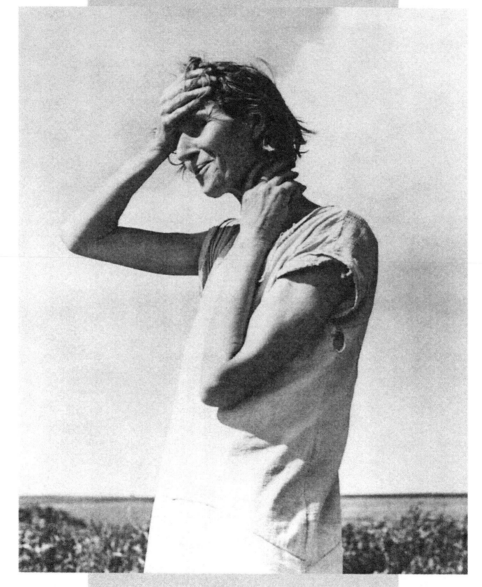

Women of the High Plains, Texas panhandle, 1938.
Source: Copyright the Dorothea Lange Collection, Oakland Museum of California, City of Oakland, Gifts of Paul S. Taylor.

United States: Social Inequality and the Burden of Poor Health

LAURA D. KUBZANSKY, NANCY KRIEGER, ICHIRO KAWACHI, BEVERLY ROCKHILL, GILLIAN K. STEEL, AND LISA F. BERKMAN

If life was a thing that money could buy, the rich would live and the poor might die
—1830s English folk song, cited by Hobsbawm (1996: 208)

The United States has the dubious distinction of ranking first among industrialized nations in inequalities in both income and wealth (Wolff 1995; Smeeding and Gottschalk 1997). Between 1974 and 1994, the top 5% of the U.S. households increased their share of the nation's aggregate household income from 16% to 21%. The top 20% of U.S. households' share of aggregate income rose from 44% to 49%, while the share among the bottom 20% shrank from 4.3% to 3.6% (DeVita 1996). Such a concentration of and disparity in wealth in the United States has not been seen since the 1920s (Wolff 1995), and these trends have continued through the late 1990s (Kawachi et al. 1999; Bernstein et al. 2000).

Growing national inequalities in income and wealth portend growing socioeconomic inequalities in health. Studies have compared data from the 1960s, the late 1970s, and 1980s and have found that even as mortality rates overall are declining in the United States, there are widening disparities in mortality by educational level (Pappas et al. 1993; Duleep 1995) and by

income level (Schalick et al. 2000). Concomitantly, the U.S. population attributable death rate due to poverty increased between the early 1970s and early 1990s, especially among black men and women (Hahn et al. 1996). Additional research suggests that these socioeconomic disparities in health may underlie many observed racial/ethnic and some gender inequalities in health (Krieger et al. 1993; Williams and Collins 1995).

Despite its greater wealth and proportion of national income spent on health care, the United States manifests poorer health than many other developed nations. The United States is ranked first in the world in the percent gross national product (GNP) spent on health care. In 1995, national health care expenditures totaled $989 billion and comprised 13.6% of the gross domestic product. Average life expectancy from birth in the United States in 1990 was, however, 75.4 years (for men and women combined), below that of 15 other World Health Organization (WHO)–participating countries. Because inequalities in health are inextricably intertwined with social inequalities, the health of the U.S. population is painfully unequal (Haan et al. 1987; Krieger et al. 1993; Williams and Collins 1995; Guralnik et al. 1996).

To date, much public health research on social inequalities has focused on who is at greatest risk for poor health outcomes. The goal has been to quantify

United States

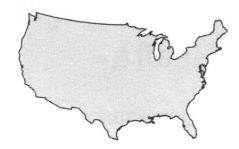

Total population (millions), 1997	271.8
Human development index, 1999	0.927
Human development index rank, 1999	3
Infant mortality rate (per 1,000 live births), 1997	7
Real GDP per capita (PPP$), 1997	29,010
Public spending on health	
as percentage of GDP, 1995	6.5

Source: UNDP 1999. [Human Development Report]

the magnitude of the effect of deprivation on health. Understanding and acting to reduce the population's burden of disease, however, requires more than estimates of risk. Also important, as suggested by what has been called a "population perspective," is distribution of risk across a population (Rose 1992). This approach takes into account both magnitude of and proportion exposed to a given risk. Those with the highest levels of risk fall in the tail of the population distribution and therefore are small in number. Those with moderate levels of risk comprise the bulk of the distribution. Rose (1992) argued that small shifts in average individual risk can lead to large population effects. Focusing solely on the ill health burden of the poor (tail of the income/wealth distribution) may underestimate the true impact of the social *gradient* in health, because each step up in the socioeconomic hierarchy is associated with better health than the level below. While Rose (1992) suggested improvements might come about by shifting the population to lower risks, a population perspective in which the distribution is altered by shifts toward the mean (e.g., reducing disparity) is also compatible with his arguments. In either case, a population perspective would consider the burden of poor health over the entire socioeconomic distribution of the population.

The importance of analyzing social inequalities in health in relation to both magnitude and distribution of risk is underscored by an increasing concern with

health equity, the idea that everyone should have an opportunity to attain their full potential for health (Calman 1997). The necessity of research on social inequalities and health is also heightened by the current focus on health as a human right (Mann et al. 1999). Adding urgency is the trend of growing economic inequalities in the United States. These economic inequalities have widened considerably over the last two decades at the same time that the social safety net of welfare and related programs has been partially dismantled (Williams and Collins 1995; Wolff 1995; Krieger et al. 1997b).

In this context, a population perspective directs attention to the importance of recognizing that different interventions may be required for a small number of people at highest risk and for the larger number of people at moderate risk for poor health outcomes. At issue is consideration of both the effect and impact of socioeconomic position on health. Measures of *effect* compare specific socioeconomic groups (such as people with a household income less than $10,000 vs. those with a household income greater than $50,000) to see how a fixed change in socioeconomic status influences some health outcome (e.g., mortality rates). Measures of *impact* compare specific socioeconomic groups in terms of their absolute differences in inequalities, taking into account the size of the groups being compared (Kunst 1997). Examination of effects of social factors can tell us who is at highest risk for adverse health outcomes (e.g., magnitude of inequality in outcome), whereas consideration of the distribution of social conditions across the population can tell us where the greatest population burden of poor health may be carried (impact). Both matter, and the simultaneous consideration of effect and impact may inform our thinking about social inequalities and health outcomes.

Conducting research on socioeconomic position and health in the United States, however, is not easy. Research on socioeconomic position has been difficult historically because of the virtual absence of adequate information on socioeconomic position in health data (Krieger and Fee 1994). Socioeconomic data typically have not been a component of published U.S. vital statistics (for a comprehensive review, see Krieger et al. 1997a). Instead, data have been stratified solely by age, sex, and what is referred to as "race" (Krieger and Fee 1994). There are a number of national surveys containing data on both socioeconomic position and health (for a detailed discussion, see Krieger et al. 1997b). These vary in the measures of socioeconomic position and health outcomes that are included, as well as in how representative they are of the U.S. population.

Thus, merging across data sets is difficult, limiting the ability of any study to be inclusive of multiple measures of both exposures and outcomes.

Conceptual Framework

Although a great deal of research has identified the effect of socioeconomic position and other social conditions on health outcomes, little attempt has been made to estimate the population burden of social inequality on poor health outcomes. Link and Phelan (1995) and others (Anderson and Armstead 1995; Kaplan 1995a) have suggested that some social factors are "fundamental causes" of disease and, as such, are critically related to health inequalities. A cause may be considered fundamental when it involves access to resources that can be used to avoid risks or to minimize the consequences of disease once it occurs. These resources, frequently distributed unevenly across society, include money, power, prestige, and various kinds of interpersonal relationships. Given the importance of these resources in structuring daily lives, the effects of fundamental causes will endure, although the intervening risk factors and, in fact, specific diseases may change over time. Investigators have suggested that social conditions as defined by socioeconomic position, race/ethnicity, and gender strongly influence individuals' access to resources and may therefore be considered social determinants of health (Standing 1997; Williams 1997).

In previous work, health effects of individual social factors have often been examined. Because social circumstances are interrelated in basic and important ways, however, their relationship to health outcomes may be understood most comprehensively by considering the joint effects of membership in two or more social categories. By *social category* we mean the various ways of classifying the different combinations of age, gender, race/ethnicity, and income groups, for example, black women with income less than $10,000 (Krieger 1994; Susser and Susser 1996). With regard to conceptualizing social determinants of health, we have opted to examine the effect and the impact of socioeconomic position on health in relation to age, gender, and race/ethnicity. Given our desire to utilize data representative of the U.S. population and based in part on the availability of data, we have chosen annual household income as a basic indicator of socioeconomic position. For the purposes of this research, we consider income to be a marker of socioeconomic position rather than a mediator of the effect of socioeconomic position on health.

Despite the numerous expressions of poor health, one of the most commonly used outcomes in work on social inequality and health is age-adjusted and sometimes age-specific mortality rates (e.g., Marmot et al. 1984; Pappas et al. 1993; Backlund et al. 1996). Although these mortality rates are the "common denominator" of health statistics because of their universal assessment across diverse populations, they are insufficient to describe the consequence of inequalities for health and well being. Of greater relevance in a context of increasing life expectancy is *premature* mortality. We all eventually die, but the relevant question is "at what age?" Additionally, as "rectangularization" of the survival curve appears in the growing elderly U.S. population (and in other countries), it becomes important to consider other critical health outcomes beyond mortality (Berkman 1988). These include functional limitations and disability related to both aging and work exposures, health among infants and young children related to developmental abilities, selected chronic conditions among adults, and mental health. Thus, to draw attention to ways that inequality both shortens and impairs people's lives, we focused on two outcomes, premature mortality and functional disability, as experienced in representative samples of the U.S. population. In this study, the measure of health inequity is the disparity in these health outcomes across race/ethnicity (restricted to blacks and whites), gender, and income group.

Methods

We present analyses framed by a population perspective to look at the effect and impact of socioeconomic inequality on two outcomes, premature mortality and functional limitations (disability). Analyses are stratified by age, gender, and race/ethnicity (restricted to blacks and whites due to sample size limitations). These analyses were conducted using data from two large-scale studies based on nationally representative samples of U.S. blacks and whites (see Box 1 for details on methods). The National Longitudinal Mortality Study (NLMS) was used for analyses of premature mortality, and the National Health Interview Survey was used for cross-sectional analyses of disability. The 1980 population estimates were obtained from the U.S. Census Bureau. These estimates were used to represent the population distribution across the adjusted 1980 income levels derived from the NLMS.

Years of potential life lost ($YPLL_{75}$) per person is a measure of premature mortality and serves as an indicator of effect in our study. The utility of a measure of

YPLL has been recognized by the U.S. General Accounting Office as the best single indicator for reflecting differences in the health status of states' populations. This office recommended that it be used to assist the distribution of federal funding for core public health functions (Selik and Chu 1997). Methods that take account of the longer life expectancy of women or whites, for example, make it more difficult to demonstrate how far short any group falls of a benchmark that we believe *should* be attainable by everyone. Thus, our method of calculating $YPLL_{75}$ does not consider known differences between groups

---

BOX 1: METHODS

Study Populations

The National Longitudinal Mortality Study (NLMS) is a long-term prospective study of mortality in the United States (Rogot et al. 1992). The study population for the NLMS consists of samples drawn from the Current Population Surveys (CPS) between 1979 and 1985. Follow-up times range from 4 to 11 years for any individual. NLMS data were obtained from the National Heart Lung and Blood Institute. Further details on the NLMS have been provided elsewhere (Rogot et al. 1992; Backlund et al. 1996).

The National Health Interview Survey (NHIS) is a continuous nationwide multistage probability design sample survey in which data about health and other characteristics of each member of the household are collected through personal household interviews of the civilian noninstitutionalized population residing in the United States. Weighted data were used for our analyses. The combined sample for 1988–1990 comprised 139,672 households containing 358,870 persons living at the time of the interview. Further description of the survey design, the methods used in estimation, and general qualifications of the data obtained from the survey are available elsewhere (Collins and LeClere 1996; National Center for Health Statistics 1997).

Determinants

Socioeconomic position was indicated by family income, as categorized by either the NLMS or the NHIS. The income categories are different in these two sources. In the NLMS, family income was adjusted to reflect 1980 dollars and was assigned to one of seven categories: $0 to $4999, $5000 to $9999, $10,000 to $14,999, $15,000 to $19,999, $20,000 to $24,999, $25,000 to $49,999, or over $50,000. In the NHIS, family income was assigned to one of four categories: under $10,000, $10,000 to $19,999, $20,000 to $34,999, or $35,000 or more (1988–1990).

Age was categorized into 5-year age groups in the NLMS. Two age groups were included in the NHIS, 45 to 65 years and 65 years and over.

Race/ethnicity included categories white and black, as reported by respondents. Neither category is exclusive of Hispanics. Other race/ethnicity categories were not included in the analyses due to unavailable data and small sample sizes.

Gender was categorized as male or female in both surveys.

Outcomes

Average $YPLL_{75}$ per person was calculated using data from the NLMS. Following methods used by the National Center for Health Statistics (National Center for Health Statistics 1997), $YPLL_{75}$ was derived using ten 5-year age groups and was not age standardized. Deaths in age groups under 25 years were not included due to instability of the data obtainable for these groups. To compute the total YPLL for each group, the number of deaths in each 5-year age stratum in race/ethnicity–gender–income group was multiplied by the years of life lost, calculated as the difference between age 75 years and the midpoint of the age stratum. For example, the death of a person 45 to 49 years of age counted as 27.5 years lost. To derive a per person YPLL in each race/ethnicity–gender–income group, this number was then divided by the number of persons in the race/ethnicity–gender–income group. $YPLL_{75}$ is an average per person per year measure. For example, 0.20 means that the average person loses approximately 2.5 months every year before the age of 75 years.

Prevalence of disability was calculated using data from NHIS and was measured as the proportion of each group that reported limitations in activities of daily living at the time of the survey. Questions were asked in reference to the last year. People were classified in terms of the major activity usually associated with their particular age group. The major activities were paid working or keeping house for those aged 18 to 69 years old and the capacity for independent living (e.g., the ability to bathe, shop, dress, or eat without needing the help of another person) for those 70 years of age and over. Each person was classified into one of two categories with regard to their performance of age-related activities: (*1*) unable to perform the major activity; or able to perform the major activity, but limited in the kind or amount of this activity; or not limited in the major activity, but limited in the kind or amount of other activities; and (*2*) not limited in any way.

Slope Index of Inequality (SII) is a measure that uses the slope of a weighted regression line to indicate the average relationship between income and individual health across the distribution of income (Wagstaff et al. 1991). Because the size of each socioeconomic group is considered, the SII represents the absolute effect on health of moving from the lowest socioeconomic position through to the highest (Preston et al. 1981).

in life expectancy, but takes an upper age limit that should be attainable (such as age 75 years) as a benchmark for everyone and shows how much we are falling short of the benchmark.

Functional disability is our second health outcome and is also an indicator of effect. Activity limitation was used to ascertain disability, which is a long-term reduction in a person's capacity to perform the average kind or amount of activities associated with his or her age group.

The slope index of inequality (SII) is a measure that takes into account both the effect and the impact of the income distribution on health. We use the SII in our analysis because it allows us to capture explicitly and clearly the gradient in health, as opposed to other measures of effect (e.g., the population attributable risk for mortality). Chapter 5 provides a full description of this measure.

Estimates of $YPLL_{75}$ per person and disability prevalence for each age–racial/ethnic–gender–income stratum (effect measures) were calculated. To demonstrate who is at highest risk and how many people bear the risk burden, we contrasted $YPLL_{75}$ per person and disability estimates with the population distribution across income categories. Slope indices of inequality for both premature mortality and disability were calculated and presented to exemplify a measure that takes account of both *effect* and *impact*.

Results

Effect of Social Inequality on Premature Mortality

Figure 1 indicates the income distribution across race/ethnicity and gender categories. In general, there is an inverse and concave relationship between income and $YPLL_{75}$ per person that is similar in all racial/ethnic–gender groups; as family income decreases, $YPLL_{75}$ increases at an increasing rate (see Table 1 and Fig. 2). At least twice as many $YPLL_{75}$ were lost per person at the lowest income levels (less than $5,000) versus the highest levels (greater than or equal to $50,000), and this ratio steadily decreases as income increases. For example, on average, black men with less than $5,000 income who are aged 50 years can expect to lose 7.75 (0.31 × 25) potential years of life, whereas black men with an income greater than $50,000 at age 50 can expect to lose 1.75 (0.07 × 25) potential years of life.

Considering both the effect of income on premature mortality and the income distribution (impact), the slope index of inequality suggests that as individuals advance from the lowest to the highest income groups, at each level of income (as defined above), on average, there is a gain of 5 days of life per person per year ($b = -0.0137$, $p < 0.01$).

Figure 1 Distribution of sample population across income levels, by race/ethnicity and gender, in the United States, 1980

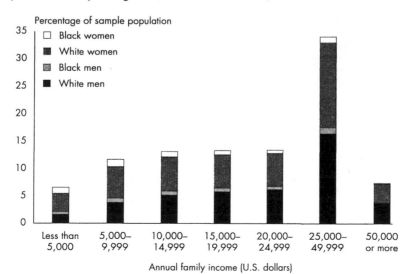

Source: Based on data from the U.S. Census Bureau.

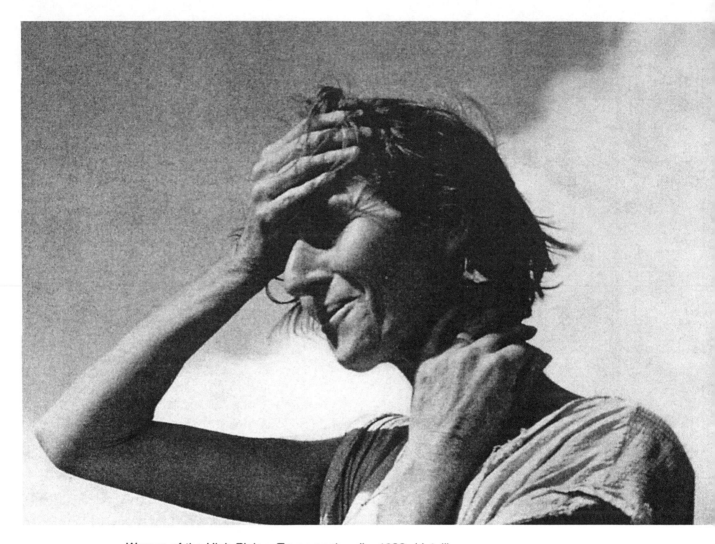

Woman of the High Plains, Texas panhandle, 1938. (detail)
Source: Copyright the Dorothea Lange Collection, Oakland Museum of California,
City of Oakland, Gifts of Paul S. Taylor.

Table 1 Premature mortality by race/ethnicity, gender, and income level in the United States, 1979–89

Family income level and social category	Population (thousands)	Share of sample population (percent)	Average years of potential life lost (YPLL$_{75}$) per person per year
Less than $5,000	7,985	6.61	0.15
Black women	1,308	1.08	0.16
White women	4,058	3.36	0.10
Black men	616	0.51	0.31
White men	2,003	1.66	0.19
$5,000–9,999	14,155	11.71	0.12
Black women	1,572	1.30	0.11
White women	6,960	5.76	0.07
Black men	975	0.81	0.21
White men	4,648	3.85	0.17
$10,000–14,999	15,947	13.20	0.10
Black women	1,146	0.95	0.10
White women	7,565	6.26	0.06
Black men	922	0.76	0.19
White men	6,314	5.22	0.12
$15,000–19,999	16,192	13.40	0.08
Black women	877	0.73	0.08
White women	7,383	6.11	0.05
Black men	832	0.69	0.14
White men	7,100	5.88	0.10
$20,000–24,999	16,300	13.49	0.07
Black women	672	0.56	0.06
White women	7,352	6.08	0.05
Black men	692	0.57	0.13
White men	7,584	6.28	0.09
$25,000–49,999	41,231	34.12	0.07
Black women	1,270	1.05	0.07
White women	18,651	15.43	0.05
Black men	1,384	1.15	0.14
White men	19,926	16.49	0.09
$50,000 or more	9,034	7.48	0.06
Black women	112	0.09	0.06
White women	4,185	3.46	0.05
Black men	153	0.13	0.07
White men	4,584	3.79	0.08

Note: Family income levels are in 1980 U.S. dollars.
Source: Based on data from the National Longitudinal Mortality Study.

Figure 2 Premature mortality by race/ethnicity, gender, and income level in the United States, 1979–89

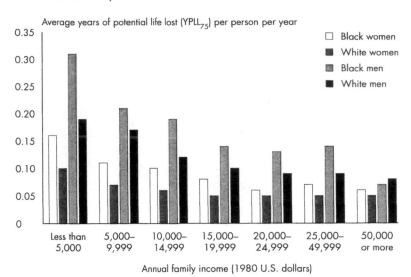

Source: Based on data from the National Longitudinal Mortality Study.

Analysis of Joint Effects

Additional analyses examined the joint effects of race/ethnicity, gender, and income on $YPLL_{75}$ (see Table 1). With regard to the effect of socioeconomic position on premature mortality (estimate of $YPLL_{75}$ per person), the overall pattern described above was largely similar in each racial/ethnic–gender group (see Figs. 2 and 3). Figure 3 is designed to juxtapose visually both the income distribution and the risk of premature mortality in each race/ethnicity and gender category. Risks were highest in the low-income group. Although the pattern was similar across subgroups, there are several differences worth noting. For instance, the population distribution of income among whites and blacks differs strikingly (see Fig. 1). For both black women and black men, the population is concentrated largely in the lower income strata, and this is particularly true for black women; 15% of blacks (19% of black women) had a family income under $5,000 compared with 6% of the white population. Because of the greater concentration of the black population at lower income levels, in terms of premature mortality, more blacks than whites experience adverse effects of low income. In addition, among the lower four income strata for both men and women, blacks are generally one and a half times more likely to lose years of life prematurely than whites. Because the proportion of the population represented by blacks is small, however, they account for a smaller percentage of the total years of life lost than whites.

With regard to gender, men lose more years of life than women in virtually all but the highest income stratum; this is true for both blacks and whites. Although the SII suggests on average a gain of 5 days of life per person per year as individuals advance from the lowest to the highest income groups, this varies across gender and race/ethnicity from as much as 11.42 days of life for black men per year to 6.21 days of life for white man per year to 6.61 days of life per black women per year to a low of 2.41 days of life for white woman per year. Thus, while patterns are similar across racial/ethnic–gender–income groups, because of distributional differences in income in the population and differences in the magnitude of effects, further insight may be gained by examining the socioeconomic gradient in premature mortality separately by gender and race/ethnicity.

Effect of Social Inequality on Disability

Similar to the patterns identified with premature mortality, there is a monotonic inverse relationship between income and disability in both age groups (see Tables 2 and 3, and Fig. 4). Among individuals age 45 to 64 years, approximately 26% had an income of less than $20,000, 26% had an income between $20,000 and $34,999, and 48% had an income greater than $35,000. In contrast, among individuals aged 65 years and over, approximately 60% had an income less than $20,000, 24% had an income between $20,000 and

Figure 3 Distribution of the burden of premature mortality across income groups, by race/ethnicity and gender, in the United States, 1979–89

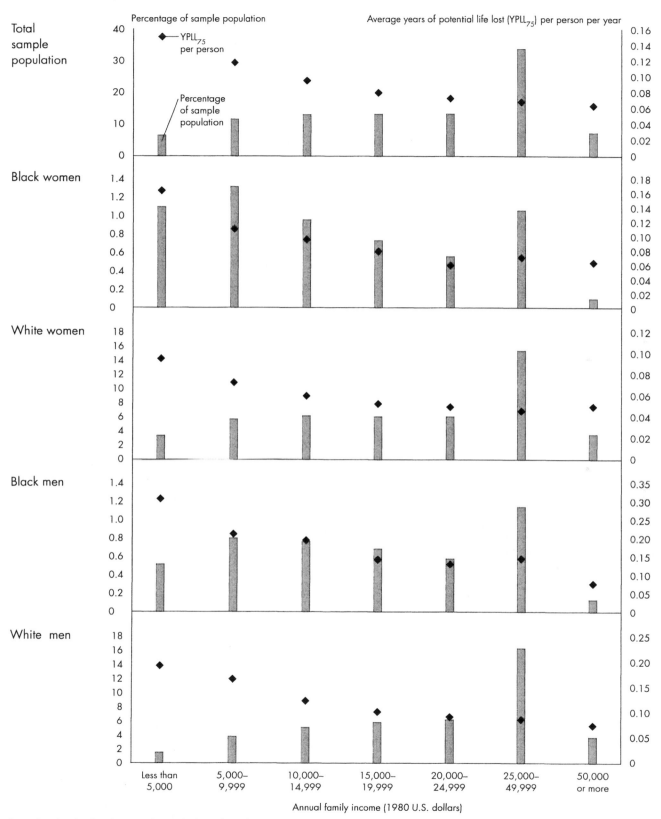

Source: Based on data from the National Longitudinal Mortality Study.

Table 2 Prevalence of disability among adults age 45–64 by race/ethnicity, gender, and income level in the United States, 1988–90

Family income level and social category	Population (thousands)	Share of sample population (percent)	Prevalence of disability (percent)
Less than $10,000	3,206	8.79	56.72
Black women	533	1.46	56.70
White women	1,511	4.14	53.90
Black men	293	0.80	60.10
White men	869	2.38	60.50
$10,000–19,999	6,262	17.18	33.36
Black women	559	1.53	31.50
White women	3,149	8.64	30.40
Black men	417	1.14	32.40
White men	2,137	5.86	38.40
$20,000–34,999	9,628	26.41	21.27
Black women	478	1.31	18.00
White women	4,580	12.56	20.90
Black men	453	1.24	21.90
White men	4,117	11.29	22.00
$35,000 or more	17,361	47.62	13.27
Black women	449	1.23	15.10
White women	7,580	20.79	13.50
Black men	500	1.37	11.00
White men	8,832	24.23	13.10

Source: Based on data from the National Health Interview Survey.

$34,999, and 17% had an income greater than $35,000. Among all subgroups aged 45 to 64 years, disability was approximately four times more prevalent in the lowest income level (less than $10,000) compared with the highest levels ($35,000 or more). Although this difference remained among individuals aged 65 years and older, the magnitude was reduced; disability was 1.7 times more prevalent among those with the lowest versus the highest incomes. Of note, the income distribution shifted for individuals aged 65 years or more so that 60% of the aged 65 years and over population had an income under $20,000 versus 26% of the aged 45 to 64 years population (see Table 3).

Among those aged 45 to 64 years, considering both the effect of income on disability and the income distribution, the SII was significant. This result suggests that as individuals advance from the lowest to the highest income groups, there is, on average, a 12% decrease in prevalence of disability ($b = -0.12$, $p < 0.05$). Among individuals aged 65 years or older the SII was significant and suggested that as individuals advance from the lowest to the highest income groups at each level of income, on average there is a 7% decrease in prevalence of disability ($b = -0.07$, $p < 0.05$).

Analysis of Joint Effects

Similar patterns are observed in each racial/ethnic–gender group, with black women again the most likely to be in the lower income strata. Although broadly comparable, these patterns nonetheless hid important distinctions among the different racial/ethnic and gender groups. In both age groups, women (black and white combined) comprised a higher percentage of the total population with an income under $10,000, than did

Table 3 Prevalence of disability among adults age 65 and over by race/ethnicity, gender, and income level in the United States, 1988–90

Family income level and social category	Population (thousands)	Share of sample population (percent)	Prevalence of disability (percent)
Less than $10,000	5,532	25.06	48.83
Black women	599	2.71	55.90
White women	3,380	15.31	46.60
Black men	296	1.34	53.40
White men	1,257	5.69	50.40
$10,000–19,999	7,642	34.62	38.88
Black women	316	1.43	45.30
White women	3,948	17.88	37.50
Black men	293	1.33	43.00
White men	3,085	13.97	39.60
$20,000–34,999	5,195	23.53	33.01
Black women	112	0.51	36.60
White women	2,582	11.70	31.60
Black men	103	0.47	32.00
White men	2,398	10.86	34.40
$35,000 or more	3,708	16.80	28.52
Black women	77	0.35	36.40
White women	1,737	7.87	29.60
Black men	70	0.32	32.90
White men	1,824	8.26	27.00

Source: Based on data from the National Health Interview Survey.

blacks (women and men combined). Given this income distribution and the effect of income on disability, women and blacks were more likely to experience disability. For example, Table 2 indicates that approximately 57% of black women aged 45 to 64 years with an income less than $10,000 are disabled. Also, although the prevalence of disability among blacks and whites was similar across men and women of similar incomes in the age group 45 to 64 years, disability was more prevalent among blacks (men and women) versus whites in the 65 years and over age group (see Tables 2 and 3). In the age 65 years and over group, black women reported the highest levels of disability across all income strata, while in the lowest income stratum white women reported the lowest levels of disability, although white women comprise a large proportion of the population with an income less than $10,000. Among individuals aged 45 to 64 years, however, dis-

ability was more prevalent among men (both black and white) than among women at each income level except the highest. This finding would suggest that a large part of the disability prevalence among women may be more strongly related to income than to gender in this age group.

Discussion

Key Findings: Effect and Impact of Socioeconomic Position on Health

In this study, we consider the health effects of socioeconomic position using a population perspective (Rose 1992). A robust effect of income on health is evident in all age, racial/ethnic, gender, and income groups and across two different markers of health status—premature mortality and disability. Those with less income

Figure 4 Distribution of the burden of disability across income groups, by age group, in the United States, 1988–90

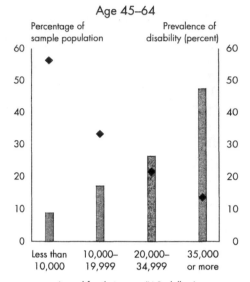

Age 45–64

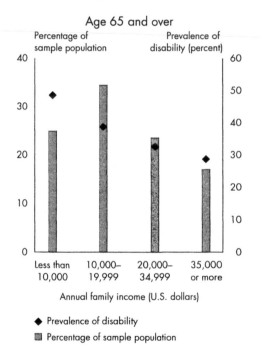

Age 65 and over

◆ Prevalence of disability

▇ Percentage of sample population

Source: Based on data from the National Health Interview Survey.

also in line with other research on socioeconomic position and race/ethnicity. For example, a recent study reported that life expectancy for whites exceeded that of blacks at every income level. Furthermore, at age 45 years, black women with an income of $25,000 or more could expect to live 3.8 years longer than those with an income of less than $10,000 (National Center for Health Statistics 1998).

As reported in other studies examining racial/ethnic and gender differences in health within socioeconomic strata (Krieger et al. 1993; Williams and Collins 1995), effects of income on premature mortality and disability varied by both race/ethnicity and gender. For example, within socioeconomic strata, blacks generally lost more years of life than whites, and men lost more years of life than women. In terms of premature mortality, black men in the lowest income stratum fared worse than any other group. In contrast, blacks and whites did not differ significantly in levels of disability within each income stratum among those aged 45 to 64 years. Among individuals aged 65 years or more, however, within each income stratum black women generally reported the highest levels of disability while white women reported the lowest levels. The pattern of findings with regard to gender also depends on which health outcome was considered. Differences between men and women across income strata were less consistent when disability rather than premature mortality was the health indicator.

An understanding of the overall influence of socioeconomic position on health is obtained by taking into account both the magnitude of the effects and the size of the group in which they occur. The slope index of inequality can be interpreted as the absolute effect of moving from the lowest to the highest income group while taking into account the actual distribution of income. This study, based on a nationally representative sample of the U.S. population, demonstrates that low income significantly increased risk of premature mortality and disability despite the fact that the lowest income groups were often composed of the fewest people.

Although the effect of socioeconomic position on health may be relatively stable, the impact will be significantly influenced by the distribution of income (or whatever marker of socioeconomic position is being considered) in the population. Given that income inequality in the United States is increasing, taking into account and tracking changes in the income distribution is particularly crucial in order to develop effective policies that address the health effects of socioeconomic position. For example, in our examination of disability in the 1988–1990 U.S. population, we find a

consistently live more disabled and less healthy lives, and die at younger ages, than their wealthier counterparts. Similar to other studies, our findings indicate that adverse health effects appear to be potentiated with increasing levels of deprivation. Our findings are marked difference in income distribution between those aged 45 to 64 years and those aged 65 years or older. A similar income distribution shift between younger and older individuals occurs in the 1980 U.S. population. More individuals aged 65 years and older were likely to have low incomes, and this is particularly true for women. Because those with low incomes are disproportionately burdened with poor health outcomes, older blacks and women, who are likely to have little income, are particularly disadvantaged. Despite the wealth of the U.S. population and the proportion of U.S. GNP spent on health care, good health eludes an unacceptably high proportion of the population, and the distribution of this disadvantage is socially determined.

Attention to both the effect and the impact of socioeconomic position on health leads to some unexpected findings. For example, previous work has suggested that women experience higher levels of disability than men in older populations (Guralnik et al. 1996). Our study indicates that men aged 45 to 64 years (both black and white) generally have higher prevalence rates of disability than women in all but the highest income stratum. Data on income distribution, however, suggest that those with low incomes are disproportionately women and that those with low incomes are more likely to be disabled. Thus, the impact of disability on 45- to 64-year-old women in low income groups is greater than for men even though male prevalence rates of disability are greater. Differences in income distribution may not be completely controlled even when socioeconomic position is included as a covariate in analyses of gender and disability. In this study, a greater understanding of the distribution of income across relevant social conditions was gained by stratifying simultaneously across race/ethnicity, gender, and age groups. Thus, studies on gender variations in disability that fail to take into account the potential confounding effect of income for men and women may be biased. Alternatively, income may be considered a mediating factor in the relationship between gender and health. Further research, however, is needed to confirm this finding while controlling more carefully for the effects of age.

Possible Biases and Limitations

The unavailability of relevant data severely constrains investigation of both the effect and the impact of socioeconomic position on health (for review, see Krieger et al. 1997b). For example, in this analysis, although we would have preferred to use more recent data, the data available for YPLL calculations were collected between 1975 and 1985. Given that income inequality has been increasing over the last decade, however, we feel some confidence that the direction of the effects we found are valid, although the magnitude may be somewhat underestimated.

Although research has suggested that family income does provide important information about social and health inequalities (Coulter and Guralnick 1959; Nagi and Stockwell 1973), there are nevertheless some concerns about the use of family income as an indicator of socioeconomic position. The family income variable does not adjust for family size or account for different family structures (single parenthood, extended family, and so forth), may fluctuate widely over time (Duncan 1996), and may be a poor proxy for purchasing power or income available to family members (Williams et al. 1997). For example, goods and services available to whites and residents of higher income neighborhoods in the United States tend to be higher quality and lower priced than those available to blacks and residents of lower income neighborhoods (Macintyre et al. 1993; Kaplan 1996).

Additional limitations may arise from the potential for racial/ethnic misclassification. Some investigators have raised concerns about the quality of race/ethnicity data (e.g., Hahn 1992; Williams et al. 1994). For example, because the distribution of a study population into different race/ethnicity categories varies depending on the assessment technique, respondent self-report of his or her race/ethnicity identification may differ substantially from an observer's assessment. Moreover, few data are available on racial/ethnic groups other than blacks and whites. It is also important to note that socioeconomic position should not be used as a proxy for race/ethnicity. Although race/ethnicity and socioeconomic position may be correlated, a number of studies have demonstrated that the effects of one cannot fully be explained by the other (Krieger and Fee 1994). As the data reported here suggest, even within each income stratum, blacks often have a worse health status than whites.

In addition, our analyses were limited because the data with regard to disability are cross sectional. As a result, some component of the association with income may be a function of reverse causation because it is likely that some people were ill or disabled and unable to work. Certainly, ill health may significantly affect income. Similarly, some of the variation in YPLL may be due to differences in access to care. Longitudinal and prospective studies of other populations, however, show that neither reverse causation nor access to care is likely to explain fully our results (Rose 1992; Seeman et al. 1994; Guralnik et al. 1996). Our findings may also be limited because our analyses of premature mortality did not take into account the age structure of the population. Many of the age-relevant differences occur at younger ages, however, which were not included in our analyses due to data limitations. In addition, we cumulated the number of years of life lost up to age 75 for each group and found the number to be consistent with other findings of differences in life expectancy between groups. Thus, we are confident that our results accurately represent the direction of the effects found.

Finally, effects of social inequality may not be uniform across all types of health outcomes. Our analyses were limited by the focus on only two health outcomes, premature mortality and disability. Social factors may affect health through multifaceted and dynamic processes, and examination of only one health outcome may result in an incomplete understanding and underestimation of their effects. Because fundamental social causes of disease involve resources that are important determinants of multiple risk factors, fundamental social causes are linked to multiple health outcomes (Link and Phelan 1995). A greater understanding of social inequality in health would be gained by considering an array of health outcomes beyond premature mortality, such as mental health, healthy aging, positive well-being, and incidence of specific diseases. Further gains may be made by examining trends in the effect and impact of the socioeconomic gradient in health over time, although at present such analyses are limited by available data.

Pathways

The manner in which socioeconomic position operates to influence health outcomes has not yet been fully elucidated (Anderson and Armstead 1995; Kaplan 1995a), although it is known that it shapes a wide array of physical, occupational, environmental, behavioral, social, and psychological factors (Krieger et al. 1993; Kaplan 1995b; Link and Phelan 1995; Ross and Wu 1995). Through efforts to understand how social inequalities influence health, we may begin to address some of these health inequalities. It is theoretically possible that the empirical link between socioeconomic position and health reflects merely a spurious association whereby underlying, genetically based factors give rise to both socioeconomic position and health outcomes. Alternatively, the "drift" hypothesis suggests that the effects of socioeconomic position on health may be due to downward mobility among persons in poor health. A variety of research has suggested, however, that these explanations are not satisfactory (Wilkinson 1986; Adler et

al. 1994). Here, we briefly review some of the mechanisms (or pathways), in addition to material deprivation, by which various aspects of socioeconomic position (measured with a variety of markers) may influence health outcomes.

Based on the assumption that education is a critical component of socioeconomic position, the cumulative advantage perspective argues that educational attainment increases resources that accumulate through life, ultimately producing a larger socioeconomic gap in health among older individuals than younger (Merton 1968; Ross and Wu 1996). Ross and Wu (1996) suggest that educational attainment influences more proximate determinants of health. For example, well-educated people are more likely to have more economic resources (full-time jobs, fulfilling work, high incomes) and more social psychological resources (high sense of personal control and social support) and to engage in better health behaviors (more likely to exercise, drink moderately, and receive preventive medical care; less likely to smoke) (Ross and Wu 1995). By accumulating health-promoting resources over time, those with more education are likely to have better health outcomes (Blane 1995; Ross and Wu 1995).

Others have argued that income inequality is itself deleterious for population health (Wilkinson 1996; Kawachi and Kennedy 1997b; Kawachi et al. 1999). In more affluent countries, what seems to predict life expectancy reliably is the extent of relative deprivation, as measured by the size of the income gap between the rich and the poor (Wilkinson 1992; Kawachi and Kennedy 1997b). One's relative socioeconomic position, rather than simply the absolute level, may also be importantly associated with health (Wilkinson 1992; Kawachi et al. 1994). A number of mechanisms by which income inequality influences health have been proposed such as underinvestment in human capital (Kaplan et al. 1996), erosion of social cohesion and social capital (Wilkinson 1996; Kawachi et al. 1997), and the potentially harmful consequences of frustration brought about by relative deprivation (Kawachi et al. 1994).

If different social groups (e.g., black men vs. white women) systematically experience differential health outcomes, it is because their options for living healthy lives are constrained by the fact of—and social processes involved in—perpetuating social inequality. These restricted options are manifested through experiences of discrimination, living and working in adverse conditions, stress, and access to medical care, as well as mediated through a range of social, psychological, cultural, and religious resources that are influenced by membership in these groups (Williams et al. 1994).

Group membership as summarized by the various social categories is associated with a social identity, a set of obligations, and accessibility of resources, which individually or jointly may influence health outcomes. To clarify *how* membership in specific social categories influences health outcomes, we will need to unpack the psychological and social ramifications of category membership and examine their effects on health. For example, psychosocial factors such as feelings of control, hostility, sense of confidence, loneliness, and isolation have shown consistent relationships with both socioeconomic position and health (Adler et al. 1994; Anderson and Armstead 1995). Certain groups (e.g., blacks) are also more likely to experience discrimination (and its attendant stresses), which is known to adversely affect physiological and psychological functioning (Anderson et al. 1989; Krieger and Sidney 1996; Williams et al. 1997). Moreover, individuals with fewer resources may be exposed to greater levels of stress or are more vulnerable to stressors and are therefore more likely to experience adverse health outcomes (Thoits 1982).

Recommendations

We have sought to integrate inequality in the social structure with inequality in health outcomes to give a sense of both the relative unfairness and the burden of poor health in the United States. According to the population perspective, the occurrence of common diseases and exposures reflects the behavior and circumstances of a whole society, and "moderate and achievable change by the population as a whole might greatly reduce the number of people with conspicuous problems . . . as many people exposed to a small risk generate more disease than a few exposed to a conspicuous risk" (Rose 1992). To implement programs that might change the distribution of risk in a population, one must understand the specifics of the population distribution across social conditions and health outcomes (Rose 1992). Our findings suggest that the burden of disease is much larger than the effect of disproportionate ill health on the very poor. Some strategies aimed at moving the entire distribution or reducing disparities may in the end be more effective than those that are focused solely on the tail of the distribution (e.g., those living in poverty). Policies that deal with the growing inequalities in income distribution, for example, may have a considerable impact on health inequalities (Kennedy et al. 1996; Kawachi and Kennedy 1997a). More informed decisions may be made when information on both effect and impact is available.

One key to documenting and evaluating systematically how socioeconomic position, race/ethnicity, gender, and age combine to produce social inequalities in health will be to improve the data available for answering these critical questions. This information will allow us to incorporate into policies an understanding that some gender and racial/ethnic differences are due to socioeconomic position differences, as well as to consider both direct and indirect effects of socioeconomic position. In a recent review, Krieger and colleagues (1997b) make a number of recommendations regarding the measurement of social class and other aspects of socioeconomic position for public health research and surveillance. Among them are recommendations to include consistent measures of socioeconomic position in all public health databases, to use theoretically grounded measures of socioeconomic position with careful consideration of measurement level, to consider contextual effects and multilevel analyses, and to consider pathways by which socioeconomic position and other social factors may influence health. Given the many pathways of influence, it is also vital that policies carefully consider early life versus adult exposures, because early childhood exposures can affect adult life dynamics in terms of achieved social status. Thus, monitoring health status in relation to socioeconomic status is key in the United States as in many other nations.

Policies may also be more effective in improving population health when they take into consideration the entire gradient in health related to family income instead of just the tail. For example, if we use estimates for a family of three in a midsized city in Massachusetts, such a family on welfare and food stamps earns $10,272 a year. The federal poverty level is $13,330. Current policies provide strong incentives to work. If the head of this household succeeds in working and earns minimum wage, then working full time and obtaining income tax credit, she or he will earn $14,017 (Gerwin 1998). Although these earnings put the family about $700 above the poverty line, working is also likely to incur additional offsetting expenses related to transportation, health insurance, and child care. Given that the family remains so near the poverty line, members of a working class family with earnings around minimum wage are still at considerable health risk. This example illustrates how focusing only on the extreme tail of the income distribution, while important, hardly solves the problem related to the observed gradient in mortality, especially among lower-middle class families. The United States lacks policy strategies enabling families to move substantially closer to the median income or even to modest standards of self-sufficiency. Public and private sector policies related to work and family issues may further enable adults to take care of dependents while maintaining long-term work commitments. Other policies related to housing, income tax, and neighborhood revitalization also hold the potential to reduce inequalities in health stemming from social inequalities. A critical next step will be to integrate policy-related disciplines with epidemiological and public health approaches.

In a time of growing income inequality in the United States and other countries, it is all the more important to document contingent inequalities in health so as to spur action to reduce these inequalities and improve health equity. A population perspective may inform research on health equity and social inequalities. Armed with this knowledge, and with a sense of who bears the burden of poor health, we may address the issue of health inequity in a targeted and comprehensive way.

References

Adler N.E., Boyce T., Chesney M.A., Cohen S., Folkman S., Kahn R.L., Syme S.L. 1994. Socioeconomic status and health: the challenge of the gradient. *American Psychologist* 49:15–24.

Anderson N.B., Armstead C.A. 1995. Toward understanding the association of socioeconomic status and health: a new challenge for the biopsychosocial approach. *Psychosomatic Medicine* 57:213–225.

Anderson N.B., Myers H.F., Pickering T., Jackson J.S. (1989). Hypertension in blacks: psychosocial and biological perspectives. *Journal of Hypertension* 7:161–172.

Backlund E., Sorlie P.D., Johnson N.J. 1996. The shape of the relationship between income and mortality in the United States. *Annals of Epidemiology* 6:12–20.

Berkman L.F. 1988. The changing and heterogeneous nature of aging and longevity: a social and biomedical perspective. *Annual Review of Gerontology and Geriatrics* 8:37–68.

Bernstein J., McNichol E.C., Mishel L., and Zahradnik R. 2000. *Pulling Apart: A State-by-State Analysis of Income Trends*. Washington DC: Center on Budget and Policy Priorities and Economic Policy Institute.

Blane D. 1995. Editorial: social determinants of health—socioeconomic status, social class, and ethnicity. *American Journal of Public Health* 85(7):903–904.

Calman K.C. 1997. Equity, poverty and health for all. *British Medical Journal* 314:1187–1191.

Collins J.G., LeClere F.B. 1996. *Health and Selected Socioeconomic Characteristics of the Family: United States, 1988–90*. Hyattsville, MD: National Center for Health Statistics.

Coulter E.J., Guralnick L. 1959. Analyses of vital statistics by census tract. *Journal of the American Statistical Association* 54:730–740.

DeVita C.J. 1996. The United States at mid-decade. *Population Bulletin* 50:2–48.

Duleep H.O. 1995. Mortality and income inequality. *Social Security Bulletin* 58:34–50.

Duncan G. 1996. Income dynamics and health. *International Journal of Health Services*. 26:419–444.

Gerwin C. 1998. How much is enough? *CommonWealth* Fall:13–14.

Guralnik J.M., Fried L.P., Salive M.E. 1996. Disability as a public health outcome in the aging population. *Annual Review of Public Health* 17:25–46.

Haan M.N., Kaplan G.A., Camacho T. 1987. Poverty and health: prospective evidence from the Alameda County Study. *American Journal of Epidemiology* 125:989–998.

Hahn R.A. 1992. The state of federal health statistics on racial and ethnic groups. *Journal of the American Medical Association* 267:268–271.

Hahn R.A., Eaker E.D., Barker N.D., Teutsch S.M., Sosniak W.A., Krieger N. 1996. Poverty and death in the United States. *International Journal of Health Services* 26(4):673–690.

Hobsbawm E. 1996. *The Age of Revolution, 1789–1848*. New York: Vintage Books.

Kaplan G. 1996. People and places: contrasting perspectives on the association between social class and health. *International Journal of Health Services* 26:507–519.

Kaplan G.A. 1995a. Where do shared pathways lead? Some reflections on a research agenda. *Psychosomatic Medicine* 57:208–212.

Kaplan G.A. 1995b. You can't get there from here: understanding the association between socioeconomic status and health requires going upstream. *Advances: The Journal of Mind–Body Health* 11:15–16.

Kaplan G.A., Pamuk E.R., Lynch J.W., Cohen R.D., Balfour J.L. (1996). Inequality in income and mortality in the United States: analysis of mortality and potential pathways. *British Medical Journal* 312:999–1003.

Kawachi I., Kennedy B.P. 1997a. Health and social cohesion: why care about income inequality? *British Medical Journal* 314(7086):1037–1040.

Kawachi I., Kennedy B.P. 1997b. The relationship of income inequality to mortality: does the choice of indicator matter? *Social Science and Medicine* 45(7):1121–1127.

Kawachi I., Kennedy B.P., Lochner K., Prothrow-Stith D. 1997. Social capital, income inequality, and mortality. *American Journal of Public Health* 87:1491–1498.

Kawachi I., Kennedy B.P., Wilkinson R.G. (eds). 1999. *Income Inequality and Health. The Society and Health Population Reader*. New York: The New Press.

Kawachi I., Levine S., Miller S.M., Lasch K., Amick B. 1994. *Income Inequality and Life Expectancy—Theory, Research and Policy*. No. 94-2. Boston: Harvard School of Public Health.

Kennedy B.P., Kawachi I., Prothrow-Stith D. 1996. Income distribution and mortality: cross sectional ecological study of the Robin Hood index in the United States. *British Medical Journal* 312(7037):1004–1007.

Krieger N. 1994. Epidemiology and the web of causation: has anyone seen the spider? *Social Science and Medicine* 39(7):887–903.

Krieger N., Chen J.T., Ebel G. 1997a. Can we monitor socioeconomic inequalities in health? A survey of U.S. health departments' data collection and reporting practices. *Public Health Reports* 112:481–494.

Krieger N., Fee E. 1994. Social class: the missing link in U.S. health data. *International Journal of Health Services* 24(1):25–44.

Krieger N., Rowley D.L., Herman A.A., Avery B., Phillips M.T. 1993. Racism, sexism, and social class: implications for studies of health, disease, and well-being. *American Journal of Preventive Medicine* 9(Suppl 6):82–122.

Krieger N., Sidney S. 1996. Racial discrimination and blood pressure: the CARDIA study of young black and white adults. *American Journal of Public Health* 86:1370–1378.

Krieger N., Williams D.R., Moss N.E. 1997b. Measuring social class in public health research. *Annual Review of Public Health* 18:341–378.

Kunst A. 1997. *Cross-National Comparisons of Socio-economic Differences in Mortality.* Rotterdam: Erasmus University.

Link B.G., Phelan J. 1995. Social conditions as fundamental causes of disease. *Journal of Health and Social Behavior* Spec No:80–94.

Macintyre S., Maciver S., Sooman A. 1993. Area, class, and health: should we be focusing on places or people? *Journal of Social Policy* 22(2):213–234.

Mann J.M., Gruskin S., Grodin M.A., Annas G.J. (eds). 1999. *Health and Human Rights: A Reader.* New York: Routledge.

Marmot M.G., Shipley M.J., Rose G. 1984. Inequalities in death: specific explanations of a general pattern? *Lancet* 1:1003–1006.

Merton R.K. 1968. The Matthew effect in science. *Science* 159: 56–63.

Nagi M.H., Stockwell E.G. 1973. Socioeconomic differentials in mortality by cause of death. *Health Services Reports* 88:449–456.

National Center for Health Statistics. 1997. *Health, United States, 1996–1997 and Injury Chartbook.* Hyattsville, MD: U.S. Government Printing Office.

National Center for Health Statistics. 1998. *Health, United States, 1998.* Hyattsville, MD: U.S. Government Printing Office.

Pappas G., Queen S., Hadden W., Fisher G. 1993. The increasing disparity in mortality between socioeconomic groups in the United States, 1960 and 1986. *New England Journal of Medicine* 329:103–109.

Preston S.H., Haines M.R., Pamuk E. (1981). *Effects of Industrialization and Urbanization on Mortality in Developed Countries.* 19th International Population Conference, Manila, Liege: IUSSP.

Rogot E., Sorlie P.D., Johnson N.J., Schmitt C. (1992). *A Mortality Study of 1.3 Million Persons by Demographic, Social, and Economic Factors: 1979–1985 Follow-Up.* Bethesda, MD: National Institutes of Health.

Rose G. 1992. *The Strategy of Preventive Medicine.* Oxford: Oxford University Press.

Ross C.E., Wu C.-L. 1995. The links between education and health. *American Sociological Review* 60:719–745.

Ross C.E., Wu C.-L. 1996. Education, age, and the cumulative advantage in health. *Journal of Health and Social Behavior* 37:104–120.

Schalick L.M., Hadden W.C., Pamuk E., Navarro V., and Pappas G. 2000. The widening gap in death rates among income groups in the United States from 1967 to 1986. *International Journal of Health Services* 30:13–26.

Seeman T.E., Charpentier P.A., Tinetti M.E., Guralnik J.M., Albert M., Blazer D., Rowe J.W. 1994. Predicting changes in physical performance in a high-functioning elderly cohort: MacArthur Studies of Successful Aging. *Journal of Gerontology: Medical Sciences* 49(3):M97–M108.

Selik R.M., Chu S.Y. 1997. Years of potential life lost due to HIV infection in the United States. *AIDS* 11:1635–1639.

Smeeding T., Gottschalk P. 1997. The international evidence on income distribution in modern economies: Where do we stand? In Neil J. (ed.) *Poverty and Inequality: The Political Economy of Redistribution.* Kalamazoo, MI: W.E. Upjohn Institute for Employment Research, pp. 79–103.

Standing H. 1997. Gender and equity in health sector reform programmes: A review. *Health Policy and Planning* 12(1):1–18.

Susser M., Susser E. 1996. Choosing a future for epidemiology: II. From black box to Chinese boxes and eco-epidemiology. *American Journal of Public Health* 86(5):674–677.

Thoits P.A. 1982. Life stress, social support, and psychological vulnerability: epidemiological considerations. *Journal of Community Psychology* 10:341–362.

United Nations Development Programme (UNDP). 1999. *Human Development Report 1999.* New York: UNDP.

Wagstaff A., Paci P., van Doorslaer E. 1991. On the measurement of inequalities in health. *Social Science and Medicine* 33(5): 545–557.

Wilkinson R.G. 1986. *Class and Health: Research and Longitudinal Data.* London, England: Tavistock.

Wilkinson R.G. 1992. Income distribution and life expectancy. *British Medical Journal* 304:165–168.

Wilkinson R.G. 1996. *Unhealthy Societies: The Afflictions of Inequality.* New York: Routledge.

Williams D.R. 1997. Race and health: basic questions, emerging directions. *Annals of Epidemiology* 7:322–333.

Williams D.R., Collins C. 1995. U.S. socioeconomic and racial differences in health: patterns and explanations. *Annual Review of Sociology* 21:349–86.

Williams D.R., Lavizzo-Mourey R., Warren R.C. 1994. The concept of race and health status in America. *Public Health Reports* 109:26–41.

Williams D.R., Yu Y., Jackson J.S., Anderson N.B. 1997. Racial differences in physical and mental health: Socioeconomic status, stress, and discrimination. *Journal of Health Psychology* 2:335–351.

Wolff E.N. 1995. *Top Heavy: A Study of the Increasing Inequality of Wealth in America.* New York: The Twentieth Century Fund Press.

CHAPTER 10

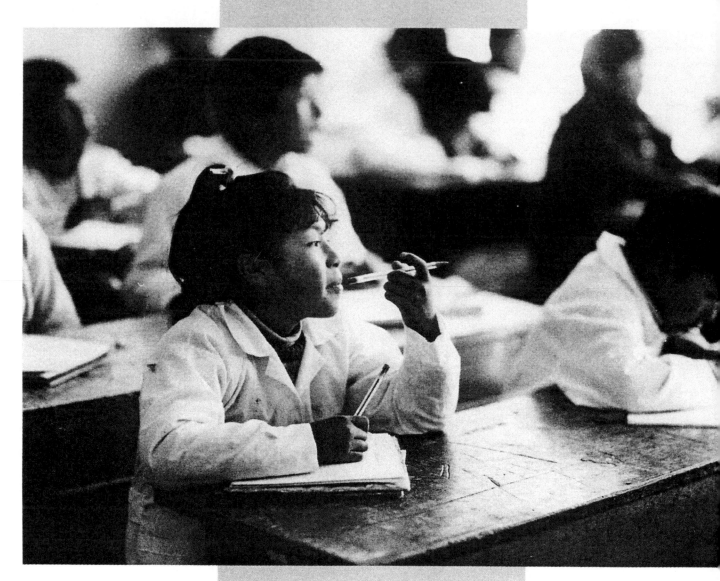

Children from rural community in their
classroom, Chile.
Source: Paul Smith/Panos.

Chile: Socioeconomic Differentials and Mortality in a Middle-Income Nation

JEANETTE VEGA, ROLF DIETER HOLLSTEIN, IRIS DELGADO,
JUAN C. PEREZ, SEBASTIAN CARRASCO, GUILLERMO MARSHALL,
AND DEREK YACH

In Chile, rapid social and economic change, combined with relatively high-quality health data, provides an important opportunity to study the relationship between socioeconomic status and mortality in a middle-income country. Although aggregate economic and social indicators are improving at the national level, there is disturbing evidence of widening socioeconomic gaps in income and health. The main hypothesis of this chapter is that, despite overall economic growth and improvement in aggregate health status, health inequalities are large and widening in Chile. This increase is temporally related to broadening income inequalities associated with the structural economic reforms and marketization over the last 15 years. Of particular relevance for broader social policies, however, the trend of widening health inequalities is tempered by the strong role of educational attainment in improving adult life expectancy. In light of the changing macroeconomic context, this chapter examines recent evidence on the factors underlying health inequalities in Chile through both individual-level and ecological-level analyses.

Economic Growth and Poverty

The Chilean economic model has been cited as an example of development to be followed by other nations because of the country's strong and sustained economic growth in the 1980s and 1990s (over 5% per year in the average annual gross domestic product [GDP] growth rate for 1991–1996) (ECLAC 1997; UNDP 1998). Not only was Chile the first country in the American region to embark on a structural economic reform process (begun in 1981), but its reform program has also been the most radical. Since the mid-1980s Chile has experienced sustained, fast-paced growth. At the same time, social expenditure as a percentage of GDP increased (from 13.1% in 1990–1991 to 13.4% in 1994–1995), and the unemployment rate diminished from 11.7% in 1980 to 7.0% in 1996. The poverty level has been halved from 45% of the population in 1987 to 23% in 1996.

Since 1980, Chile has been administratively decentralized into 13 political and administrative regions from north to south, which are subsequently divided into provinces and counties (of which there are 335). A Governor named by the President and a council with representatives from different community and regional organizations constitute the local government in each of these regions. The mission of the regional government is to promote the social, cultural, and economic development of the region and to administer the annual budget that is allocated as a percentage of the national government's budget. In addition, each region receives annually a percentage of the total budget for public investment, which constitutes the Regional Development Fund.

Chile

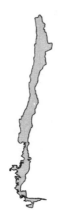

Total population (millions), 1997	14.6
Human development index, 1999	0.844
Human development index rank, 1999	34
Infant mortality rate (per 1,000 live births), 1997	11
Real GDP per capita (PPP$), 1997	12,730
Public spending on health as percentage of GDP, 1995	2.3

Source: UNDP 1999. [Human Development Report]

Those critical of the Chilean model point to increasing inequalities in income distribution. There has been a slow but persistent erosion in the income share of the poor. In 1996, the poorest decile of the population earned 1.4% of the total income while the richest claimed over 40% of the total income. Thus, despite economic growth and declining poverty rates, the skew in income distribution has worsened considerably since the onset of reforms. Thus, the high levels of income inequality prevalent in the mid-1980s have persisted, while a significant decline in poverty is derived mainly from economic growth (UNDP 1998).

Education and Employment

With the demise of Pinochet's military government and the arrival of democracy in 1990, education became the foremost priority on the social agenda. Social consensus was reached on the importance of educational reform, both as a mechanism to equalize social opportunities and as means to increase Chile's international competitiveness. Since 1990, the government has doubled its spending on public education and has restructured the educational curriculum to decrease the gap in the educational quality between public and private schools. For example, national standardized examinations were implemented after the fourth and eighth grades in a representative sample of public and private schools, and computers (and, later, Internet access) were brought into the schools. Private schools in Chile currently account for only 8% of the total, while 57% are municipal and 35% are private schools subsidized by the government, usually in areas where the municipal government cannot meet the educational demands of its population.

Data from the periodic national household survey of a nationally representative sample, CASEN (Encuesta de Caracterizacion Socioeconomica Nacional), indicate that between 1987 and 1994 both the relative and absolute differences in mean educational attainment for the extreme income quintiles decreased. Mean educational attainment (in years of education) in the poorest quintile increased by 12.3% over this period, while the richest quintile improved by 5.2%. Nonetheless, it should be recognized that in 1994 the poorest quintile achieved only 7.3 years of formal schooling while the richest had almost double that at 12.2 years.

Currently, 40% of the population are economically active. Of these, 94% are employed and 6% are unemployed. Since the mid-1980s the duration of employment has increased to 4.5 years on average, and the length of time unemployed has decreased to 3 months, suggesting more employment stability. Most of those unemployed are concentrated in the poorest income quintile, among women, and in the younger age groups.

A strong correlation between education, occupation, and income has been documented in Chile. A recent analysis of the periodic household survey (CASEN 1996) demonstrated a close correlation between mean income and years of formal education. Additionally, increases in income level were more pronounced upon completing high school and upon leaving the university. Education is also closely associated with occupational category; each occupational category has a specific educational profile, which is, in turn, associated with income level.

Health Status in Chile

Half of Chile's population is concentrated in two of the country's 13 political and administrative regions—Valparaíso and metropolitan Santiago—which represent only 4% of the national territory. The population density is lowest in the extreme north and south of the nation. The average annual population growth was

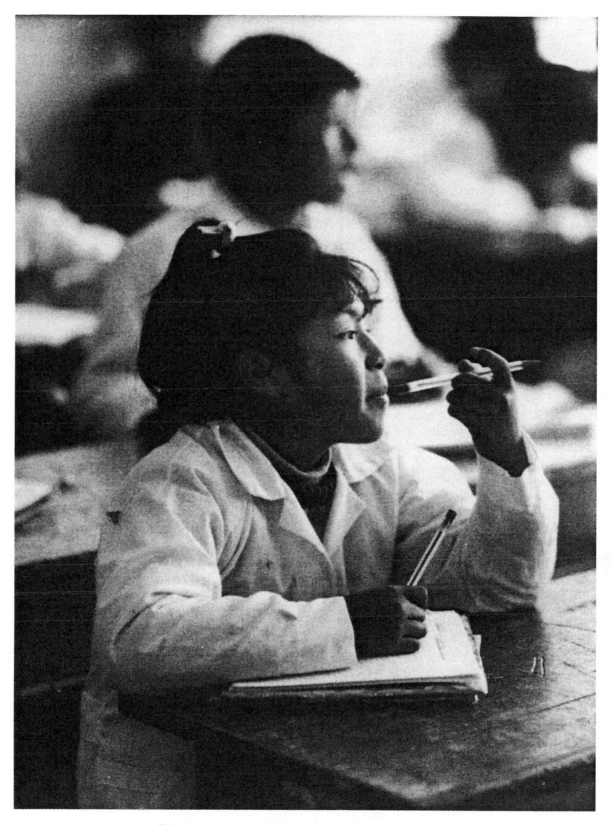

Children from rural community in their classroom, Chile.
Source: Paul Smith/Panos.

1.7% during the period 1985–1990 and 1.6% for the period 1990–1995, a decrease due mainly to lower fertility coupled with low immigration.

Overall health indicators, such as life expectancy and infant mortality rate, have consistently improved in the last 20 years. Infant mortality rate has decreased from 32 per 1000 live births in 1980 to 11.1 per 1000 live births in 1996 (INE 1998a,b) and life expectancy has increased from 67.4 years in 1980 to 74.4 in 1996. It is, however, unclear whether all socioeconomic groups have benefited equally from these improvements.

The leading causes of mortality are diseases of the circulatory system, which taken together account for 58% of all deaths. Malignant neoplasms rank second overall and first among women. Mortality from infectious diseases and perinatal complications has declined over time, as have the rates for metabolic, endocrine, and nutritional disorders, mainly due to the decrease in diabetes mortality. Injuries, accidents, and violence have become increasingly serious problems and now rank high among the causes of death and hospitalizations. The chronic diseases most often reported by the population are cardiovascular diseases, especially arterial hypertension, rheumatic diseases (particularly back problems and joint disease), diabetes mellitus, chronic bronchitis, mental disorders, peptic ulcer, and epilepsy (MINSAL 1998).

The objective of this study is to examine the extent to which educational attainment functions as a causal mechanism distributing the burden of premature mortality and stratifying life expectancy. By using both individual analysis as well as ecological analysis, the study incorporates a multilevel design. The study design is a comparison of national "unlinked" cross-sectional mortality studies for three periods and ecological analysis of life expectancy by county for the period 1988–1996. The analysis that follows examines trends in life expectancy and mortality based on individuals grouped by educational level, using comparable estimates from three points in time. The study subsequently develops an ecological analysis of life expectancy by county level and sex for the period 1988–1996.

Results

Individual Analysis:
Education and Life Expectancy

The average number of years of education attained has increased in the adult Chilean population between 1985 and 1996. As Table 1 shows, there has been an increase in the relative share of the population in the upper two education groups for males and females. Accounting for the increase in the population size, the absolute number of people in the upper three education groups increased, while the group without education decreased in both relative and absolute terms. Comparing males and females over the period, does not provide clear evidence of a systematic gender gap in education in Chile.

Table 2 shows the temporary life expectancy between ages 20 and 69 years for males and females by educational level (see Box 1). Life expectancy between 20 and 69 years of age has increased for both sexes over the period, 0.4 years for women (47.4 to 47.8 years) and 0.5 years for men (45.1 to 45.6 years). Less-educated persons have a lower temporary life expectancy than better-educated persons, and these differences have progressively increased from 1985–1987 through 1994–1996: from 6.3 to 8.7 years for men and from 3.6 to 4.5 years for women (see Table 2). In general, temporary life expectancy in higher educational groups increased with time and declined in the lower educational groups. For males in the group without education, it decreased by 2.0 years, while the highest educated groups advanced by 0.4 years. Female temporary life expectancy in the group without education decreased by 0.3 years, while this measure for the more educated group increased by 0.6 years. Put another way, males in the lowest educational group suffered a decline in this indicator more than six times that of females in the lowest educational group over the period measured.

Gender differentials in temporary life expectancy are actually much higher at lower levels of education (see

Table 1 Adults age 20 and older by education level in Chile, 1986, 1991, and 1995

(percent)

Years of schooling	1986	1991	1995
Men			
0	6.1	4.8	3.9
1–8	50.2	45.6	41.7
9–12	32.7	25.5	37.4
13 or more	11.0	14.1	17.0
Women			
0	7.2	5.8	4.7
1–8	50.8	46.5	42.5
9–12	33.1	34.8	35.6
13 or more	8.9	12.9	17.2

Source: National Institute of Statistics, Chile.

Table 2 Temporary life expectancy among adults age 20–69 by education level in Chile, selected years, 1985–96
(years)

Years of schooling	1985–87	1990–92	1994–96	Change 1985–96
Men				
0	41.5	40.7	39.5	–2.0
1–8	44.8	44.7	44.7	–0.1
9–12	45.1	45.4	45.6	0.5
13 or more	47.7	47.8	48.1	0.4
Total	45.1	45.4	45.6	0.5
Gap between groups with most and least education	6.3	7.2	8.7	2.4
Women				
0	44.9	44.5	44.6	–0.3
1–8	47.3	47.5	47.6	0.3
9–12	47.9	47.9	47.9	0.0
13 or more	48.5	48.7	49.1	0.6
Total	47.4	47.5	47.8	0.4
Gap between groups with most and least education	3.6	4.2	4.5	0.9

Source: National Institute of Statistics, Chile.

BOX 1: METHODS USED IN THE INDIVIDUAL ANALYSIS

Cause of death data based on the International Classification of Disease (version nine) for the period 1985–1996 along with annual population projections based on the censuses from 1982 and 1992 (INE CELADE 1995) were used to assess age-, sex-, and cause-specific death rates for the population 20 years and older for three periods, 1985–1987, 1990–1992, and 1994–1996. These period death rates were linked to "years of education attained" (none, 1–8, 9–12, and 13 or more) (National Institute of Health Statistics). People under the age of 20 years were excluded from this study because of the dynamic level of the education variable in the school-going population.

Based on these mortality rates, probability of dying, life expectancy at different ages, temporary life expectancy between ages 20 and 69 years, and mortality rates directly ad-

justed to the 1992 Chilean male and female populations were computed for persons over 20 years of age (Reed and Merrell 1975). Abbreviated life-tables were calculated based on an initial cohort of 100,000 survivors as recommended by Greville (1946) and (1984). Temporary life expectancy (e20–69) can be interpreted as a function of the probability of dying between the ages of 20 and 70 years (Shkolnikov et al. 1998). It represents the average number of years that a fixed population, between ages 20 and 70 years, is expected to live, assuming its current age-specific death probabilities. Its value is less than life expectancy at age 20 years given that it does not take into account those who live and die after age 70 years. The use of temporary life expectancy, however, allows for international comparisons with countries where life expectancy is not as high as it is in Chile.

Table 3 Female-male gap in temporary life expectancy among adults age 20–69 by education level in Chile, selected years, 1985–96 (years)

Years of schooling	1985–87	1990–92	1994–96	Change 1985–96
0	3.44	3.87	5.11	1.67
1–8	2.51	2.78	2.90	0.39
9–12	2.74	2.46	2.27	–0.47
13 or more	0.82	0.89	0.96	0.14
Total	2.27	2.11	2.24	–0.03

Source: National Institute of Statistics, Chile.

Table 3). There is a 5.1 year gender gap in 1994–1996 among those without education compared with a 1 year difference for those with 13 or more years of approved education. With the exception of the 9 to 12 year educational strata, the gender gap in health for each educational level has also increased over time. Because of the shift of the population distribution to more highly educated groups, which in turn have smaller gender gaps, the total gender gap in health is more or less constant. This increasing educational inequality in health for both men and women over time is illustrated in Figure 1 (see also Box 2). There is a clear inverse relationship between educational level and life expectancy which becomes more accentuated in the last period. Furthermore, the disproportionate health gains for women at high levels of education and the sharp declines for men without education are readily apparent in the Figure 1.

Age-specific causes of death and their contributions to explaining the life expectancy gap between the highest and lowest educational strata are presented in Figures 2 and 3. These figures depict both males and females in the first and final time periods of this study, 1985–1987 to 1994–1996. Among men, external causes are the leading contributors to the life expectancy differences in all ages up to the 55–59 year

---

BOX 2: MEASURES OF HEALTH INEQUALITY

Both absolute and relative measures of health inequality are used: the life expectancy rate difference (LERD) of lowest versus highest educational level and the population attributable life lost index (PALL %) (Shkolnikov 1998; Mackenbach and Kunst 1997). The population attributable life lost index, conceptually equivalent to the population attributable risk (PAR) (see chapter 5), can be interpreted as the proportional increase in overall life expectancy that would occur in the hypothetical case in which everyone experiences the life expectancy of the highest educational or occupational group.

To further compare differences across groups, life expectancies corresponding to different education levels were plotted against the midpoint for the relevant percentile of the subgroup, with the population ordered from low to high educational status (Pappas et al. 1993; Wagstaff et al. 1991). The lowest educational level is plotted at the midpoint on the abscissa of the graph. The proportion of the population in each higher education group is added and plotted at the respective midpoints. For example, the lowest educational level among males for the period 1985–1987 comprises 6.2% of that group, and its life expectancy (47.5 years) is therefore plotted at 3.1 on the x-axis. The proportion of the population in each higher educational group is added and plotted at the respective midpoints (Pappas et al. 1993; Wagstaff et al. 1991). With this procedure it is possible to plot on the same scale the distributions and ranges of education that differ both for the study periods and between subgroups of the population (see Fig. 1). The plots make adjustments for increasing units of educational attainment by creating a relative scale for each subgroup to assure that changes in population size alone are not responsible for an apparent increase in inequality. To measure the effect of education on general mortality and cause-specific mortality, the Arriaga method of analyzing life expectancy by age and cause was utilized (Arriaga 1984; see also chapter 5). The method allows the splitting of differences in life expectancy between extreme socioeconomic—in this case, educational—groups into contributions of different ages and causes.

Figure 1 Life expectancy at age 20 by education level in Chile, selected years, 1985–96

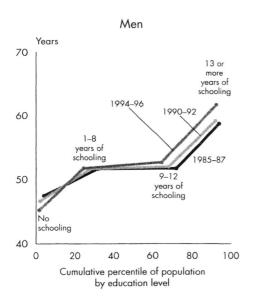

Men

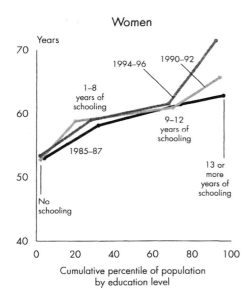

Women

Note: To compare differences across groups, life expectancies corresponding to different education levels are plotted against the midpoint for the relevant percentile of the subgroup, with the population ordered from low to high education status (Pappas and others 1993; Wagstaff and others 1991). The lowest education level is plotted at the midpoint on the abscissa of the graph. The proportion of the population in each higher education group is added and plotted at the respective midpoints. The plots make adjustments for increasing units of educational attainment by creating a relative scale for each subgroup to ensure that changes in population size alone are not responsible for an apparent increase in inequality. (For a full explanation see Box 2.)
Source: National Institute of Statistics, Chile.

age group in 1985–1987, contributing 46% of the total gap in life expectancy by educational level. The same is true in 1994–1996, when external causes are also the main cause of life expectancy inequality at all ages among men except the 65–69 year age group (see Fig. 3). Motor vehicle accidents account for the gap in life expectancy due to external causes and have increased over the time period in all educational groups, especially in the lower educational strata. In contrast, suicides and homicides decreased in frequency in all educational groups. Respiratory causes are the second largest contributor to the gap in life expectancy for both periods at younger ages (up to 44 years of age), replaced by digestive at middle ages (45–54 years of age) and cardiovascular in men older than 54 years.

The absolute difference in number of years of life expectancy between extreme educational groups increased for all causes during the period, except for neoplasms and ill-defined causes. The increase is more accentuated for cardiovascular, from 0.37 to 0.62 year of life expectancy difference, and digestive, from 0.45 to 0.79 year of life expectancy difference.

For women, external causes are also a leading factor accounting for the gap in life expectancy by educational level (at *younger* ages during 1985–1987 and at *all* ages for the period 1994–1996) (see Figs. 2 and 3). The main contributor to the *total* gap in life expectancy at all ages in the first period, however, was cardiovascular disease (18%). In the first period, external causes contributed only 9% of the *total* gap in life expectancy by educational level. By 1994–1996, however, external causes accounted for 15% of the total difference in life expectancy between extreme groups, becoming the leading cause of inequality in life expectancy among women. The contribution of external causes to the difference in life expectancy between educational groups more than doubled from 0.3 to 0.7 year. This increase is mainly related to the increase in motor vehicle accidents in the three lower educated strata and a decrease in the most educated level. "External" as the leading cause was followed by respiratory causes at younger ages, neoplasms at middle ages (35–40 years) and cardiovascular diseases after 45–49 years of age. Gall bladder and cervical cancer are the most important contributors to the overall educational gap in life expectancy for cancers and stroke for cardiovascular causes.

In summary, the analysis of the gap in temporary life expectancy by cause highlights several important trends (see Figs. 3 and 4) in Chile: First, external causes are becoming an increasingly important stratifier of adult life expectancy in both men and women; second, overall differentials in mortality between extreme educa-

Figure 2 Cause-specific decomposition of difference in temporary life expectancy between adults with the most and least education, by sex and age group, in Chile, 1985–87

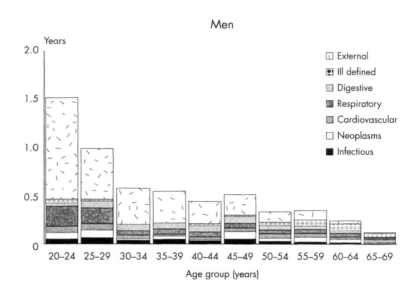

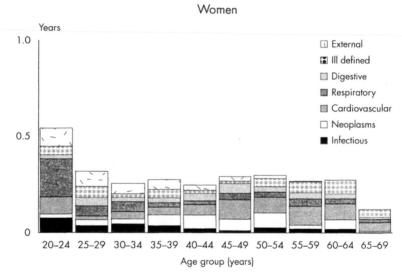

Note: Total difference in temporary life expectancy between the education groups is 6.25 years for men, 3.63 years for women.

Source: National Institute of Statistics, Chile.

tional groups are attributable largely to gaps at younger ages, particularly in men; and finally, cardiovascular disease contributes surprisingly little to the overall gap between educational groups for men, whereas for women it is significant, particularly at middle ages.

Table 4 presents several measures of life expectancy distribution by sex and educational strata for the periods 1985–1987, 1990–1992, and 1994–1996. While

the overall life expectancy improved over these years, all measures of inequality *increased* in both males and females for the extreme groups. The temporary life expectancy rate difference increased from 6.3 to 8.7 years between periods for men and from 3.6 to 4.5 years for women. The population attributable life lost index, or PALL % (a measure of the absolute rate of increase in the overall life expectancy that would occur when

Figure 3 Cause-specific decomposition of difference in temporary life expectancy between adults with the most and least education, by sex and age group, in Chile, 1994–96

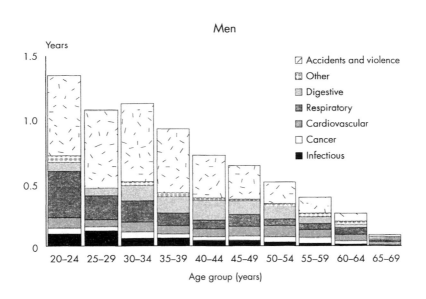

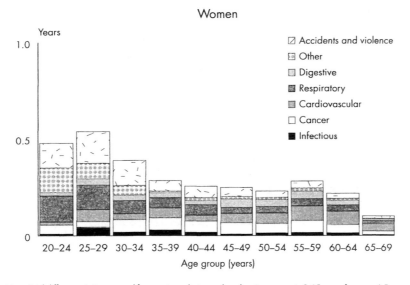

Note: Total difference in temporary life expectancy between the education groups is 8.65 years for men, 4.5 years for women.

Source: National Institute of Statistics, Chile.

everyone has the life expectancy of the highest educational group), increased from 2.8 to 3.4 years for men and from 1.4 to 1.8 years for women. In other words, if everyone had the life expectancy of the highest group in the population, then overall life expectancy would have increased by 3.4 years for men and 1.8 years for women for the period 1994–1996 compared with 2.8 and 1.4, respectively, for the earlier period, 1985–1987.

Ecological Analysis

Our ecological analysis allowed the comparison of counties with regard to inequalities in socioeconomic conditions and health status (see Box 3). The analysis of life expectancy at the county level reveals that male life expectancy at birth ranges over a span of 19.6 years, from 64.1 to 83.7 years. For females, life expectancy

Figure 4 Distribution of counties by average life expectancy at birth by sex in Chile, 1988–96

(239 counties and county clusters)

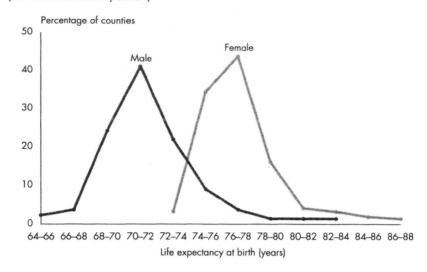

Source: National Institute of Statistics, Chile.

ranges over a span of 14.4 years, from 73.3 to 87.7 years. The range of life expectancy is greater for males than for females, a phenomenon that has been documented in the United States as well (Murray et al. 1998). It is striking that even within the same city there are counties in which the average life expectancy is 8.5 years shorter than that in a neighboring affluent county. Counties with a high life expectancy are either the most affluent, with a very small percentage of population below the poverty line, or are closed, isolated rural communities. Counties with the lowest life expectancy have very high levels of poverty, and in counties with low female life expectancy, a higher than average percentage of the population is indigenous.

Table 5 presents the results of regression models fitted to explain variance in life expectancy at birth for males and females.

Results show that the models that best describe inequalities in life expectancy for men and women include the following variables: percentage of the population economically active, percentage of the population that is rural and mean years of education. The predictive values are quite high: an R^2 of 0.478 for females and an R^2 of 0.415 for males. The beta values associated with education are higher than those of the other predictor variables, including occupational status. In other words, the average number of years of education is a strong predictor of county inequality in mortality.

Table 4 Summary measures of inequality in temporary life expectancy among adults age 20–69 by education level in Chile, selected years, 1985–96

	Men			Women		
Indicator	1985–87	1990–92	1994–96	1985–87	1990–92	1994–96
Temporary life expectancy (years)	45.1	45.4	45.6	47.4	47.5	47.8
Temporary life expectancy rate difference (years)[a]	6.3	7.2	8.7	3.6	4.2	4.5
Population attributable life lost index (percent)	6.0	7.0	7.0	2.0	3.0	4.0
Population attributable life lost (years)	2.8	3.0	3.4	1.4	1.5	1.8

a. Shows the difference in life expectancy between the groups with the most and least education.
Source: National Institute of Statistics, Chile.

Table 5 Coefficients from linear regression analysis of life expectancy, by sex, in Chile, 1988–96

(239 counties and county clusters)

Explanatory variable	Male life expectancy at birth	Female life expectancy at birth
Constant	52.48 (35.01)	62.11 (52.07)
	1.499	1.193
Percentage economically active	0.214 (7.4)	0.164 (7.1)
	0.029	0.023
Percentage rural	0.056 (7.8)	0.032 (5.6)
	0.007	0.006
Mean years of education	0.844 (7.6)	0.752 (8.5)
	0.112	0.089
R^2	0.415	0.478

Note: Coefficients show the relationship between the explanatory variable and life expectancy. The t-values are in parentheses. The standard errors are given below the coefficients.
Source: Authors' calculations.

BOX 3: METHODS USED IN THE ECOLOGICAL ANALYSIS

Ecological, or small area analysis, was performed using data from the 335 Chilean counties to assess the relative importance of various living conditions and social context variables in explaining variance between counties in life expectancy at birth. Life-tables by county and sex were calculated using the mortality files for the 9 year period 1988–1996. Small counties (less than 11,000) persons were merged with adjoining areas leading to 239 counties and county clusters, each with its own life-table. The following variables reflecting county-level social context were derived from the 1992 census and the annual household survey (CASEN 1996):

- Percent of population economically active
- Percent of population that is rural
- Ratio of the percentage of the population over 65 years to the percentage of the population less than 15 years
- Percentage of households in extreme poverty (defined as a lack of basic needs and more than three dependents per worker younger than 45 years old and with no more than

8 years of education; or more than three dependents per worker older than 45 years old and with no more than 2 years of education)
- Average (mean) education level—derived from the total number of years of education attained among those aged 20 years and older and divided by the total number of persons aged 20 years and older
- Percentage of households with unmet basic needs (defined by any of the following: overcrowding; no running water, electricity, or sewage facilities; lack of proper floor or walls)
- Percentage of population without education, with 1 to 8 years, 9 to 12 years, or 13 or more years of approved education

These indicators of county-level social context were used as independent variables in a model of county-level life expectancy using ordinary least squares regression techniques. County age structure was incorporated into the regression model in order to control for its confounding effect.

Discussion

Before the main findings of this study are discussed, several important methodological issues should be noted. First, the fact that the data on socioeconomic position used to calculate the numerator and denominator for specific mortality rates come from two different sources—death certificates and census data—may lead to a numerator–denominator bias. Such a bias results from the fact that the classification of educational or occupational level varies systematically according to the source, a problem that has been widely discussed elsewhere in the literature (Shkolnikov et al. 1998). As in other countries, there is a tendency in Chile to overestimate the level of education in both the census data and death certificates (Solis 1990), with a larger overestimation in the latter. Therefore, this bias would have the effect of underestimating the relationship between educational level and mortality risk. The knowledge that the probability of bias can be minimized using aggregated categories (Shkolnikov et al. 1998) led us to aggregate our data into four broad educational categories and 3 year time periods. In Chile, the classification of educational categories does not differ between the census and the death certificates, with a similar percentage of under-registration of population and deaths (1.4%), a fact that also minimizes the biases that can arise from using different data sources.

Next, we address our choice of social stratifier—education. In Chile, education is a better predictor of health status than occupation at the individual and aggregate levels in part because of the much better quality of educational data. Preliminary analyses of our data showed that the Chilean national mortality databases are not adequate for valid analyses of mortality by occupational class on an individual level. Therefore we did not use occupational categories for the analysis of individual deaths.

Finally, it is important to note that our ecological analysis did not include a health service variable. Our preliminary analyses did not show a correlation between health outcomes and variables related to medical care, such as the number of annual medical visits per 1000 inhabitants, distribution of public and private insurance, and coverage of vaccination and Pap smears. These findings are in agreement with what has been previously reported by Concha and Aguilera (1999).

Summary of Main Findings

From the results of the individual-level analysis, it can be seen that in Chile, as in many other countries, longevity in adults is strongly linked to level of educational attainment. In all three time periods studied, there is a strong stepwise improvement in survival probability with increasing educational attainment. Moreover, this gradient, or level of educational inequality, appears to be increasing with time. The adult life expectancy gap across extremes in educational achievement increased from 6.3 to 8.7 years for men and from 3.6 to 4.5 years for women between 1985 and 1996.

A closer look at the nature of the increasing gaps reveals that, distressingly, the adult life expectancy of those with the lowest levels of educational attainment actually fell. As such, longevity benefits are disproportionately concentrated in the highest educational classes. This divergence between extreme educational groups has previously been documented in Russia by Shkolnikov et al. (1998). In fact, it is the shift in the distribution of the population to higher education levels that accounts for this apparently paradoxical effect. If the education distribution were held constant over the study period, then overall life expectancy would also have remained constant (Vega et al. 2000).

This finding has profound implications, for it suggests that education is an effect modifier in the relationship between life expectancy and income. If, hypothetically, the education level of the Chilean population had remained the same, a much lower improvement in life expectancy would have occurred despite economic growth and an increase in the absolute income of all groups. In fact, between 1985–1987 and 1994–1996 temporary life expectancy (20–69) increased by 0.40 and 0.44 year for women and men, respectively. If the educational distribution is held constant during that period, however, the increases are only 0.22 and 0.07 year, that is, 44% and 84% less, respectively, than it would have been without adjustment.

More fundamentally, however, it is worth considering why, in the context of Chilean macroeconomic reforms, aggregate health outcomes are improving while inequalities in health are increasing. Integral to our analysis is the understanding that inequalities in health indicators reflect not just inequalities in *health care*, but the *entire conjunction of socioeconomic factors* that lead to health and disease. In the language of Diderichsen's conceptual framework (see chapter 2), it is clear that the "social context" in Chile has changed considerably. As described at the beginning of this chapter, macroeconomic reforms have been successful in expanding the economy, halving the rate of poverty, and maintaining constant levels of public expenditure for social programs. A major exception to this trend has been the priority accorded to education as exemplified by a doubling of public expenditure and the implementation of major reforms in the last 9 years. As shown in Table 1, this investment has been associated with a relative and absolute shift toward higher levels of education in the population. Other things equal, it is reasonable to assume that these are macro trends that have helped to improve population health. In fact, the county-level analysis supports the particular importance of mean educational levels and higher employment as important predictors of higher county life expectancy. Notably, poverty levels and percentage of the population with unmet needs did not explain variation in county life expectancy. This raises the possibility, as suggested elsewhere in the literature (Kawachi et al. 1997; Kennedy et al. 1998; Wilkinson 1992, 1994, 1997), that declines in relative poverty, rather than absolute poverty, may be more strongly related to health.

It is clear that the macroeconomic reforms in Chile were accompanied by increasing income inequality; however, it is unclear what, if any, health impact may have arisen from this trend. Macroeconomic processes of reform (economic, health, welfare, and educational) have swept through Chile in the last decade. In this contextual framework (see chapter 2) only educational policy has been an exception in the implementation of marketization-dominated policies. In the last two democratic governments, education has been the top priority on the social agenda. The government has doubled the public expenditure on education over the last 9 years and has implemented a major reform of the public education system. The effect of the structural reform in the country has been the widening of income disparities. The improvement of the educational distribution has, however, offset the potentially adverse health effects of increasing economic inequities. This issue has strong policy implications, which are considered below.

Although untangling the balance of social contextual factors and their relative contributions to health will require further analysis, this study through individual and ecological analysis unambiguously establishes that education, whether measured at the individual or the community level, is a very strong predictor of longevity. This association between education and health has long been recognized, yet an understanding of the precise mechanisms by which education affects health remains somewhat of a mystery. Educational attainment, especially that of women, affects many aspects of life that, in turn, influence the risk of mortality. Health and education are linked through family income, reproductive patterns, employment status, use of health services, healthy lifestyles (including nutrition, tobacco use, and exercise), and a greater sense of empowerment. In other words, education is a critical building block of what is referred to as "human capital" (Anand and Ravallion 1993).

Beyond conjecture, however, the decomposition of the educational extremes in life expectancy provides some insights into the health hazards of lower educational attainment and the health dividends of higher attainment. The first observation is that the education effect does not respect different causes of death, but rather trespasses with abandon. An inverse gradient between education level and age-specific mortality was found for all major causes of disease. Second, the education gap in life expectancy is highest for young men and women and decreases progressively with age. This reflects, in part, the very strong age association with external causes of death (primarily motor vehicle accidents), which is the major explanation for the gap between high and low educational groups' mortality rates for both men and women. Third, the increase in the overall gap from 1985–1987 to 1994–1996 is reflected across all major causes of death except neoplasms and ill-defined causes.

These observations of the pervasive and growing ill effects of low educational attainment argue for a hypothesis of generalized susceptibility, as opposed to one of differential exposures (see chapter 2). It may be, however, that the greater susceptibility of the poorly educated is related to a cluster of specific exposures—environmental, behavioral, psychosocial, and limited access to services.

Education, Gender, and Health

Inequality by gender reveals that even though females have a higher life expectancy than males, the difference in the average life expectancy of men and women is decreasing. When looking at the differences between extreme educational groups it is clear that inequality in life expectancy is much wider for males. In other words, the gradient in health outcomes is flatter for women than it is for men. Furthermore, inequality in life expectancy is increasing for both sexes, but for different reasons. For women, inequality in life expectancy is increasing primarily due to the improvement of life expectancy in the highest socioeconomic level, with the lowest educational level decreasing in life expectancy of 0.3 year during the period. For men, inequality in life expectancy is increasing mainly because of the greater reversal in life expectancy in the two lowest educational groups (−2.0 years for those with no education and −0.1 year for those with 1 to 8 years of education). These complex changes deserve further scrutiny in terms of the disease-specific causes that underlie the gaps in adult life expectancy between educational groups.

Gender-specific analysis of causes of death are also important markers for policy. Contrary to what is generally perceived, the contribution of cardiovascular diseases to educational inequalities in life expectancy appears to be relatively high for Chilean women. This may be due to the high prevalence of hypertension in the female population in Chile. Hypertension has been found in a population-based study in Valparaiso, Chile, to be related to socioeconomic conditions (Vega et al. 1998). The study showed that while the global prevalence of hypertension in the general population aged 25 to 64 years was 11.4%, the prevalence was 14.2% in the lowest socioeconomic level (compared with 9.3% in the highest socioeconomic group). This represents a 52% higher risk of hypertension associated with marginal socioeconomic conditions. The high relative levels of cardiovascular disease in women of middle ages and the relatively large contribution of respiratory illness in young males provide a highly specific analysis of the components of the gap in temporary life expectancy with important links to public health intervention possibilities.

Policy Implications

Addressing social context
If Chilean reforms are to succeed in improving the quality of life of all inhabitants, they must take into account income inequalities in the design and implementation of social policies in education, health, and other sectors. Social policies must be oriented so as to overcome the direct effect of increasing income inequalities. The evidence in this chapter points to the highly significant role of education in mediating income inequalities and protecting against even wider health inequalities than those that have emerged. The fact that education has been identified as such a critical mediating social variable in Chile is highlighted by the plight of those with no education—a group that is actually faring worse in terms of premature mortality than they were 10 years ago. The identification of the decrease in health status in less educated groups should guide policy and resource allocation toward improving education and facilitate access to care among more uneducated groups, especially in the younger population. Furthermore, although occupational gradients were not measured in this study, the role of labor policies and unemployment protections should not be overlooked when addressing social context and policy.

Modifying individual behavior
Specific risks related to unhealthy behaviors, such as smoking and alcohol use, were not directly assessed in this study due to their absence in the type of routine data available in the vital statistics. The cause of death analysis, however, points to potential points of entry for further research or pilot projects to reduce behavioral risks. It is quite clear that motor vehicle accidents are the leading contributors to deaths by external causes in both sexes in Chile (INE 1998a,b; MINSAL 1998). This finding should promote the development of policies oriented to reduce the incidence of road traffic accidents, with a particular focus on younger age groups.

The findings that neoplasms are the greatest contributor to the gap in life expectancy in middle aged women and that cardiovascular diseases are the main contributor to the gap in older males and females should lead to better targeted policies of screening and treatment for both. Prevention and treatment programs should also focus on the leading cancers in women, gall bladder and cervical, and on preventive measures such as screening and early detection of hypertension and other risk factors for cardiovascular diseases in both genders.

Monitoring counties and rethinking allocation formulas
Changes in health status and health inequalities in Chile will require policies that affect the combination of individual *and* contextual factors. The identification of geographical inequalities in small areas should guide equity-oriented policies at the municipal and regional level to decrease the unacceptable health status differences that persist despite aggregate gains. From this point of view, it is important to continue undertaking analyses at the county level, especially in light of the progressive decentralization process in Chile, a process that has included the reallocation of resources for health care and education. Educational programs aimed at decreasing the existing educational gap among counties are of particular importance, given the strong relationship between education and health status that has been found at both the individual and aggregate level. Policies to redress inequities might include the allocation of resources for health and education based on equitable formulas that take into account social disparities and the development of specific policies to reinforce their local governments. Such resource alloca-

tion schemes have been implemented in the United Kingdom and Sweden (Diderichsen et al. 1997). Periodic (or continuous) monitoring of those counties with higher needs will track progress toward or away from greater equity.

The future equity research agenda for Chile includes further elucidation of the pathways through which social position, inequalities in education, occupation, and income influence health outcomes. Furthermore, the relationships among these factors, and in particular the influence of social context and social position on individual risk factors, deserve further study.

References

Anand S., Ravallion M. 1993. Human development in poor countries: on the role of private incomes and public services. *Journal of Economic Perspectives* 7(1):133–150.

Arriaga E. 1984. Measuring and explaining the change in life expectancies. *Demography* 21(1):83–96.

CASEN. 1996. *Resultados de la Encuesta de Caracterización Socioeconómica Nacional.* Santiago, Chile: Ministerio de Planificación.

Chiang C.L. 1984. *The Life Table and its Applications.* Malabar, FL: R.E. Krieger.

Concha M., Aguilera X. 1999. Enfoque epidemiológico de la desigualdad en Salud. *Revista Chilena de Salud Pública* 1:43–52.

Diderichsen F., Varde E., Whitehead M. 1997. Resource allocation to health authorities: the quest for an equitable formula in Britain and Sweden. British Medical Journal 315:875–878.

ECLAC (Economic Commission for Latin America and the Caribbean). 1997. *The Equity Gap: Latin America, the Caribbean and the Social Summit.* Santiago, Chile: United Nations.

Greville T.M.E. 1946. *United States Life Tables and Actuarial Tables 1939–1941.* Washington, DC: United States Department of Commerce, Bureau of the Census.

INE (Instituto Nacional de Estadísticas). 1998a. *Compendio Estadístico.* Santiago, Chile: INE.

INE. 1998b. *Anuario de Demografía y Causas de Muerte.* Santiago, Chile: INE.

INE CELADE (Instituto Nacional de Estadísticas, Centro Latinoamericano de Demografía). 1995. *CHILE: estimaciones y proyecciones de población por sexo y edad. Total País: 1950–2050,* LC/DEM/R.217, Serie OI No. 97, Santiago, Chile: INE CELADE.

Kawachi I., Kennedy B., Lochner K., Prothrow-Stith D. 1997. Social capital, income inequality and mortality. *American Journal of Public Health* 87(9):1–8.

Kennedy B.P., Kawachi I., Glass R., Prothrow-Stith D. 1998. Income distribution, socioeconomic status, and self-rated health in the United States: multilevel analysis. *British Medical Journal* 317: 917–921.

Mackenbach J.P., Kunst A.E. 1997. Measuring the magnitude of socioeconomic inequalities in health: an overview of available measures illustrated with two examples from Europe. *Social Science and Medicine* 44:757–771.

MINSAL (Ministerio de Salud). 1998. *Tarjeta de Presentación Situación de Salud.* Santiago, Chile: MINSAL.

Murray C., Chen L. 1993. In search of a contemporary theory for understanding mortality change. *Social Science and Medicine* 36(2):143–155.

Murray C.J.L., Michaud C.M., McKenna M.T., Marks J.S. 1998. *U.S. Patterns of Mortality by County and Race: 1965–1994.* Centers for Disease Control and Harvard School of Public Health. Cambridge, MA: Harvard Center for Population and Development Studies.

Pappas G., Queen S., Hadden W., Fisher G. 1993. The increasing disparity in mortality between socioeconomic groups in the United States, 1960 and 1986. *New England Journal of Medicine* 329(2):103–109.

Reed J., Merrell M. 1975. *Un método rápido para la construcción de una tabla de vida abreviada.* CELADE. Serie D, No. 49, Santiago, Chile: CELADE.

Shkolnikov V. 1998. Class-based measurement of inequalities in length of life. Paper presented at the Global Health Equity Initiative Workshop on Measuring Inequalities in Health, Oxford, England.

Shkolnikov V.M., Leon D.A., Adamets S., Andreev E., Deev A. 1998. Educational level and adult mortality in Russia: an analysis of routine data 1979 to 1994. *Social Science and Medicine* 47(3): 357–369.

Solis F. 1990. Mortalidad por causas en los servicios de salud del país y factores de nivel de vida asociados. Tesis para obtar al grado de Magister en Bioestadística, Escuela de Salud Pública, Universidad de Chile.

UNDP (Programa de las Naciones Unidas Para el Desarrollo). 1998. *Desarrollo humano en Chile 1998. Las Paradojas de la Modernización.* Santiago, Chile: Editorial Trineo.

United Nations Development Programme (UNDP). 1999. *Human Development Report 1999.* New York: UNDP.

Vega J., Hollstein R., Delgado I. 2000. *Social Science and Medicine* (in submission).

Vega J., Jadue L., Escobar M.C., Espejo F., Delgado I., Garrido C., et al. 1998. Hipertensión arterial en Chile: resultados encuesta de base programa CARMEN. *Revista Médica de Chile.*

Wagstaff A., Paci P., van Doorslaer E. 1991. On the measurement of inequalities in health. *Social Science and Medicine* 33: 545–557.

Wilkinson R.G. 1992. Income distribution and life expectancy. *British Medical Journal* 304:165–68.

Wilkinson R.G. 1994. The epidemiological transition: from material scarcity to social disadvantage. *Daedalus* 123(4):61–77.

Wilkinson R.G. 1997. Health inequalities: relative or absolute material standards? *British Medical Journal* 314:591–595.

CHAPTER 11

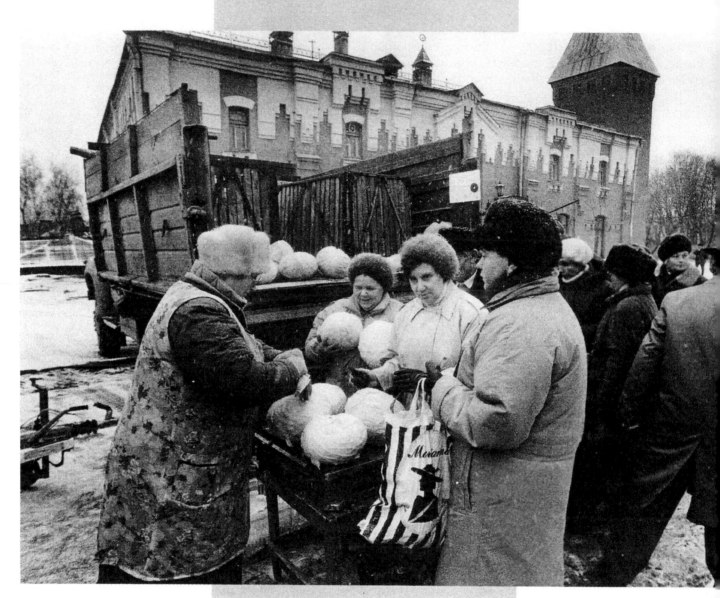

Selling cabbages directly to consumers,
Old Market, Kostroma, Russia.
Source: Heidur Netocny/Panos.

Russia: Socioeconomic Dimensions of the Gender Gap in Mortality

VLADIMIR M. SHKOLNIKOV, MARK G. FIELD, AND EVGUENIY M. ANDREEV

Old women there were lots, but few old men.
The things that bent old women broke old men.

Boris Slutsky (1999)

In Russia, the historical widening of the gender gap in mortality was associated with a radical reduction in infectious diseases and infant deaths from the beginning of the twentieth century to the mid-1960s. There was a particularly rapid reduction in mortality in the decade after World War II, due in large part to the introduction of antibiotics and subsequent reduction in mortality due to infection. Between 1896 and 1964 the difference in life expectancy at birth between men and women increased from 2 to nearly 9 years, while life expectancy at birth increased from 31 to 64 years for men and from 33 to almost 73 years for women (Shkolnikov and Meslé 1996). As in other countries, this major change was related to a reduction in women's health hazards, which had characterized the low social status of women in Russian society, namely, high fertility, low hygienic standards, and poor maternal and medical care.

Since 1965, however, overall mortality in Russia has increased. This unusual pattern is due to rising mortality rates among adults, both men and women, from cardiovascular diseases, external causes of death (acci-

dents and violence), and lung cancer (Meslé and Shkolnikov 1995). By 1996, life expectancy at birth in Russia had dropped below 60 years for men and below 73 years for women. The gaps in life expectancy at birth between Russia and the West have widened to 12 to 13 years for men and 7 to 8 years for women due in part to continuous progress in the West and in part to significant deterioration in Russia.

Although both sexes in Russia have experienced an obvious worsening of their health status since 1965, the rise in mortality has been substantially steeper among men. The gender gap in life expectancy at birth had exceeded 13 years by the mid-1990s and was at a level approximately double that of other industrialized countries and about 4 years greater than it was in Russia in the 1960s.

This chapter provides a systematic analysis of data on temporal, socioeconomic, and spatial variations in gender-specific mortality indices of the Russian population from 1965 to 1996. It covers two rather different periods of recent Russian history. During the first period, a time of "stagnation" between 1965 and 1984, socioeconomic growth in Russia was continuing (albeit slowly) in terms of industrial production, population incomes, and consumption. This development, however, coincided with gradually increasing problems in public health and a slow decrease in life expectancy at birth associated with a variety of factors including med-

Russia

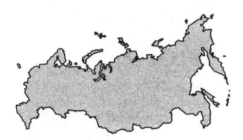

Total population (millions), 1997	147.7
Human development index, 1999	0.735
Human development index rank, 1999	71
Infant mortality rate (per 1,000 live births), 1997	17.2
Real GDP per capita (PPP$), 1997	4071
Public spending on health	
as percentage of GDP, 1995	4.3

Source: UNDP 1999. [Human Development Report]

ical care, peculiarities of socioeconomic policies, and health behaviors (Okolski 1993; Field 1995). A further strain on the economy and the well-being of the population was an enormous increase in defense expenditures at the expense of the civilian sector after the 1964 removal of Nikita Khrushchev. From 1952 to 1959 according to recent CIA estimates, the annual percentage increase in Soviet defense spending was 0.4. From 1960 to 1969 that figure increased to 5.7, a more than 14-fold jump. From 1970 to 1974 it was 3.3 (Firth and Noren 1998).

The second period, between 1985 and 1996, was especially remarkable because of three extraordinary events in Russian society; the anti-alcohol campaign of 1985 (Shkolnikov and Nemstov 1997), the disintegration of the Soviet Union in 1991, and the "shock" liberalization of prices in 1992 followed by other market-oriented changes in socioeconomic policies. These events were associated with striking changes in Russian mortality patterns.

The government of Secretary General Mikail Gorbachev launched an ambitious anti-alcohol campaign in May 1985 consisting of a set of administrative, economic, judicial, and medical measures that led to a forced, rapid decrease in the production and consumption of alcoholic beverages. A twofold drop in officially registered alcohol sales and a 25% to 30% reduction of alcohol consumption were achieved between 1985 and 1987 (Nemtsov 1995; Treml 1997).

In December 1991, the presidents of Russia, Ukraine, and Belarus declared that the Soviet Union had ceased to exist. Fifteen new countries were formed. Several lo-

cal wars and armed ethnic conflicts occurred between 1990 and 1996 in former Soviet regions. Soviet industry was decentralized, and many economic links were truncated, causing long-lasting negative consequences for the economies of the newly independent states.

The liberalization of prices and termination of state subsidies in many sectors of the economy were launched by the Government of Prime Minister Egor Gaidar at the beginning of 1992, in the midst of an acute crisis of Russia's command economy. Liberal monetary and macroeconomic measures were not balanced by satisfactory social policies. In a short period, these measures led to galloping inflation, an explosive rise in consumer prices, and abrupt labor market shocks. This led to a twofold drop in real income, significant declines in consumption of goods and services, the almost complete liquidation of people's savings, the spread of poverty, and a rise in income inequalities. Our analysis will show which "responses" in the mortality of Russian men and women were associated with these social experiments.

Highly significant differences in sociocultural backgrounds, behaviors, and living conditions among different social groups are associated with the higher or lower risks of dying among men and women from various causes (Whitehead and Diderichsen 1997). A consideration of these multiple differentials enables us to see the gender gap in mortality rates from a variety of angles and to suggest factors underlying the overall and gender-specific worsening of health in Russia.

This chapter is divided into three sections. The first describes general trends in life expectancy at birth for men and women for the period 1965 to 1996. It shows how they diverge from the trends observed in other countries and explores the pattern of ages and causes of death responsible for widening the gender gap in life expectancy at birth in Russia. The second section focuses on the mortality of men and women by socioeconomic and sociodemographic group (education, occupation, and marital status) for the years around the population census of 1989 and the microcensus of 1994. It analyzes the variations across these groups in terms of overall levels of mortality, length of life, and gender. The third section examines the steep increase in mortality in the early 1990s. It considers changes in the structure of the gender gap in mortality with respect to causes of death and educational, regional, and urban/rural divisions of the Russian population. Finally, we summarize and discuss the findings, addressing the reasons for such a high gender gap in mortality in Russia, given the fact that both men and women tend to be exposed to the same general macroscopic conditions, whether political, social, or economic.

Data and Methods

The present study relies on a variety of statistical data, including results of censuses, particularly of the last all-Soviet Union census of 1989 and the all-Russia microcensus of 1994. In Russia population data are recorded through routine statistics. The Goskomstat, or State Statistical Committee of the Russian Federation, produces these data on an annual basis and includes differences in mortality and life expectancy by residence (urban vs. rural population) and among 84 (out of the total of 89) administrative regions ("oblasts" or autonomous republics of the Russian Federation).

The state statistical system permits a study of differentials in mortality according to educational, occupational, and marital status using only population censuses (or representative microcensuses). When calculating death rates, the numbers of those who died during a calendar year classified by sex, age, and social group (from death certificates) are used as the numerator, and corresponding population numbers (from population censuses) are used as the denominator.

This approach to evaluating mortality indices by social strata has an important shortcoming. It does not guarantee a fully accurate correspondence of the data on the population with the data on deaths because the mortality information, received from the relatives of a deceased person, may differ from self-identification on the census questionnaires (Valkonen 1993). Despite the potential problem of numerator–denominator bias, however, the method of "unlinked" estimation has been used productively to further our understanding of socioeconomic differences in mortality in many countries, including the United States (Buell et al. 1960; Kitagawa and Hauser 1973; Christenson and Johnson 1995), New Zealand (Pearce and Howard 1986), Finland (Nayha 1977), Hungary (Valkonen 1989), and Poland (Brajczewski and Rogucka 1993). The problem of the numerator–denominator bias has been extensively studied in Britain, with its history of decennial analyses of occupational and social class mortality. Comparisons have been made of the magnitude of social class differences derived from this approach and those derived from a longitudinal, record linkage study based on a 1% sample of the population of England and Wales enumerated at the 1971 and subsequent censuses. These comparisons have shown that such biases as may exist are unlikely to seriously distort estimates of the social class effects (Goldblatt 1989). This is particularly so when a few broad socioeconomic categories are used (Marmot and McDowall 1986). Such aggregation thus seems to be one way to reduce numerator–denominator bias, as has been done for Hungarian data (Carlson 1989).

In the present study, we use very broad categories for education and occupation, classifying the population into those who have received university and secondary specialized education (upper educational class) and those who have secondary, incomplete secondary, and lower level education (lower educational class). For occupational analysis, the population is divided into those who are nonworking and working. The latter category is divided, in turn, into white-collar and blue-collar workers. The range of ages under consideration is restricted to the age intervals of 20 to 69 years for education and 20 to 64 years for occupation.

Another concern may be related to a problem of the validity of "male-oriented" occupational categories for women. Although the data available in Russia do not give an opportunity to use alternative classifications for women's sociooccupational positions (e.g., according to husband's status), we argue that this type of bias in Russia is likely to be smaller than that in western countries.

Life expectancies within respective ranges of ages or "temporary" life expectancies (for details, see Arriaga 1984) and probabilities of surviving from lower to upper age limits of the same intervals are used as aggregate mortality measures for sociodemographic groups.

The "component analysis" method is used to estimate contributions of ages and causes of death to overall differences in life expectancy between genders or population groups (Andreev 1983; Arriaga 1984; Pressat 1985). We also use simple correlation statistics to measure the strengths of associations between variations of life expectancies, or of changes in life expectancies, by region.

Results

General Trends and Gender Differences in Life Expectancy

Table 1 traces temporal changes in the life expectancy at birth in Russia, Eastern Europe, the European Community, and the United States since 1970. Continuous progress in Western Europe and the United States clearly contrasts with long-term stagnation (or very little progress) in Eastern Europe and deterioration in Russia. Between 1970 and 1984, the life expectancy at birth in Russia decreased by 1.3 years for men and by 0.5 year for women. Between 1985 and 1987, there was a remarkable short-term increase in life expectancy by just over 3 years for men and just over 1 year for women due to the anti-alcohol campaign (Shkolnikov and Nemtsov 1997). Between 1988 and 1991, life expectancy decreased gradually, remaining at an unusu-

Table 1 Life expectancy at birth in Russia, Eastern Europe, the European Union, and the United States, selected years, 1970–96

(years)

Year	Russia		Eastern Europe		European Union		United States	
	Male	Female	Male	Female	Male	Female	Male	Female
1970	63.0	73.5	66.3	71.9	68.6	74.9	67.1	74.7
1980	61.4	73.0	66.8	73.6	70.7	77.5	70.0	77.4
1984	61.7	73.0	67.1	74.1	71.8	78.6	71.2	78.2
1987	64.9	74.3	67.2	74.0	72.6	79.3	71.5	78.4
1991	63.6	74.4	66.8	74.9	73.2	80.0	72.0	78.9
1992	62.0	73.8	66.9	75.1	73.5	80.3	72.3	79.1
1993	59.0	71.9	67.2	75.3	73.6	80.3	72.2	78.8
1994	57.5	71.1	67.2	75.4	74.0	80.6	72.4	79.0
1995	58.2	71.8	67.3	75.6	74.0	80.7	72.6	78.9
1996	59.8	72.5	67.5	75.6	74.4	81.0	73.1	79.1

Eastern Europe comprises Albania, Bulgaria, the Czech Republic, Hungary, Poland, Romania, Slovakia, and the former Yugoslavia (Bosnia-Herzegovina, Croatia, Macedonia, Serbia and Montenegro, and Slovenia).

Source: For Russia, authors' analysis; for Eastern Europe and the European Union, World Health Organization 2000; for the United States, Centers for Disease Control and Prevention, 2000.

ally high level before dropping sharply between 1992 and 1994 to below 58 years for men and 71 years for women. Between 1995 and 1996, there was some recovery, and life expectancy increased to values characteristic of the early 1980s.

The gap in life expectancies between Russia and western countries has widened dramatically since the 1970s. Indeed, comparing male and female life expectancies at birth in Russia in 1970 and 1994, with the U.S. or average values of the European Community

countries, one can see that in 1970 the difference was 4 to 5 years for men and 1 to 1.5 years for women, while by 1994 it had grown to 15 to 16 years and 8 to 9 years, respectively. A comparison of life expectancy trends of Russian men with those of Russian women is, in fact, a comparison of two very unfavorable evolutions—both show an unprecedented deterioration, unique in the industrialized world.

Figure 1, however, also shows a steady increase in the gender gap in life expectancy from the early 1960s

Figure 1 Gender gap in life expectancy in Russia, 1961–96

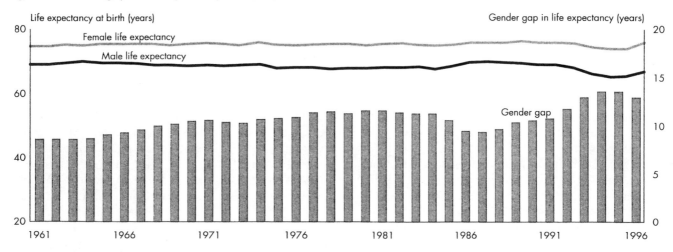

Source: Goskomstat 1997; authors' analysis.

Figure 2 Life expectancy at birth, by sex, and GNP per capita in selected countries, 1995–96

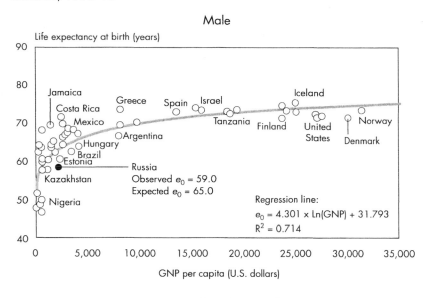

Male

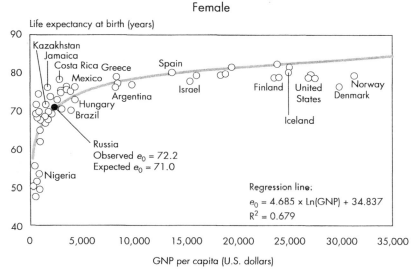

Female

Note: e_0 is life expectancy at birth.
Source: Buchet 1997.

onwards, a considerable short-term reduction in the gap attributable to Gorbachev's anti-alcohol campaign in 1985–1987, and then a steep increase in the gap that reached its apogee in 1995. Between 1965 and 1984, the widening of the gap was primarily a result of a worsening of male life expectancy, whereas female life expectancy remained at approximately the same level. The most recent abrupt deterioration was very substantial for both sexes, although much greater for males than for females. The decrease in life expectancy between 1991 and 1994 for women (just over 3 years) was about half of that for men (nearly 7 years).

In Figure 2, male and female life expectancies at birth are plotted against per capita gross national product (GNP) in 1995–1996 for 52 countries. It is well known that the relationship between these two variables across countries is a classic logarithmic function (Preston 1976; United Nations 1982). For men, the Russian position is worse than expected on the basis of per capita GNP because the observed value of the life expectancy at birth is 59 years, while the expected value is 65 years. The observed value of life expectancy at birth for women, however, is slightly better than expected (72.2 vs. 71 years; see Fig. 2). This suggests that women's life expectancy corresponds to the relatively poor level of overall "development" in Russia, while the men's figure is substantially worse than one might expect. In 30 years, the overall gender gap grew from 9 to 13.5 years, due largely to steeper increases in male mortality rates from ages 20 to 70 years, while the role of gender differentials in mortality rates among children and the elderly was much less marked. Among those of working age, the ratios of male to female mortality rates were three- to fivefold in the early 1990s. In terms of causes of death, the greatest contributions to the overall gender gap in life expectancy at birth were cardiovascular diseases (middle and older aged) and accidents and violent causes (younger adults). Excess mortality of men from cancers also contributes considerably to the overall gender gap; however, the widening of the gap over time does not result significantly from cancer (for more details, see Shkolnikov et al. 1996).

Social Gradients in Mortality and the Gender Gap

Education

Table 2 shows life expectancies between the ages of 20 and 69 years for four educational categories. At the time of the census of 1989, the gap in life expectancy between the upper educational class (combining university, incomplete university, and secondary specialized educational levels) and the lower educational class (combining secondary, incomplete secondary, and lower educational levels) was about 4 years for males and about 1 year for females. The gap between the two extreme limits of the range, that is, university educa-

tion versus incomplete secondary, primary, and lower education, was greater than 5 years for males and about 2 years for females. In 1989, these differentials are equivalent to a 9% reduction in the male mortality rate and a 7% reduction in the female mortality rate for each additional year of education (Shkolnikov et al. 1998b).

Interestingly, mortality rates among Russian people with university education 20 to 69 years of age are close to mortality rates for general western populations. For example, in 1989, life expectancy within the age range of 20 to 69 years was nearly 46 years in Russia for men with higher and incomplete higher education and nearly 46 years for the general male population in France. A comparison of age- and cause-specific components of the educational differential in life expectancy for the age range of 20 to 69 years within the Russian male population (university education vs. lower education) with respective components of the gap between the general French and Russian male populations suggests that the educational differential within Russia is in many ways similar to the intercountry differential. Not only are the magnitudes of the gaps the same (4.8 and 4.7 years), but the structures of the gaps by age and cause of death are also rather similar. The structure of the Russian educational gap in life expectancy for age 20–69 is shown in Figure 3. As is true in the France and Russia comparison, the role of accidents and violence is overwhelming among adults under age 45 years, while among those aged 45 to 69 years chronic diseases play the main role.

Gender differences in life expectancy in Russia vary inversely with the level of education (see Table 2). In the population as a whole, the gender gap in life ex-

Table 2 Temporary life expectancy among adults age 20–69 by education level and sex in Russia, 1989
(years)

Education level[a]	Women	Men	Difference
University and			
incomplete university	48.04	45.60	2.44
Secondary specialized	47.69	44.14	3.55
Secondary	46.33	40.76	5.57
Incomplete secondary, primary,			
and incomplete primary	45.65	39.44	6.21
Total	47.04	42.01	5.03

a. Higher (university) and incomplete higher education is 13–17 years in length, secondary specialized education is 12–14 years, secondary education is 10–11 years.
Source: Shkolnikov, Leon, Adamets, Andreev, and Deev 1998.

Figure 3 Difference in temporary life expectancy (age 20-69) between men with university education and men with secondary and lower education by age and cause of death in Russia, 1989

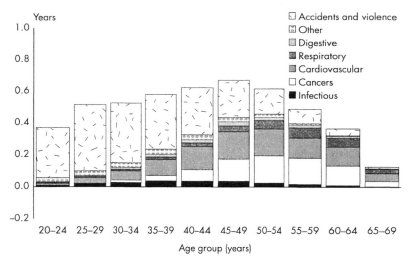

Note: Total difference is 4.8 years.
Source: Goskomstat 1997; authors' analysis.

pectancy (ages 20 to 69 years) was 5 years in 1989; among those in the upper educational class (university and incomplete university, and secondary specialized education), it was only 3 years, while for the lower educational class (secondary and incomplete secondary, primary, and incomplete primary), it was almost 6 years. This suggests that excess mortality of men is concentrated to a large extent among the least educated population groups.

Occupational groups

Table 3 presents the life expectancies within the range of ages 20 to 64 years by occupational category for 1988–1989. The group of nonworking people has an extremely high mortality rate. According to the 1989 census, this group constituted 14% of the working-age population. In the late 1980s, there was no official unemployment in Russia and real unemployment, although it existed, was very low. In the 1980s for those under the retirement age (60 years for men and 55 years for women), chronic diseases, disability, and early retirement due to difficult working conditions were the main reasons for not working for the state. This finding corresponds with the fact that in 1989 the difference in mortality rates between working and nonworking people was much smaller in the 20- to 24-year-old age group than at older ages (due to a greater number of students aged 20 to 24 years). A more detailed analysis of causes of death (not given here) shows that high mortality in the nonworking population was due primarily to chronic diseases such as cancers, circulatory and infectious diseases, while external causes

Table 3 Temporary life expectancy among adults age 20–64 by occupational category and sex in Russia, 1988–89

(years)

Occupational category	Women	Men	Difference
White collar	44.19	42.72	1.47
Blue collar	43.14	39.77	3.37
Not working	38.96	30.23	8.73
Total	43.41	40.15	3.26

Source: Goskomstat 1997; authors' analysis.

(accidents and violence) played a relatively minor role. Overall, it is likely that the very high mortality rate among nonworking people in 1988–1989 was due largely to the fact that many of them were not working because of health problems.

The difference in mortality rate between white- and blue-collar workers is also large (see Table 3). From 1988 to 1989 the gap in life expectancy between exact ages 20 and 65 years was 3 years for men and 1 year for women. For both men and women, the majority of the gap in life expectancy between white-collar and blue-collar workers (aged 20 to 64 years) was due to accidents and violence at ages 20 to 50 years. This contrasts considerably with the gap between working and nonworking people, which was primarily due to chronic diseases.

As expected, in 1988–1989, the gender gap in life expectancy between exact ages 20 to 65 years was the smallest for the white-collar workers (1.5 years). It was far smaller than the gender gap for the blue-collar workers (3.4 years) and for the nonworking population (8.7 years).

Marital status

As in many other countries, the most notable mortality difference in Russia in 1988–89 occurred between those married and those never married (Table 4). The magnitude of this difference is probably linked to the high prevalence of marriage in Russia (82% of men are married, although this proportion declines for women to 48% by age 70 years, due to widowhood). Those not conforming to this norm may not have married due to health reasons.

The next highest mortality rate is observed among the widowed. Death rates are extremely high among those widowed at ages 25 to 29 years, and especially ages 20 to 24 years, when widowhood is rare. At these ages, widowhood and death are probably caused by the same event: an accident in which one spouse dies and the other lives only a short time longer. The difference in mortality between those married and those divorced is very significant for men and *not* significant for women.

The age-specific contributions to the overall differences between the married and the other marital status categories are at a maximum at ages 55 to 59 years for men and at ages 60 to 64 years for women. The difference in temporary life expectancy between married and divorced women is an exception because the maximum is not very pronounced and occurs at ages 50 to 54 years. Hence, mortality differences, linked to marital status, are wider among older age groups compared with the differences by educational level or occupational category.

In 1988–1989, the gender gap in mortality was greatest for the widowed and those never married (a difference of 9.4 years of life expectancy between exact ages 20 and 70 years for both groups), followed by the divorced (7.1 years), and then the married (4.1 years).

Steep Increase in Mortality in the Early 1990s

The life expectancy at birth in Russia decreased by 6.5 years for men and by 3.5 years for women between 1989 and 1994, mostly in the period 1992–1994. Analyses of changes in mortality patterns in the early 1990s tend to focus on a consideration of their links with prior trends and particularly with the short-term improvement due to the anti-alcohol campaign of 1985 (Meslé and Shkolnikov 1995; Shkolnikov et al. 1996; Leon et al. 1997; Avdeev et al. 1997). Other studies discuss possible reasons for and mechanisms of the re-

Table 4 Temporary life expectancy among adults age 20–69 by marital status in Russia, 1988–89 (years)

Marital status	Women	Men	Difference
Married	47.44	43.31	4.13
Never married	43.97	34.62	9.35
Widowed	45.48	36.08	9.40
Divorced	47.16	40.05	7.11
Total	47.11	42.52	4.59

Source: Goskomstat 1997; Shkolnikov et al. 2000.

cent health crisis (Field 1995; Shapiro 1995; Nemtsov 1995; Ryan 1995; Cornia 1997; Shkolnikov et al. 1998a). In summary, these findings suggest that the mortality upsurge cannot be attributed to absolute deprivation, collapse of the health system, or environmental degradation. Instead, psychological stress caused by the shock of an abrupt and painful economic transition most likely played a major role, largely mediated by the adverse health effects of alcohol abuse (Shkolnikov et al. 1998a; Shkolnikov and Cornia 2000). More specific knowledge about the origins of the stress and the mechanisms of its influence has not been achieved, however, mainly because detailed individual-level data are lacking.

Let us consider several particular aspects of the recent mortality increase, examining structural similarities and dissimilarities of changes in male and female mortality indices by age, principal cause of death, sociodemographic group, urban and rural residence, and region.

Changes by cause of death in the early 1990s

It has already been noted that between 1989 and 1994 the decrease in the life expectancy of men was almost twofold greater than that of women. Consequently, the gender gap in life expectancy at birth grew from 10 years to almost 14 years between 1989 and 1994 (see Fig. 1). In 1994, an overwhelming part of this gap was due to the differences in mortality rates between men and women aged 20 to 65 years from accidents and violent (external) causes and from cardiovascular diseases (Fig. 4). By comparing the causes of death associated with the gap due to excess mortality of males from different causes in 1989 to the equivalent causes in 1994, one can see that the contribution of external causes has increased from just over 3 years to nearly 5 years, and the contribution of cardiovascular diseases has also increased from 3 to 5 years. In proportional terms, the relative contribution of cardiovascular diseases in the total gender gap in life expectancy at birth was stable (about 33%), the contribution of cancers decreased from 18% to 12%, and those of respiratory (8%), digestive diseases (3%), infectious diseases (2.5%) and residual causes (3.5%) were approximately constant, whereas the contribution of accidents and violent causes increased substantially from 32% to 38% between 1989 and 1994.

The patterns of male–female differences in age-specific mortality rates for the years 1989 and 1994 are shown in proportional terms (Fig. 5) and in absolute terms (Fig. 6). Surprisingly, the male–female ratios of age-specific mortality rates do not differ much between 1989 and 1994. They are somewhat higher in 1994 for ages 45 to 75 years and somewhat higher in 1989 for young adults aged 20 to 30 years. Overall, this means that proportional increases in mortality rates were rather similar for both sexes, a puzzling observation first reported by Leon et al. (1997). This contrasts with a striking increase in gender gap in life expectancy in 1992–1994 and can be explained by the nature of life expectancy as an aggregate mortality measure. Life expectancy is much more sensitive to the same proportional increases in higher age-specific mortality rates (males) than in lower age-specific mortality rates (females). In terms of standardized mortality rates (standardized to the WHO European Standard Population), the increase in overall mortality in 1992–1994 for men was somewhat greater than that for women: 36% versus 24%, respectively. Figure 6 shows clearly that the absolute difference in age-specific mortality rates between men and women grew very significantly between 1989 and 1994. Certainly, it led to a widening of the gender gap in life expectancy and in absolute numbers of deaths.

Changes with respect to social groups in the early 1990s

One of the most important questions is whether the steep increase in mortality in Russia between 1992 and 1994 affected all sections of the population equally, regardless of social status. The fact that a full census has not been conducted since 1989 makes answering this question quite difficult. In February 1994, however, a microcensus was conducted that covered a representative 5% sample of the Russian population. From this, it has been possible to obtain estimates of the population denominator by education, although only for the age group "16 and over." Using these data to provide a midperiod denominator for deaths occurring in 1993–1994, we have estimated mortality rates by educational class and compared them with equivalent estimates for 1988–1989 (based on the 100% census in 1989). Adjusting for age, mortality in the upper and lower educational classes among those aged 16 years and older was found to have increased between 1988–1989 and 1993–1994, although the increase among both men and women was largest in the lower educational group (see Table 5). Therefore, the results given in Table 5 cannot be directly compared with the above results obtained with the help of direct standardization. Here the indirect method of standardization is utilized to yield the standardized mortality ratios. It appears that during the period of momentous change in Russia, including the collapse of the Soviet Union in 1991

Figure 4 Female-male difference in life expectancy at birth by age and cause of death in Russia, 1989 and 1994

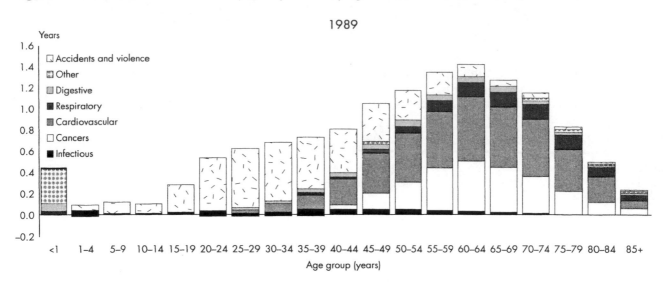

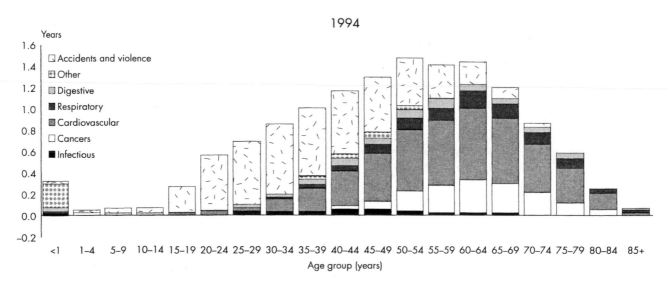

Note: Total difference in 1989 is 10.4 years, and in 1994, 13.5 years.
Source: Goskomstat 1997; authors' analysis.

and the beginning of the "shock" reforms toward a market economy, educational differences in mortality widened very significantly for both men and women. Indeed, if the level of mortality of the overall male population in 1988–89 is taken as 100, then the difference between upper and lower educational groups increased from 43 in 1988–89 to 82 in 1993–94. For females this educational gap increased from 32 in 1988–89 to 58 in 1993–94.

Table 5 also shows a remarkable dissimilarity between men and women with respect to mortality in-creases in the upper educational class. The increase for women was moderate (8%), while the equivalent increase among men was as large as 35%, although it was significantly smaller than that among men with lower education (57%). Overall, the mortality increase in the early 1990s was concentrated among the least educated, and the degree of this concentration was probably greater among women.

This finding is in line with another piece of evidence, based on an analysis of 450,000 death certificates issued in Moscow between 1993 and 1995 (Chenet et al.

Figure 5 Ratio of male to female age-specific mortality rates in Russia, 1989 and 1994

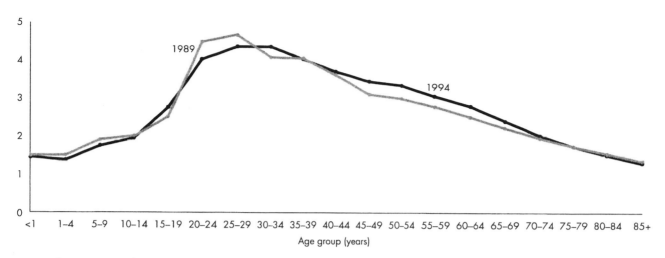

Age group (years)

Source: Goskomstat 1997; authors' analysis.

1998). Significantly elevated proportions of deaths due to accidents, violence, and alcohol-related causes were associated with lower educational and occupational status for both men and women. For women, however, these socioeconomic gradients were steeper. This analysis permits an assumption that in the early 1990s the *relative* increase in mortality among women with lower status was greater than that among men with lower status.

Changes with respect to the urban/rural divide in the early 1990s

The long-term increase in mortality in Russia between 1965 and 1980 was greater among men living in rural areas (Table 6). Because of this, the difference between urban and rural male life expectancies grew from 1.5 years at the end of the 1960s to 3 years by the end of the 1970s. For women, the urban/rural difference remained comparatively small, although there was a

Figure 6 Male-female difference in age-specific mortality rates in Russia, 1989 and 1994
(per 100,000)

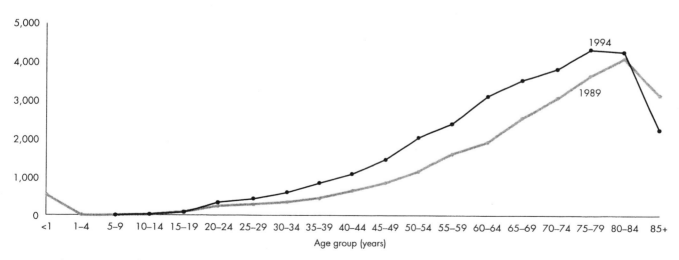

Age group (years)

Source: Goskomstat 1997; authors' analysis.

Table 5 Age-standardized mortality ratios among adults age 16 and over
by education level and sex in Russia, 1988–89 and 1993–94

(index: overall sex-specific mortality rate in 1988–89 = 100)

	Men			Women		
Period	Higher education[a]	Lower education[b]	Total	Higher education[a]	Lower education[b]	Total
1988–89	68	111	100	72	104	100
1993–94	92	174	149	77	135	124

a. Includes incomplete higher and secondary specialized education.
b. Includes secondary, incomplete secondary, primary, and incomplete primary education.
Source: Shkolnikov et al. 2000.

slightly lower life expectancy among the rural population (0.2 to 0.5 year in favor of urban residents). Consequently, the gender gap in life expectancy at birth
was greater in rural areas.

In the 1970s, the growth of alcoholism was one of
the most painful social problems in Russian villages.
The decrease in alcohol consumption in the mid-1980s
due to the anti-alcohol campaign led to a slight reduction in the gap in life expectancy between urban and
rural men (2.2 years in 1987), largely due to a steeper
decrease in alcohol-related deaths in rural areas. Between 1988 and 1991, the mortality of rural men was
increasing at a speed somewhat greater than that of
their urban counterparts. In 1992, however, this trend
unexpectedly reversed, and the gap between urban and
rural male life expectancies began to decrease. Between
1991 and 1995, the urban/rural difference in life expectancy for men decreased from 2.4 years to only 0.5
year. This was largely due to an accelerated rise in death
rates in urban areas. The male–female gap in urban areas had become almost as large as in rural areas (13.3
years vs. 13.8 years in 1994).

Table 6 Life expectancy at birth by sex and urban or rural residence
in Russia, selected years, 1958–96

(years)

	Male			Female		
Year	Urban	Rural	Difference	Urban	Rural	Difference
1958–59	63.0	62.9	0.1	71.5	71.3	0.2
1969–70	63.5	62.0	1.5	73.3	73.1	0.2
1979–80	62.3	59.3	3.0	73.1	72.6	0.5
1987	65.4	63.2	2.2	74.5	74.5	0.0
1990	64.4	62.0	2.4	74.4	73.9	0.5
1991	64.1	61.7	2.4	74.3	73.9	0.4
1992	62.5	60.7	1.8	73.8	73.5	0.3
1993	59.3	57.9	1.4	72.0	71.5	0.5
1994	57.7	56.9	0.8	71.0	70.9	0.1
1995	58.4	57.9	0.5	71.7	71.7	0.0
1996	60.1	58.6	1.5	72.7	72.0	0.7

Source: Shkolnikov, Cornia, Leon, and Meslé 1998.

The increase in mortality in the early 1990s was steeper in towns. Moreover, the decrease in life expectancy of men was slightly greater in metropolitan cities than in the residual urban population. Indeed, in the regional capitals of the Russian Federation between 1990 and 1994, male life expectancy at birth decreased by 7 years, and in other towns it decreased by 6.3 years. For women, the respective difference was negligible. The narrowing of the urban/rural gap between 1992 and 1995 was a unique phenomenon in the pattern of mortality rates in Russia over the last 40 years. In 1996, it began to increase, and the urban/rural gap again widened.

An examination of the difference between urban and rural populations in life expectancy at birth by age and cause of death in 1996 (not shown here) suggests that the advantage of living in a city rather than a village was equal to 1.5 years for men and 0.7 year for women. A major part of this difference for men, but not for women, was due to excess countryside mortality rates from accidents and violence among those aged 20 to 30 years.

Changes with respect to regions
in the early 1990s

For much of the twentieth century, the northern and eastern parts of Russia tended to experience higher mortality rates than those in the south and the west. Mortality rates were higher in the European North, Ural, Siberia, and the Far East and lower in the Northern Caucasus, Volga, and the Central Black-Soil regions. Even in the late 1970s, the regional variation in life expectancy fully corresponded to the traditional pattern of a northern and eastern disadvantage in mortality. The anti-alcohol campaign altered this pattern, however, because between 1985 and 1987 increases in life expectancy at birth were greater in those regions where its starting level was lower. Thus, during the anti-alcohol campaign, many territories in the east and in the north of Russia improved their relative positions according to the level of life expectancy at birth.

Ranking regions according to their life expectancy shows that the increase in mortality in the early 1990s led to a partial restoration of the traditional regional pattern characteristic of 1979–1980 (Shkolnikov and Cornia 2000). This finding also confirms the observation by Avdeev et al. (1997) that in many regions where the mortality decline between 1985 and 1987 was greater, the subsequent increase in the early 1990s was also greater. This association was, however, stronger for female than for male life expectancies. For women,

the correlation coefficient between regional increases in life expectancy between 1985 and 1987 and decreases for the same regions between 1987 and 1994 was 0.7, while for men the equivalent coefficient was 0.5. The correlation coefficient between regional life expectancies in 1989 and 1994 was 0.82 for women and 0.6 for men.

In 1994 the regional pattern of male mortality rates differed from the traditional pattern. For example, male life expectancy at birth in the Central, North-Western, and East Siberian economic regions has become relatively worse, while it has improved in the Volga-Vyatka and Ural economic regions. Perhaps the best examples of this asymmetrical decrease and the subsequent increase in mortality can be found in two metropolitan Russian cities. Moscow and St. Petersburg are both cities where the increase in life expectancy for men between 1985 and 1987 was comparatively small (1 and 1.7 years, respectively) while the decrease in life expectancy between 1988 and 1994 was very large (9.1 and 7.5 years, respectively).

Ecological analyses have shown that decreases in male life expectancy by region in the early 1990s were associated with certain socioeconomic indicators (Cornia 1997; Walberg et al. 1998). The strongest association was found with labor turnover (number of fired employees plus number of hired divided by the total number of employees), which can be considered a proxy for the magnitude of changes in the labor market or the pace of economic reform.

Regional variation in the gender gap in life expectancy is driven mostly by the life expectancy of men rather than women (as in other industrialized countries [Vallin 1990]). In 1994, the correlation coefficient of the gender gap in life expectancy with the regional life expectancy of Russian men was -0.52, while the equivalent coefficient for the life expectancy of women was only 0.19.

Interpreting the Findings

As clearly shown by our data, over the last three decades the Russian population has experienced unfavorable trends in overall mortality and life expectancy at birth. This is thought to be largely a result of general conditions such as relatively low living standards, underfinancing of the health system and other social services, and lack of emphasis on values and human rights in policy. These factors begin to explain the widening of the gap in life expectancy between Russia (as well as other former Soviet countries) and the West.

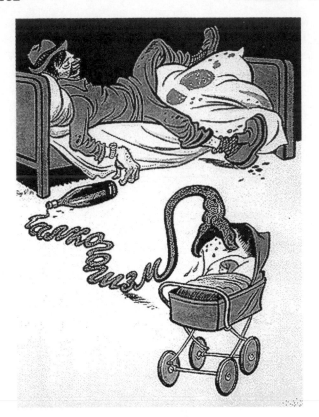

Russian anti-alcohol campaign poster, with snake spelling "Alcoholism". 1985–1989.
Source: http://yuricle.design.ru/alco

However, mortality trends in Russia are comparatively worse for men than for women. This can be explained by the excess male mortality at working ages due to accidents, violence, and premature cardiovascular diseases, as well as relatively high rates of alcohol abuse and smoking among Russian men. The success of the anti-alcohol campaign in the mid-1980s was reflected in a substantial decrease in the difference between male and female life expectancy at birth, demonstrating the size of the burden of excess deaths (mostly among men) associated with alcohol in Russia.

The analysis of social and gender gradients in mortality sheds light on possible explanations for the Russian health crisis and on the protective mechanisms perhaps more characteristic of women. Health selection explained only a small proportion of the high mortality rates in 1989. Overall, the differentials in mortality associated with educational level, occupational class, and marital status in Russia in 1989 appear to have been at least as large as those in western countries (for further details, see Shkolnikov et al. 1998a,b). In this respect, the similarity between the communist Russia of the 1980s and the capitalist West is quite unexpected because the relationship between income and educational or occupational category is not as strong in Russia as in the West. This argues for the relatively stronger influence of sociocultural and behavioral factors rather than the direct effects of economic inequalities in Russia compared with the West. There are certainly links, however, between these two types of factors. Indeed, in relation to health equity, there is a strong body of evidence from Western Europe documenting the way in which individual behaviors are influenced by the socioeconomic environment in which people live and work (for reviews, see Blaxter 1990; Graham 1993; Whitehead 1994, 1995; Dahlgren 1997).

One of the most important findings of this study is that while the gender gap in mortality is considerable in all socioeconomic and sociodemographic groups, it is always smaller for men and women in higher social positions than in the lower ones. The same conclusion can be drawn from urban/rural and regional comparisons. In all cases, disadvantaged groups tend to experience greater gender gaps in mortality. Social, regional, or residential gradients in male mortality are steeper than in female mortality, and female mortality is lower than male mortality even in relatively unfavorable situations such as living in the countryside or in a remote region and having a lower education or manual occupation. These patterns are similar to those found in Western European countries (Vallin 1990, 1995).

One possible contributory factor is that within lower socioeconomic groups men may be exposed to higher risks than women due to their higher involvement in heavy and primary industries, transport, and all types of hard manual labor, as well as being more likely than women to adopt unhealthy lifestyles.

There is a gender differential in the effects of marital status on mortality. Although the protective effect of marriage is very clear, the elevation of risk associated with the status of divorce is almost negligible among women, while among men it is very pronounced. Alcohol abuse among men is a frequently cited reason for divorce and also raises the risk of death in divorced men. This may partially explain why the difference in mortality between divorced and married men is so much greater than that for women.

Unfortunately, very little direct information about men's and women's health practices and behaviors in Russia is available. There are even fewer sociological data related to sociocultural factors, particularly attitudes toward individual health and the body. Nevertheless, it is possible to mention several informative results concerning alcohol consumption and smoking.

A survey of the drinking habits of men and women in Moscow documented large gender disparities (Shurygina 1996). Women tended to drink less, consuming mostly wine, while men drank much greater amounts and preferred vodka and other hard liquors. Men drank more often with their friends, while women drank more frequently with their husbands and other family members. Most interestingly, alcohol consumption was lower in groups of men with higher education, but, paradoxically, it was somewhat greater in the equivalent group for women. (Certainly in all educational groups, male alcohol intake is greater.) A relatively small group of women with low education levels and engaged in hard manual labor were found to be similar to men in their drinking habits (higher alcohol consumption with a large proportion of vodka).

Smoking is quite widespread among Russian men and relatively rare among Russian women, especially at middle and old ages. Almost 60% of men aged 15 to 65 years smoked in 1996, while the proportions of smokers among women were 15% to 20% for those aged 15 to 45 years, 5 to 10% for those aged 40 to 55 years, and 1% to 2% for those over 55 years (Zahoori et al. 1999; McKee et al. 1998). For both men and women, the prevalence of smoking is somewhat lower in small towns and villages than in big cities, higher among divorced people than among those of any other marital status, and higher among people without a university education.

The steep mortality increase after the collapse of the Soviet Union in 1991 and liberalization of prices in 1992 has attracted much attention. The existing evidence suggests that the health crisis of the early 1990s can be related to certain socioeconomic and sociopsychological factors such as labor market shocks and stresses, growing income inequalities and relative deprivation, lack of law and order, and lack of social cohesion and social capital (Shapiro 1995; Cornia 1997; Shkolnikov et al. 1998; Walberg et al. 1998; Kennedy et al. 1998).

The mortality crisis of the early 1990s produced unequal effects on male and female mortality in Russia. Although proportional increases in female mortality rates were rather close to those in male mortality rates, absolute levels of mortality rates, numbers of excess deaths and losses in life expectancy between 1990 and 1994 were much greater for men than for women. There is some evidence suggesting that women with higher levels of education, unlike men in the same educational group, experienced only a very modest mortality increase in the early 1990s. Changes in regional patterns of mortality suggest that for women this increase was closer to a simple return to the old mortality patterns that existed before the anti-alcohol campaign, while for men significant new elements due to adverse effects of socioeconomic shocks were detected.

One sociological explanation of the difference between men and women in coping with such stresses is related to differences in sex roles (Watson 1995). According to this hypothesis, Russian men may tend to identify more strongly with their occupational and political roles, which may be a source of frustration and anomie, while women may focus more on the household, family, children, spouse, and parents. Although women generally report poorer health than men, they tend to take better care of themselves and to spend more money on pharmaceuticals. Thus, unemployment and the transition from a command to a market economy may be stressful for men in different ways than for women. Men and women certainly seem to cope with stress in different ways: Compared with women, men are more likely to abuse alcohol, engage in violent or suicidal behavior, smoke more, and eat less healthily. It is true that mortality among Russian women is very high compared with western standards, but, as we have seen, in their own socioeconomic context they are doing better than men in certain ways. A great part of excess male mortality in Russia is associated with behavioral and sociocultural risk factors. The extent to which these are also associated with socioeconomic conditions such as absolute poverty, relative poverty, or inadequate access to effective health care is not known. The critical question, however, is whether social and health policy measures directly targeted at behavioral, sociocultural, and sociopsychological changes could be effective even with limited resources and independent of major improvements in the Russian economy. Such policies might include development of educational modules on lifestyle and health, systematic anti-tobacco and anti-alcohol policies (through taxation, health education in schools, media campaigns, restrictions in trade, quality controls), promotion of sports and exercises, and strengthening of law and order. Although the analysis of the Russian mortality crisis is an oft-cited and dramatic example of the differential health effects of economic transition, the policy question of how best to remedy the situation in the Russian and other post-Soviet state contexts remains unresolved.

References

Andreev E.M. 1983. Metod komponent v analize prodolzjitelnosti zhizni [The component method in analysis of life expectancy]. *Vestnik Statistiki* 3:42–47.

Arriaga E. 1984. Measuring and explaining the change in life expectancies. *Demography* 21(1):83–96.

Avdeev A., Blum A., Zakharov S., Andreev E. 1997. Réaction d'une population hétérogène à une perturbation. Un modèle d'interprétation des évolutions de mortalité en Russie. *Population* 1:7–44.

Blaxter M. 1990. *Health and lifestyles*. London: Routledge.

Brajczewski C., Rogucka E. 1993. Social class differences in rates of premature mortality among adults in the City of Wroclaw, Poland. *American Journal of Human Biology* 5:461–471.

Buchet M. 1997. Tous les pays du monde. *Population et Sociétés*. 20:Août.

Buell P., Dunn J.E., Breslow L. 1960. Occupational–social class risks of cancer mortality in men. *Journal of Chronic Diseases.* 12:600–21.

Carlson E. 1989. Concentration of rising Hungarian mortality among manual workers. *University of South Carolina, SSR* 73(3):119–128.

Centers for Disease Control and Prevention. National Center for Health Statistics (http://www.cdc.gov/nchs/fastats/pdf/4728t12.pdf). Nov 7, 2000.

Chenet L., Leon D., McKee M., Vassin S. 1998. Deaths from alcohol and violence in Moscow: socio-economic determinants. *European Journal of Population* 14:19–37.

Christenson B.A., Johnson N.E. 1995. Educational inequality in adult mortality: an assessment with death certificate data from Michigan. *Demography* 32:215–229.

Cornia A.G. 1997. Labour Market Shocks, Psychosocial Stress and the Transition's Mortality Crisis. Paper presented at the Project Meeting on Economic Shocks, Social Stress and the Demographic Impact, April 17–19, in Helsinki.

Dahlgren G. 1997. Strategies for reducing social inequities in health—visions and reality. In: Ollila E., Koivusalo M., Partonen T. (eds), *Equity in Health Through Public Policy*. Helsinki: STAKES, pp. 23–53.

Davis C. 1993. The health sector in the Soviet and Russian economies: from reform to fragmentation. In: *The Former Soviet Union in Transition*, pp. 852–872. Washington, DC: Government Printing Office.

Field M. 1995. The health crisis in the former Soviet Union: a report from the "Post-War" zone. *Social Science and Medicine* 4(11):1469–1178.

Goldblatt P. 1989. Mortality by social class, 1971–85. *Population Trends* 56:6–15.

Goskomstat. 1997. *Rossiyskiy statisticheskiy yejegodnik 1996 [Russian Statistical Annual 1996]*. Moscow: Goskomstat.

Graham H. 1993. *When Life's a Drag: Women, Smoking and Disadvantage*. London: HMSO.

Kennedy B.P., Kawachi I., Brainerd E. 1998. The role of social capital in the Russian mortality crisis. *World Development* 26(11): 2029–2044.

Kitagawa E.M., Hauser P.M. 1973. *Differential Mortality in the United States: A Study in Socioeconomic Epidemiology*. Cambridge, MA: Harvard University Press.

Leon D.A., Chenet L., Shkolnikov V.M., Zakharov S., Shapiro J., Rakhmanova G., Vassin S., McKee M. 1997. Huge variation in Russian mortality rates 1984–1994: artefact or alcohol or what? *Lancet* 350:383–388.

Marmot M.G., McDowall M.E. 1986. Mortality decline and widening social inequalities. *Lancet* 2:274–276.

McKee M., Bobak M., Rose R., Shkolnikov V., Chenet L., Leon D. 1998. Patterns of smoking in Russia. *Tobacco Control* 7:22–26.

Meslé F., Shkolnikov V.M. 1995. La mortalité en Russie: une crise sanitaire en deux temps. *Revue d'Etudes Comparatives Est-Ouest* 4:9–24.

Nayha S. 1977. Social group and mortality in Finland. *British Journal of Preventive and Social Medicine* 31(4):231–237.

Nemtsov A.V. 1995. *Alkogolnaya situatsiya v Rossii. [Alcohol Situation in Russia]*. Moscow: Foundation on Health and Environment.

Okolski M. 1993. East–West mortality differentials. In: Blum A., Rallu J.-L. (eds), *European Population*, vol 2. Paris: Institut National d'Etudes Démographiques, pp. 165–189.

Pearce N.E., Howard J.K. 1986. Occupation, social class and male cancer mortality in New Zealand, 1974–78. *International Journal of Epidemiology* 15:456–462.

Pressat R. 1985. Contribution des écarts de mortalité par âge à la différence des vies moyennes. *Population* 40(4–5):766–770.

Preston S.H. 1976. *Mortality Patterns in National Poulations*. NY, London: Academic Press.

Ryan M. 1995. Alcoholism and rising mortality in the Russian Federation. *British Medical Journal* 310:646–648.

Shapiro J. 1995. The Russian mortality crisis and its causes. In: Åslund, A. (ed), *Economic Reform at Risk*. London: Pinter, pp. 149–178.

Shkolnikov V.M., Andreev E.M., Maleva (eds) 2000. *Neravenstvo i smertnost v Rossii [Inequality and Mortality in Russia]*. Moscow: Signal.

Shkolnikov V.M., Cornia A.G. 2000. Population crisis and rising mortality in transitional Russia. In: Cornia A.G., Paniccá R. (eds). *The Mortality Crisis in Transitional Economies*. Oxford: Oxford University Press, pp. 253–279.

Shkolnikov V.M., Cornia A.G., Leon D.A., Meslé F. 1998. Causes of the Russian mortality crisis: evidence and interpretations. *World Development* 26(11):1995–2011.

Shkolnikov V.M., Leon D.A., Adamets S., Andreev E., Deev A. 1998b. Educational level and adult mortality Russia. *Social Science and Medicine* 17(3):357–369.

Shkolnikov V.M., Meslé F. 1996. The Russian epidemiological crisis as mirrored by mortality trends. In: DaVanzo J. (ed), *Russia's Demographic Crisis*. Santa Monica, CA: RAND, pp. 113–162.

Shkolnikov V.M., Meslé F., Vallin J. 1996. Health crisis in Russia. *Population: An English Selection* 8:123–190.

Shkolnikov V.M., Nemtsov A.V. 1997. The anti-alcohol campaign and variations in Russian mortality. In: Bobadilla J.-L., Costello C., Mitchell F. (eds), *Premature Death in the New Independent States*. Washington, DC: National Academy Press, pp. 239–261.

Shurygina I.I. 1996. Razlitchiya v potreblenii alkogolya mejdu mujchinami i jenschinami v Moskve [Differences between men and women in alcohol consumption in Moscow]. *Sotsiologicheskii Jurnal* 1–2:169–175.

Slutsky B. 1999. "Old women and old men." In: Smith G.S. (ed, transl), *Things that Happened*. Moscow: Glas Publishers.

Treml V. 1997. Soviet and Russian statistics on alcohol consumption and abuse. In: Bobadilla J.-L., Costello C., Mitchell F. (eds), *Premature Death in the New Independent States*. Washington, DC: National Academy Press, pp. 220–238.

United Nations. 1982. *Levels and Trends of Mortality Since 1950*. New York: United Nations.

United Nations Development Programme (UNDP). 1999. *Human Development Report 1999*. New York: UNDP.

Valkonen T. 1989. Adult mortality and level of education: a comparison of six countries. In Fox J. (ed), *Health Inequalities in European Countries*. Aldershot: Gower, pp. 142–162.

Valkonen T. 1993. Problems in the measurement and international comparisons of differences in mortality. *Social Science and Medicine* 36:409–418.

Vallin J. 1995. Can sex differentials in mortality be explained by socio-economic mortality differentials? In: Lopez A.D., Caselli G., Valkonen T. (eds), *Adult Mortality in Developed Countries: From Description to Explanation*. Oxford: Clarendon Press, pp. 179–200.

Vallin J. 1990. Quand les variations géographiques de la surmortalité masculine contredisend son évalution dans le temps. *Espace, Populations, Sociétés* 3:467–478.

Walberg P., McKee M., Shkolnikov V.M., Chenet L., Leon D.A. 1998. Economic change, crime, and mortality crisis in Russia: regional analysis. *British Medical Journal* 317:312–318.

Watson P. 1995. Explaining rising mortality among men in Eastern Europe. *Social Science and Medicine* 41(7):923–934.

Whitehead M. 1994. Counting the human costs: opportunities for and barriers to promoting health. In: Levin L., McMahan L., Ziglio E. (eds), *Economic Change, Social Welfare and Health in Europe*. WHO Regional Publications European Series No. 54. Copenhagen: WHO, pp. 59–75.

Whitehead M. 1995. Tackling inequalities: a review of policy initiatives. In: Benzeval M., Judge K., Whitehead M. (eds), *Tackling Inequalities in Health: An Agenda for Action*. London: King's Fund, pp. 22–52.

Whitehead M., F. Diderichsen. 1997. International evidence on social inequalities in health. In: Drever F. and Whitehead M. (eds), *Health Inequalities—Decennial Supplement*. DS Series No 15. Stationery Office, pp. 45–69.

World Health Organization. 2000. Health for All. Statistical Database for Personal Computer. World Health Organization Office for Europe, Copenhagen. http:/www.who.dk/country.htm.

Zohoori N., Henderson K., Gleiter K., Popkin B. 1999. *Monitoring of Health Conditions in the Russian Federation: The Russia Longitudinal Monitoring Survey 1992–98.*, University of North Carolina at Chapel Hill, North Carolina: Carolina Population Center.

CHAPTER 12

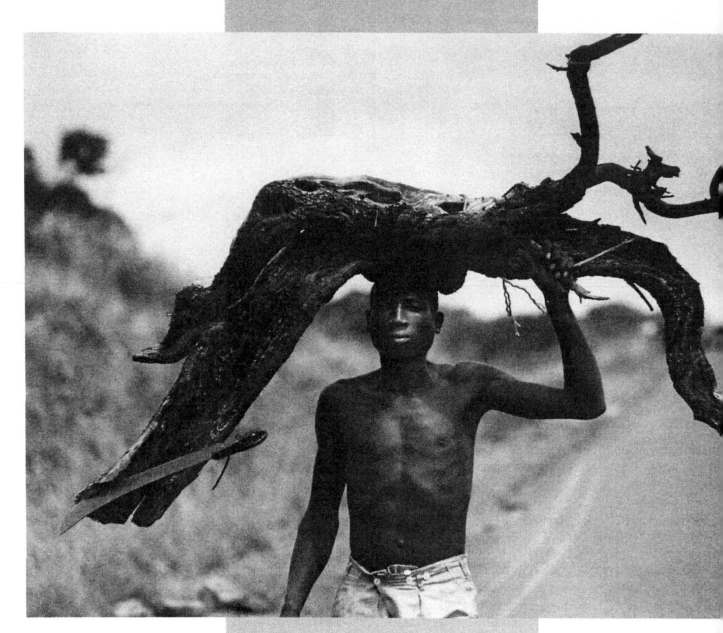

Rwandese refugee gathering firewood in Benaco camp, Tanzania.
Source: Heldur Netocny/Panos.

Tanzania: Gaining Insights into Adolescent Lives and Livelihoods

VINAND M. NANTULYA, AVE MARIA SEMAKAFU,
FLORENCE MULI-MUSIIME, AUGUSTINE MASSAWE, AND
LAWRENCE MUNYETTI

Adolescents: Inequities in Lives and Livelihoods

Adolescence is the period of transition from childhood to adulthood, involving not only physiological changes but also psychological and social development. According to the World Health Organization's definition, adolescence covers the 10- to 19-year-old age group and includes a large and growing proportion of the world's population. Globally, there are over 1 billion young people, with 85% of them living in developing counties (Auer 1999). In Tanzania, over half of the country's total population of 31 million is under 18 years of age, and almost one-third of the population falls into the adolescent age range of 10–19 years (Tanzania Bureau of Statistics 1996; Tanzania/UNICEF 1999).

Adolescents represent a large proportion of the population in developing countries, yet within these countries policy rarely addresses their particular needs. Challenges to the health and development of the young have impacts not only for their current well being but also for their life chances in adulthood and the well-being of their children (Tarantola and Gruskin 1998). Despite this, many developing countries lack a strategy for addressing adolescents as a specific sociodemographic group. Furthermore, adolescents are not given the opportunity to participate in the design and implementation of the policies and programs that affect their own lives and livelihoods. This exclusion means that their concerns may not be adequately taken into account. Failing to address the health and other needs of adolescents will have lifelong consequences for their well being.

Young people from low-income families are particularly vulnerable and more profoundly affected by the inadequacy of government policies. Adolescence is a critical stage of life when inequities in lives and livelihoods are established or reinforced. The life chances of adolescents in Tanzania are jeopardized by both poverty and low levels of education. In 1979, when primary and secondary school education was free, Tanzania had one of the highest literacy rates in Africa, with primary school enrollment rates approaching 100%. Today primary school enrollment stands at 77%, with 30% to 40% of children, mostly from low-income families, dropping out before the seventh year of education, in part due to the introduction of cost-sharing in education, initiated by the implementation of Structural Adjustment Programs (SAPs) in the early 1980s. The

157

Tanzania

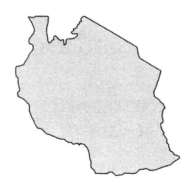

Total population (millions), 1997	31.4
Human development index, 1999	0.421
Human development index rank, 1999	156
Infant mortality rate (per 1,000 live births), 1997	92
Real GDP per capita (PPP$), 1997	580
Public spending on health as percentage of GDP, 1995	2.5

Source: UNDP 1999. [Human Development Report]

poorest rural regions have dropout rates as high as 70%. Secondary school enrollment is also low, currently standing at 15%. Children from low-income families suffer both from material and educational disadvantage, casting a long shadow over their future.

In Tanzania there is a tendency to regard adolescents as sources of free labor and income. Increasing urbanization, the intensification of rural poverty, as well as the resulting intensification of unpaid agricultural labor at home (Shao et al. 1992; Mbilinyi and Semakafu 1995) have been accompanied by an increase in the migration of adolescents from rural to urban areas. These young migrants are ill equipped for gainful employment, and homelessness, prostitution, street vending, and child labor are commonplace. Both male and female adolescents are earning income through dangerous and exploitative menial occupations in plantations and mines, as well as through prostitution in urban centers. In a discussion of the role of economic change on the behavior of adolescents and youth in Tanzania, Lugalla (1995) showed clearly how the behavior of adolescents from poor families carried a higher health risk than those from higher income families. It is difficult to determine both the magnitude of rural/urban migration as a cause of internal displacement of adolescents and its impact on their lives. In his study, Lugalla (1995) estimated that there were 70 new arrivals from the countryside per day in Dar es Salaam alone. There

is no doubt that rural/urban migration by adolescents is growing, and it is beginning to attract the concern and attention of the public (Lugalla 1995; Luena et al. 1996; Livigha and Mekacha 1997).

In addition to the socioeconomic pressures placed on adolescents, cultural influences may exacerbate the problems. There is great diversity within Tanzania in cultural practices of socializing adolescents into adulthood, ranging from taboos against premarital sexual encounters to encouragement of child indulgence in preadolescent sex (Tumbo-Masabo and Liljeström 1994; Mabala 1995). In some tribes, for example, adolescent girls are taken out of school at puberty for seclusion and training in sexual and other related issues. This undermines the education of girls, leading to gender inequities in an important determinant of adolescent livelihood. Thus, culture is a very important determinant of livelihood not only in adolescence but also later in adulthood.

The aim of this study was to shed light on previously ignored aspects of adolescent lives which are of major public health significance in Tanzania and elsewhere. Complementary methods, including a literature review, survey and group discussions, and policy analysis, were used to gain information on the needs and circumstances of adolescents in Tanzania. The chapter endeavors to develop a deeper understanding of the life chances and opportunities for good health of Tanzanian adolescents, particularly vulnerable adolescents, in order to inform policy developments in this important area.

The first section looks at what information on adolescents can be gleaned from the routine statistical sources and literature. The second section presents further insights gained from our interviews and discussion groups with vulnerable adolescents, for example, those working in mines and on plantations, commercial sex workers, street children, refugees, and other children living in difficult circumstances. The third section assesses current national policies related to adolescence. Policies are viewed in the light of the understanding gained from the previous phases of research. The final part of the chapter draws lessons for future research and policy development in Tanzania.

Findings

Information from Routine Statistics and Literature

The review of basic population statistics revealed that approximately 45% of the Tanzanian population is under 15 years of age (see Box 1). Women constitute

50.5% of the population. Approximately 80% of the population live in the rural areas, but with increasing urbanization estimated at 4% per annum, this picture is likely to change. Attempts to probe more deeply into the health and socioeconomic circumstances of different age groups in the population, particularly adolescents, have proven extraordinarily difficult. Crucial databases such as the Demographic Health Surveys and routine health statistics fail to focus on adolescents as a sociodemographic group with specific development needs. In the Health Statistics Abstracts (Tanzania Ministry of Health 1997b), for example, all Tanzanians are classified into two age groups: children, aged zero to 5 years, and adults (the rest). From the data it is impossible to identify the social background, residence, and health status of various age groups among the "adult" category.

From the available routine data, there is no doubt that Tanzanian children under 5 years of age are at severe risk of ill health and death. The under-5 year mortality rate is estimated at 144 deaths per 1000 live births (World Bank 1998–99; World Bank 1999) and an estimated 31% of those under 5 years are underweight (below two standard deviations from weight for age) (Tanzanian Bureau of Statistics 1996; Tanzania/UNICEF 1999). There is no reason to believe, however, that the period of high risk ends at age 5 years. Indeed, the poor health status of the under-5 years population would suggest the need for extra vigilance concerning the plight of older children.

Much-needed information on adolescents, however, is sparse, and what exists tends to be concentrated narrowly on reproductive aspects and sexually transmitted diseases and thus predominantly focused on girls. Most of the statistics are silent about the health of adolescent boys and young men. Available data indicated high rates of adolescent marriage and childbearing, child and adolescent labor, and female genital mutilation (Shao et al. 1992). The 1994 Tanzania Knowledge, Attitudes, and Practice Survey, for instance, notes that between 17% and 35% of teenage girls have already begun childbearing or are pregnant with their first child. As shown in Figure 1, by age 15 years, just over 1% had started childbearing, whereas by age 19 years, over 60% had started childbearing (Tanzania Bureau of Statistics 1996).

Female genital mutilation is a widespread traditional practice among many tribes in Tanzania, resulting in serious health consequences for adolescent girls. It has been estimated that the genital mutilation rates are around 10% in urban areas, rising to 20% in rural areas. The Northern highlands and central zones report the highest rates, at 64% and 49%, respectively (Institute of Adult Education 1990).

There are disturbing data related to sexually transmitted diseases among adolescents. For example, it is estimated that 7% of pregnant girls test positive for the human immunodeficiency virus (HIV), that 68,000 of those under the age of 15 years are infected with HIV/AIDS (acquired immunodeficiency syndrome), and that 520,000 adolescents have lost their mother or both parents to AIDS (Tanzania Ministry of Health 1997a; Tanzania/UNICEF 1999). Having a sexually transmitted disease in Tanzania can lead to exclusion and marginalization (Resnick et al. 1997), with further implications for health and livelihoods. Substance abuse among adolescents is believed to be widespread and increasing. In their study on school-based health promotional pilot surveys, Mbatia and Kilonzo (1996) found that among students aged 11 to 20 years who were interviewed and admitted to being on drugs, 71% reported that they sniffed petrol, while alcohol was

---

BOX 1: REVIEW OF ROUTINE DATA SOURCES AND LITERATURE

Routine data on adolescent health and social circumstances were reviewed including program reports from government and international agencies, United Nations (U.N.) agencies, bilateral aid agencies, and nongovernmental organizations, as well as special research and intervention projects. A number of statistical reports were reviewed, including the Tanzania Health Statistics Abstracts (various years); the 1996 Tanzania Demographic and Health Survey; the 1994 Tanzania Knowledge, Attitude, and Practice Survey; African Medical and Research Foundation (AMREF) reports; UNICEF reports; a United Nations Population Fund (UNFPA) study on youth sexuality; reports of the reproductive health study group at the University of Dar es Salaam; Ministry of Health Statistical Abstracts (various years); Urban Health Project for Dar es Salaam reports; National Family Planning Program reports; National AIDS Control Program reports; Mental Health in Tanzania reports; and the reports of the Tanzania–Netherlands Project to Support HIV/AIDS Control in Mwanza Region (TANESA) and the Adult Morbidity and Mortality Project. A special focus was placed on information related to age, sex, place of origin (rural and urban), level of education, marital status, being in school versus out of school, occupation, and types of services for adolescents.

Figure 1 Adolescent girls who have begun childbearing or first pregnancy in Tanzania, 1996

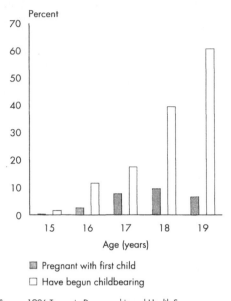

Source: 1996 Tanzania Demographic and Health Survey.

imbibed by 43%. The reasons given for drug use included sociability, curiosity, and relief of psychological stress related to the pressures of economic hardships.

There is a lack of services and programs for adolescents provided by national government and international aid agencies alike. The data from specific programs and projects, such as the Adult Morbidity and Mortality Project (AMMP), the Tanzania Essential Health Intervention Project (TEHIP), and UNICEF programs, focus on the under-5 year age group and adults, neglecting preadolescents and adolescents. This inadequacy has undoubtedly hindered recognition of, and programming for, the special needs of these groups.

Among Tanzania's main health programs—Maternal and Child Health (MCH), family planning, and AIDS control—the adolescent component is limited in scope, with the focus predominantly on girls and their reproductive role. Male children are almost entirely neglected. The programs also tend to focus on adolescents in school and exclude those who have dropped out of school, yet those who drop out are the poorer and more vulnerable group of adolescents. School health programs are also inadequate and underfunded.

Oppong-Odiseng and Heycock (1997) carried out a descriptive study to investigate adolescents' knowledge and use of local health-related services. The main finding of the study was that services and programs do not adequately reach adolescents. Adolescents prefer confidentiality in health services, a feature that is missing in public health facilities. Moreover, adolescents are not regarded as a social category, and thus are "unfairly excluded" from enjoying their basic rights to health and health care services. The authors concluded that adolescents are a group with particular needs and should be the target of specific policy interventions, as are the under-5 year olds.

Insights from the Group Discussions

In the group discussions conducted in our study (see Box 2), many of the adolescents who had dropped out of school—both those who were unemployed and those

---

BOX 2: SURVEY AND GROUP DISCUSSIONS WITH SELECTED VULNERABLE GROUPS

Adolescents, both those in school and drop-outs, were recruited for an interview survey and group discussions from four areas: a mining area (Mirerani, in Arusha), a sugar plantation (Kilombero, in Morogoro Region), an urban center (Dar es Salaam), and a rural area (Kigoma). Study sites were chosen with the aim of reaching specific vulnerable groups of adolescents. Hence, the mining center (Arusha) and sugar plantation (Kilombero) were selected for their potential to provide insights into the coping strategies for adolescents engaged in employment for which they were officially too young. Dar es Salaam was selected because it is a rapidly growing urban center with high in-migration of poorer adolescents from the rural areas (Livigha and Mekacha 1997; Lugalla 1995). Kigoma was included because it is a remote, low-income, rural area with high population migration dynamics due to movement of refugees and business people from neighboring countries and the high numbers of adolescents living without parents in refugee camps.

The selection methods used to recruit participants to the survey and discussion groups had to be adapted to suit the varied circumstances in which the different groups of adolescents could be found. To interview those who were attending schools, the local primary and secondary schools were identified in each area and the advice sought of those in charge about the characteristics of the schools and their pupils. Schools were selected if their student population was representative of the socioeconomic backgrounds typical of the area. Permission was sought from the school authorities, and self-completion questionnaires were administered to all pupils aged 13 to 19 years who were in school on the day of the interview.

Adolescents who had dropped out of school were more difficult to locate. Because it was important that the initial contact with the adolescents be neutral, it became necessary to use reconnaissance methods to identify the most appropriate and nonthreatening entry point for each specific group of adolescents. This method enabled us to identify both the formal and informal leaders, establish a rapport with them, explain the objectives of the study, and enlist their participation and that of other adolescents. Their involvement was particularly important in identifying and engaging the urban groups, those who were the street children, commercial sex workers, drug users, and children in conflict with the law.

A total of 713 adolescents completed the questionnaire: 224 in the mining area, 329 in the sugar plantation area, 100 in the urban area of Dar es Salaam, and 60 in the refugee area. The questionnaire asked about their age, sex, family situation, school attendance, living arrangements, employment (if any), episodes of illness in the past 3 months, and use of health services.

Participants for more in-depth group discussions were then selected from among the respondents to the questionnaire. Groupings were based on common and shared experiences, especially with regards to their occupation/engagement. The group discussion participants are described in Table 1. Note that in one area, Kilombero, discussion

Table 1 Characteristics of group discussion participants

Area and sex	Age range (years)	Type of group	Occupation or life circumstance	Number of groups
Kilombero				
Male	17–19	Dropped out of school	Cane cutters	2
Male	14–19	In school	Students	1
Female	13–19	In school	Students	1
Female	13–18	In school	Students	1
Male and female	18–20	Dropped out of school	Jobless	2
Female	42–50	Parents	Villagers	1
Male and female	48–60	Parents	Villagers	1
Male and female	35–45	Guardians	Secondary school teachers	1
Male and female	27–55	Parents and guardians	Employed	1
Kigoma				
Male and female	14–18	In school	Students	2
Male	13–18	In school	Refugees	1
Male	17–19	Dropped out of school	Jobless	2
Male and female	15–19	Dropped out of school	Refugees	2
Arusha				
Male	10–13	Dropped out of school	Miners	6
Female	13–16	In school	Students	1
Dar es Salaam				
Female	13–19	Dropped out of school	Commercial sex workers	2
Male and female	11–16	Dropped out of school	Street children	2
Male	13–19	Dropped out of school	Jobless	3
Female	14–19	Dropped out of school	Jobless	1
Male and female	14–19	Dropped out of school	Drug pushers	1

Source: Authors' observations.

groups for parents and teachers were also arranged through the schools. The discussions took place 2 to 3 days after the scheduled interview. The Kiswahili language was used as the medium of communication during the discussions. A total of 33 discussion groups were organized, with the average group consisting of six to eight randomly selected participants. Each session lasted an average of 1 hour. To ensure confidentiality, the discussions were undertaken in private. For example, the in-school discussions took place in the school compounds after school hours, away from teachers and parents. For the out-of-school adolescents, the choice of venue depended on the type of group involved, with participants themselves helping to identify an acceptable venue. Each discussion was led by a senior member of the research team and assisted by a technical assistant. To stimulate discussion, questions were asked regarding attitudes and beliefs about adolescence, sources of livelihoods, living conditions, experiences of ill health, sexuality and sexually transmitted diseases, and access to health services.

in some form of gainful employment—commonly described their experiences in terms of severe hardship:

"To be an adolescent is like living in hell. If we do not go out to look for any jobs, our parents, brothers, and sisters back home will suffer."

"It is a tough experience being an adolescent: You are expected to provide for yourself, yet the economic situation is tough even for our parents."

"We cannot be employed because we are under age, and yet we need to provide for our own survival the hard way."

"People refer to us as *wahuni* (thugs); whatever effort we make to survive, they criticize. To be an adolescent from a poor family and out of school, you are automatically a lay-about, a prostitute, a *bhang (marijuana)* smoker, and all sorts of filthy titles."

Those in school concurred thus: "Adolescence is tough especially if one is idle. For us in school, things are not easy, but for those out of school, life is very hard." "*Wanaipata joto la jiwe*" is a Swahili expression meaning that life for those out of school is as calamitous as "holding a hot stone in one's hand."

These sentiments capture some of the dilemmas and challenges that adolescents face in Tanzania. There are serious issues affecting their lives and livelihoods, including intra- and intergroup inequities that are rarely captured and taken into consideration when programs are developed. The following are "snapshots" of the day-to-day lives of some of the vulnerable adolescents in our study, as recounted to the researchers during the group discussions. The aim is to help give a more complete picture of how pervasive adolescent health threats are in Tanzania and to show how the more vulnerable adolescents are profoundly affected by lack of policy action to enhance their lives and livelihoods.

The life of an adolescent miner

Most of the adolescents working in mine pits were primary school drop-outs, all of them boys. All were in migrants, coming from as far away as Kigoma, Mbeya, Mwanza, Dodoma, Kilimanjaro, and Tanga. The boys were recruited directly by the supervisors of different pits and became members of that pit. The contracts obliged the pit owner to provide one meal per day, but without any wage. The mine owners were not obliged to provide accommodation to the boys, and so they spent their nights in the compressor shed in the field. During the cold and windy season, they were forced to spend the night down in the pits.

After being used to explode rocks, the compressor would be switched off by the pit supervisor to save fuel. The boys would immediately descend into the pits despite intense dust emanating from the exploded graphite rock. Any rock dust brought to the surface was given to the pit supervisor to harvest all the precious stone he could lay his hands on. Thereafter, the boys scavenged for the leftovers. Any lucky find was left to the so-called miners, to constitute their wage. Each miner could only scavenge his own dust. The boys reported that they experienced tremendous cash flow problems.

There was also an acute shortage of water, and the miners normally went for 3 or more months without bathing. The nearest stream was 10 kilometers away, and, because they were not paid a regular wage, the miners preferred to maximize their working hours and increase their chances of getting Tanzanite stones. They normally worked as miners for a maximum of 10 years.

The main health problems they faced working under these dusty conditions were tuberculosis and upper respiratory infections. Sexually transmitted diseases were also a problem. Prostitution was rampant in the satellite village Mirerani, which stands only 5 kilometers away from the fields. When the young men fell sick, they had to take care of themselves. All health care facilities in Mirerani were privately owned, and most of them were drug shops. Self-prescription was the order of the day. Work-related injuries and deaths were common. The pit owners did not have modern equipment, and collapse of the mine pits was a common occurrence. While this chapter was being prepared, in fact, one such collapse occurred in the study area, with the loss of close to 100 lives. Inevitably, there must have been some adolescents among the casualties.

The life of young sugar cane cutters

The sugar cane cutters we interviewed were groups of youths recruited from the neighboring regions (Iringa and Mbeya) in the southern highlands. According to our study, more than 50 of them were below age 20 years, and most were school drop-outs. They were housed in dormitories in camps for workers and slept on papyrus mats on a cement floor. The daily assignment for each cane cutter was to harvest 3.5 tons of sugar cane. To complete the assignment, the boys reported that they had to wake up at 5:00 A.M. They worked long hours in the hot sun in a swampy environment heavy with the herbicides and fertilizers used on the plantation. They described their experiences as work "so demanding, it is like doing a long, difficult physical exercise." They said that due to the severe physical demands of the work, most of them took a break for two seasons before accepting a second contract. They said it was difficult to work continuously for more than 3 years.

The cane cutter's life was closely linked with life in the neighboring village. During the weekends, the camp was almost empty, as a significant number of cane cutters had girlfriends in the village. Sexually transmitted diseases were reported to be one of their major problems. Other health problems cited by the cane cutters were malaria, chest infections, skin diseases, diarrhea, and stress. Cholera outbreaks were reported to be a common occurrence. Work injuries, including snakebites and machete accidents, were also common among the cane cutters.

From the group discussions, it was evident that there was lack of accurate health information about sex and sexuality. Some participants believed that abstaining from sex for more than 2 weeks could lead to loss of virility. Money was usually in short supply, and they often shared concubines to "save" their virility. The cane workers complained bitterly about these concubines, describing the situation as "impossible to survive." To cut down on costs, many resorted to going with schoolgirls from the village who charged less. This was corroborated by the schoolgirls in scheduled interviews, who further confessed to starting sexual involvement with cane cutters as early as 10 years of age. Homosexuality among the cane cutters was also re-

vealed, with older cane cutters having allegedly enticed the younger ones to accept the relationships.

Life in a refugee camp

The United Republic of Tanzania is a union between the former Republic of Tanganyika (the mainland) and Zanzibar. It shares borders with eight countries—Burundi, Kenya, Malawi, Mozambique, Rwanda, Uganda, Zaire, and Zambia. Most of these countries, particularly those on its western and northwestern borders, have high levels of political instability and military insecurity. As a result, there are about 350,000 refugees in western Tanzania, mostly from Burundi and the Democratic Republic of Congo.

The study area, the Mtabila refugee settlement in Kigoma, western Tanzania, had a significant adolescent population. Most of them had fled their country of origin while they were in school. They had no parents, and subsequently the administration of the camp created artificial families made up of five girls or boys. The members of each group managed their lives as a family.

According to our interviews, the major problems were related to sexuality, mental health, and uncertainty about their future. Some of the adolescent refugees had become discreet prostitutes. Moreover, rape cases were on the increase, with the offenders reported to be fellow refugees and men from the neighboring communities. Both boys and girls reported being lonely and depressed. They feared for their future, and those who were in school did not expect to go further in their studies. Because they needed clearance to go outside the settlement, their integration into the local communities was restricted. Below is an account of Karenzo, a refugee girl from Burundi:

Karenzo is the eleventh child in a family of 13 children. She found herself at the Tanzania border in 1995, after she and her fellow students were forced to flee while in school. They arrived at the border and were taken to the reception center, a local sports stadium, and after 2 weeks moved to a refugee camp. Because most of them were students, they were divided into groups of five and registered as a family. There were several such families at the camp.

The major problem for Karenzo has been loneliness. She misses her parents, brothers, and sisters and has been admitted to the camp dispensary several times with a mental breakdown. When she left home, she was in class six, but in the camp, she no longer attends school. She hopes that one day she might rejoin her family.

She has been raped twice. Although she reported the matter to camp authorities, the culprits have yet to be arrested. The first time she was raped, it was by a fellow refugee who fled the camp after the incident. The second culprit is still not known. She sustained injuries during the first rape and had an infection with discharge after the second.

Life on the streets of Dar es Salaam

Among the adolescents living on the streets of Dar es Salaam are the unofficial commercial sex workers (bar maids and housemaids), overt commercial sex workers, street children, street vendors, and others in conflict with the law. All those interviewed were in-migrants. Some had moved into the city with their parents, while a significant number had migrated on their own in search of opportunities.

The girls lived in shared overcrowded rooms. One room could sometimes accommodate more than eight girls who slept on mattresses spread on the floor. The boys, on the other hand, often slept in abandoned broken-down vehicles, at bus stops, and in bars. They bought food from food vendors in the slums popularly known as the *mama ntiliye*, and the food in most cases consisted of a fried piece of cassava and boiled beans. One meal a day was the norm. When they fell sick, they had to look after themselves and prescribe their own medication. Substance abuse was rampant. One said that "*bhang* [kat or marijuana] smoking gives confidence to endure tough jobs and long days without food."

The adolescents also used other substances like heroine and petrol. Some described a concoction they called a "cocktail." This was a mixture of heroine, lime, and petrol or a mixture of *bhang (kat)* and heroine. They said cocaine was not regularly included in the cocktail because it was very expensive, but they occasionally used it.

Most of the adolescents we interviewed on the streets were registered in school but confessed that their attendance was irregular. Some of the adolescents in the streets, however, had dropped out of school largely for economic reasons. For the adolescent boys, the only opportunity to earn money was in the markets and at bus stops as park boys. Very few managed to get employed as street vendors to sell locally made juices, biscuits, and water. The girls began as housemaids or barmaids—essentially disguised commercial sex workers—and ultimately ended up as full time sex operatives. The following response from one key informant gives further insight into life on the streets:

When asked about his health and future, Iddi said that he understood the problems of drug abuse, but for him it was a means of survival. "Without drugs, there is no hope. There is nobody to care for me." He would not consider going back to the village, however, because "life is tougher out there!"

Adolescent views on health care services

Our study also revealed how the adolescents perceived the accessibility and acceptability of health services in both the urban and rural study locations. None of the public health facilities mentioned seemed to offer any specific services tailored to the health needs of adolescents, whether outpatient or inpatient. The adolescents said that they were expected to attend clinics meant for adults and to share the inpatient and outpatient facilities, including the wards. Adolescent girls, as young expectant mothers, were also expected to share Maternal and Child Health, as well as Family Planning, services with their parents and other adults. This arrangement was not culturally sensitive, and, as a result, adolescent mothers tended to shy away from the services even though the services were free.

Moreover, the adolescents interviewed complained that clinic staff were rude and often did not show any understanding of the adolescents' situations. This had the effect of excluding from the public health facilities even those adolescents who were able to access them. Despite the fact that public health facilities were very widely distributed and geographically accessible, the cultural barriers and inattentiveness to adolescent needs rendered these clinics inaccessible to the adolescent population.

Assessment of Current National Policies

With insights gained from our study, we analyzed the current national policies that potentially impacted the lives of adolescents (see Box 3). The policy analysis revealed several gaps and contradictions inherent within and between policies and policy guidelines. First, the 1990 National Health Policy states that its overall objective is "to improve the health and well-being of *all* Tanzanians, with a focus on those most at risk, and to encourage the health system to be more responsive to the needs of the people." Of the six specific objectives given, however, none addresses adolescents. The policy also recognizes the need to improve and develop urban health services, but specific provisions are not made to meet the challenge of the large influx of adolescents into urban centers. Furthermore, there is little evidence of any awareness of adolescents as a population group with special needs.

The recent government guidelines regarding user charges for health services attest to this. According to the guidelines, children under 5 years of age are exempt from payment of the fees and, by government pro-

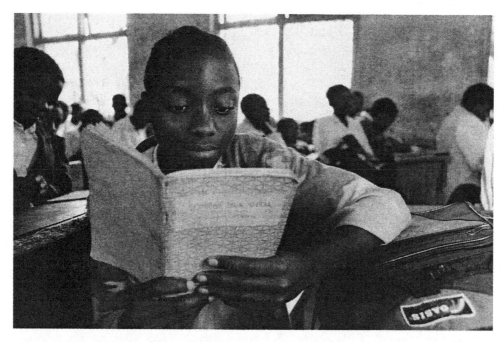

Mwenge Primary School where parents must pay for the school building due to cost-sharing, Shinyanga, Tanzania. *Source:* Crispin Hughes/Panos.

nouncements made at the celebrations to mark the International Day for the Aged in 1999, those aged 65 years and above are to receive free health care. Those above the age of 5 years, including preadolescents (6 to 10 years) and adolescents, are not exempt regardless of their social circumstances. This is a major source of inequity, as it adversely affects those from low-income families and in other vulnerable circumstances. This is tantamount to an unfair denial, by the state, of the right of vulnerable groups of adolescents to health care.

The 1992 National Population Policy, on the other hand, decries the migration of youth from rural to urban centers and the declining labor and productivity in both rural and urban areas. It sets forth four goals:

1. Preparing young people before marriage to become good, responsible parents

2. Educating the public on benefits of women marrying and bearing children after 18 years of age
3. Developing the labor force by expanding primary school enrollment, technical education, and other training
4. Reducing the rate of rural/urban migration

These are noble goals, but there are no strategic programs to achieve them. The policy also assigns the Ministry of National Education and Culture to incorporate Family Life Education into primary, secondary, and teacher education curricula and into all education activities of the various ministries. Six years down the road, however, this is still at the pilot stage. The policy further mandates raising the minimum age of marriage for girls from 15 years, set by the marriage act of 1971, to 18 years, a change that has yet to be achieved. Furthermore, there is no marriage age minimum for adolescent males.

BOX 3: ANALYSIS OF NATIONAL POLICIES CONCERNING ADOLESCENTS

Our study analyzed nine major national policies, selected because of their likelihood to affect adolescent lives and opportunities for good health, either directly or indirectly. Their central objectives and strategies for achieving those objectives were assessed for their likely impact on the issues that emerged from the findings of the earlier phases of this study.

In this context, the following government policies were appraised: National Health Policy (1990), National Population Policy (1992), Education and Training Policy (1995), National Youth Development Policy (1996), Policy on Community Development (1996), Cultural Policy (1997), National Policy on HIV/AIDS/STD (draft 1995), Proposals for Health Sector Reforms (1994), and Health Sector Reform Plan of Action (1996–1999).

The Education and Training Policy of 1995 is explicit about its focus on increasing access to quality education for women and other disadvantaged groups and areas in the country. Ironically, the policy prescribes a reduction in subsidies concurrently with the introduction of cost recovery and cost sharing measures, which may be partly responsible for the high rates of nonenrollment of children in school in the poor rural districts throughout the country. Moreover, the quota system for selecting students for public secondary schools, introduced and applied to ensure district and gender parities, is said to have outlived its original purpose. It is to be phased out, creating room for further inequities based on income status.

The National Youth Development Policy of 1996, along with the Education and Training Policy and the Population Policy, acknowledges that youths, defined as those aged 15 to 24 years, are economically active and engaged in several productive sectors, but they also constitute up to 60% of the unemployed labor force in the country. The Youth Development Policy thus implies that young people constitute a large potential work force, and development of this population category should focus on their effective participation in economic production in the future as adults as well as in their current status as youth.

While the National Youth Development Policy recognizes youth as a labor force, the Community Development Policy of 1996 places responsibility on communities to identify and discard the customs and traditions that have deleterious effects on children and young people. These include treating children as part of the labor force, charging a bride price (ostensibly as compensation for lost labor), discriminating against girls when it comes to distributing the proceeds of the household's economic activities, and denying girls the right to inherit property. Children and young people, as well as elderly and disabled people, are delineated as population groups requiring special care. The policy is clearly not in consonance with the National Youth Development Policy, which recognizes youth as a labor force. It does not make any reference to international conventions on child labor, however, thus opening an avenue for child exploitation, especially in mines, on plantations, and as domestic labor.

According to the Cultural Policy of 1997, one of the objectives of culture is the promotion of community by upholding good habits and discouraging "evil" practices such as drug abuse, sexual abuse, drunkenness, laziness, sloppiness, loitering and sexual promiscuity, as well as discrimination on the basis of gender. The policy then decries the erosion of traditional child rearing practices brought about by the interaction with other cultures and the tendency for some parents to leave child guidance to teachers in schools. The National Policy on HIV, AIDS and sexually transmitted diseases (STDs), however, advocates a departure from this position. The policy advocates the introduction of education on condom use, human sexuality, and other reproductive health issues into the curricula of schools and training institutions. Additionally, it promotes free access to information about HIV, AIDS, and STDs for women of all ages. These provisions are clearly not in line with traditional childrearing practices and the minimization of teacher responsibility for child guidance advocated by the Cultural Policy. Although the National Policy on HIV, AIDS, and STDs does pay some attention to the youth in school, it is clearly more focused on girls, who are identified specifically for education about their own bodies and human sexuality. The policy does not, however, address their reproductive rights. Again, boys are not included in the discussion. Moreover, the policy is completely silent about the sizeable proportion of adolescents not in school.

The topic of health education and health promotion in schools has become a thorny issue. In some quarters, it is recognized that preparation for adult life is not all about sex and sexuality. Adolescents need information to enable them to make choices concerning their lives and livelihoods. Adolescents are products of the society in which they live and are affected not only by social forces but also by physical ones, such as the common causes of morbidity and mortality in the community. The task of educating adolescents was to be addressed countrywide by the national school health program, but, due to funding constraints, the program is currently not in operation. Moreover, because of the declining enrollment of children in schools, the program may miss the large proportion of adolescents and preadolescents who are not in school. School health programs, however, represent a vital opportunity for the re-entry of preadolescents and adolescents into the health system following their exit after the prescribed immunization schedule at age 5 years.

The National Policy Guidelines and Standards for Family Planning Services, Delivery and Training, first published in 1992 and revised in 1994, asserts that

- All males and females of reproductive age, including adolescents, irrespective of their parity and marital status, shall have the right of access to family planning information, education, and services
- Adolescents shall be provided with information, education, and counseling on family planning
- Sexually active adolescents who seek family planning services shall be counseled and provided with family planning methods that are appropriate to them.

The policy, however, is silent on the specific training needed to enable service providers to deal with adolescents as well as the actual provision of education and services to adolescents.

The Strategy for Reproductive Health and Child Survival (1997–2001) is a framework that aims to provide guidelines on priority areas in reproductive health in order to improve the quality of health of Tanzanian citizens of all ages. The policy recognizes maternal morbidity and mortality as a major problem and sets as a goal the reduction of both rates by 50% by the year 2001. Surprisingly, the special vulnerability of adolescent mothers is not recognized, and no specific measures are recommended to address their plight. The policy sets out to introduce and expand user-friendly services into clinics and facilities. To date, however, there has been no movement toward this goal.

Unlike the National Policy Guidelines and Standards for Family Planning Services Delivery and Training, the Strategy for Reproductive Health and Child Survival further recognizes the shortcomings of health providers and sets out a strategy to increase the capacity of reproductive health providers. The resources set aside for reproductive health services do not, however, match the good intentions of the policy. Overall, only a paltry 0.87% of the proposed budget for implementing the strategy is earmarked specifically for adolescent/youth-targeted activities. Moreover, the strategy follows the general trend of focusing only on reproductive health services specifically for girls.

The National Youth Development Policy of 1996 cautions against the mistaken assumption that adolescents, as a group, enjoy good health—an assumption it blames for the absence of "specific plans for youth health services." The policy identifies five health problems:

- HIV/AIDS/STD
- Poor nutrition
- Drug abuse leading to promiscuous behavior
- Harmful traditional practices
- Childbearing at an early age

It charges the Ministry of Health with ensuring the availability of health services to youth without fees, intimidation, or discrimination of any kind and with improving sexual health education. The policy also instructs the Ministry of Education and Culture to provide Family Life Education at all levels of education. The provision of free health care services is not, however, in conformity with the Health Sector Reform Policy of 1994, which boldly declares that health care will no longer be provided free and then proceeds to recommend amendment of the health policy accordingly. The policy makes the provision that "the poor, disadvantaged and vulnerable groups will be given special attention." This, however, does not include adolescents regardless of their socioeconomic circumstances.

The Health Sector Reform Plan of Action (1996–1999) envisions a health sector that will be efficiently managed, well organized, and restructured following the reform process. The required drugs and medical supplies will be available at all the health facilities at a "reasonable price," a sustainable health financing mechanism will have evolved, and the health care workers will be motivated and productive. Of particular relevance to the youth is the provision for a national school health program. The school health program is seriously underfunded, however, and its planned activities have been abandoned due to lack of funds. Moreover, the plan makes no reference to adolescents who have dropped out of school. The health sector plan does not address adolescent problems holistically, let alone attempt to bring in the issue of policy rationalization. It should also have touched on the question of the preadolescent, both in and out of school, but it ignores this issue.

Toward Greater Equity in Adolescent Health

This critical evaluation suggests that there are discrepancies between the needs of adolescents and the relevant policies and programs currently being implemented. First and foremost, adolescent health needs are not known or documented, and thus it is not surprising that their needs are not met. For the few needs that are recognized by policy makers, such as family planning, either the strategies for implementation are inadequate or the programs are stalled due to insufficient funding. As a result, the existing policies are skewed toward the sexual health of girls, neglecting not only adolescent boys but all girls who are not in school and all nonsexual health needs such as nutrition, substance abuse, and accident prevention.

Tanzanian authorities seem to be responding to the challenge by formulating more and more policies. The multiplicity of policies that make reference to the lives and livelihoods of adolescents in a piecemeal way, however, result in glaring contradictions. Youth should work and yet are told not to work, and there is supposed to be access to free care, yet user fees are introduced. The perceptions of the adolescents themselves, as revealed in our interviews and group discussions, can be summed up as follows: "The big problem is that it seems society and the government in general do not have any special plans for us."

Insights from the study indicate that health hazards, poor education, lack of participation in development planning, and lack of access to and/or poor utilization of life opportunities by adolescents are the result of underlying socioeconomic inequities (in particular, poverty) in society and unhealthy adult behaviors that are socially imposed on these young people. As a transition stage from childhood to adulthood, adolescence represents a critical window of "vulnerability." Exposure to health-damaging situations and lifestyles may have a particularly powerful effect in determining the future life chances of adolescents, especially those born into or who find themselves in impoverished circumstances.

Whether adolescents are exposed to or protected from factors that are harmful at this stage may influence their life chances for many years to come. For example, adolescents who are able to stay in school and gain an education are protected from unemployment or dangerous working conditions. They are more likely to be on a "road to health," a path that leads to a life of opportunities and life choices in adulthood.

On the other hand, groups of adolescents can be identified who, during this critical period, may be set on a downward course. Dropping out of school, for instance, not only jeopardizes their future earning capacity and living standards directly but also may lead to deteriorating socioeconomic circumstances, such as child labor, migration away from family and social support, earning a living on the streets (sometimes in the sex trade), and so forth. Such disadvantages at an early age will have a myriad negative effects throughout their adult lives. This is ample justification for special attention to be paid to the developmental needs of this life stage. Yet, from the insights gained by this multifaceted study, it is clear that vulnerable groups of adolescents in Tanzania continue to face a bleak future.

Four Suggested Steps Forward

Four practical pointers emerge from this study for future research and policy in relation to adolescent health equity in low-income countries such as Tanzania. First, this study draws attention to two major policy inequities (1) the relative neglect of adolescent health needs relative to other age groups and (2) the health and social system insensitivity to the diverse needs of vulnerable groups within the adolescent population.

Adolescence must be seen as a critical stage in the life cycle that cannot be dissociated from the broader socioeconomic environment. Such an approach avoids the all too common trend of policy of seeing adolescents as reproductive and sexual threats. Allowing adolescents a voice in crafting more appropriate policies is an important mechanism for ensuring that programs and policies are well matched to the needs of all adolescents and particularly the most vulnerable. The group discussion methodology employed in this study brought out the voices of some of these most marginalized adolescents.

Second, our study highlights the gaps and inadequacies of available population data. The issue of improving the routine data collection needs to be brought to the planning table in the context of both national information systems and data collection controlled by the international aid agencies. As a way forward, certain databanks should be re-analyzed because the results may uncover important insights into the magnitude and dynamics of issues facing adolescents and preadolescents in Tanzania. Such databanks include the longitudinal community-based Adult Morbidity and Mortality Project (AMMP) studies, the 1997 Statistical Abstract, and the 1996 Demographic and Health Survey. Data collection and analysis must be made more sensitive and responsive to adolescents and their needs.

As emphasized above, however, the health problems of adolescents must be understood in the larger socioeconomic context. As Cocksey (1994) observes, "a substantial amount of primary data, for example, the 1988 population census, which could be used with relative confidence to chart certain aspects of national patterns of poverty, has not been analyzed within a poverty perspective. Further analysis of this data set could still be done."

Third, our findings show that there is a much broader range of health-damaging factors to which Tanzanian adolescents are exposed than is typically recognized. The special health needs of groups such as miners and refugees call for much broader thinking on how to address vulnerable adolescents' lives and livelihoods. The findings of such qualitative research should influence the approaches taken by outside aid agencies. A "lives and livelihoods" approach to adolescents implies that the antecedents of poor health need to be tackled in the broader economic and social sphere—going well beyond a focus on adequate provision of medical care.

Fourth, adolescents should not be perceived as mere objects to be addressed by interventions. They should be viewed as active participants in shaping their own lives and communities. Adolescents are struggling not only for integration into society but also for a role to play in their society. They need more than the incessant reminder that they are the "future leaders"—a common phrase in most societies. The paradox is that the choices and opportunities made available to them, to enable them to move in that direction, are often not reflected in development planning, especially in poor countries.

Our study sets the stage for a critical review of the position of adolescents in Tanzania's development agenda. The boys and girls are crying out for attention, not rhetoric. They are calling for an all-inclusive process for developing a realistic, comprehensive development strategy that has measurable objectives. Action-oriented research is now needed in order to inform policy review. The process for policy review and rationalization should be fully participatory and involve the following stakeholders: the government, government agencies, nongovernmental organizations, U.N. agencies, parents, teachers, and, above all, the adolescents themselves. The findings described here indicate the need for pilot studies in a variety of developing country contexts to demonstrate how adolescents can be engaged and involved in programs addressing their needs.

This study was funded by the Swedish International Development Agency (SIDA).

References

Auer B. 1999. *Issues and Concepts of Youth Development.* Paper presented at the Global Meeting of Generations, January 1999, Issues 4. http://www.idc.org/gmg/Youth Paper.htm.

Cocksey B. 1994. Who is poor in Tanzania? A review of recent poverty research. In: Bagachwa M.S.D. (ed), *Poverty Alleviation in Tanzania. Recent Research Issues.* Dar es Salaam: Dar es Salaam University Press, pp. 57–90.

Institute of Adult Education. 1990. *Female Circumcision.* Unpublished Report. Dar es Salaam, Tanzania.

Livigha A., Mekacha R. 1997. Youth Migration and Poverty Alleviation: A Case Study of Petty Traders (*wamachinga*) in Dar es Salaam. Unpublished report of the Research on Poverty Alleviation Project, University of Dar es Salaam, Dar es Salaam, Tanzania.

Luena O., Mwingira M., Angwazi A., Semakafu A. 1996. *Towards Greater Empowerment of Women in Tanzania.* National nongovernmental preparatory conference report for the U.N. World Conference on Women, Beijing, 1995. Dar es Salaam: AMREF.

Lugalla J. 1995. *Crisis, Urbanization and Urban Poverty in Tanzania: A Study of Urban Poverty and Survival Politics.* Lanham, Maryland: University Press of America.

Mabala R. 1995. Today's Girl, Tomorrow's Woman. Unpublished research report. Dar es Salaam, Tanzania: UNICEF.

Mbatia J., Kilonzo G.P. (eds). 1996. *Drug Abuse Prevention. A Handbook for Education in Tanzania.* Dar es Salaam, Tanzania: Mehata Publications.

Mbilinyi M., Semakafu A. 1995. Gender and employment on sugarcane plantations in Tanzania. Sectoral Activities Working Papers, Industrial Activity Branch, Geneva: ILO.

Oppong-Odiseng A.C.K., Heycock E.G. 1997. Adolescent Health Services—Through Their Eyes. Unpublished research report, Derbyshire Queen's Hospital, Department of Pediatrics.

Resnick M.D., Bearman P.S., Blum R.W., Bauman K.E., Harris K.M., Jones J., Tabor J., Beuhring T., Sieving R.E., Shew M., Ireland M., Bearinger L.H., Udry J.R. 1997. Protecting adolescents from harm. Findings from the National Longitudinal Study on Adolescent Health. *Journal of the American Medical Association* 278(10):823–832.

Shao I.F., Kiwara A.D., Makusi G.J. 1992. *Structural Adjustment in a Socialist Country: The Case of Tanzania.* Harare, Zimbabwe: SAPES Books.

Tanzania. Bureau of Statistics. 1996. *Demographic and Health Survey 1996.* Calverton, MD: Macro International.

Tanzania. Ministry of Education and Culture. 1997. *Education and Training Policy.* Dar es Salaam: Government Printer.

Tanzania. Ministry of Health. 1990. *National Health Policy.* Dar es Salaam: Government Printer.

Tanzania. Ministry of Health. 1994. Guidelines for the Implementation of Cost Sharing. Unpublished.

Tanzania. Ministry of Health. 1994. *National Policy Guidelines for Family Planning Services, Delivery and Training.* Dar es Salaam: Government Printer.

Tanzania. Ministry of Health. 1997a. *National Control Program HIV/AIDS/STD Surveillance of 1996.* Epidemiology Unit, National Aids Control Program Report No. 11. Dar es Salaam: Government Printer.

Tanzania. Ministry of Health. 1997b. *Tanzania Health Statistics Abstract.* Dar es Salaam: Government Printer.

Tanzania. Ministry of Health. Undated. *Strategy for Reproductive Health and Child Survival 1997–2001.* Dar es Salaam: Government Printer.

Tanzania/UNICEF. 1999. *Women and Children in Tanzania.* Dar es Salaam: Government Printer.

Tarantola D., Gruskin S. 1998. Children confronting HIV/AIDS: charting the confluence of rights and health. *Journal of Health and Human Rights* 3(1):60–86.

Tumbo-Masaba Z., Liljeström R. 1994. *Chelewa, Chelewa: The Dilemma of Teenage Girls.* Uppsala, Sweden: Scandinavian Institute of African Studies.

United Nations Development Programme (UNDP). 1999. *Human Development Report 1999.* New York: UNDP.

The World Bank. 1998–99. *World Development Report: Knowledge for Development.* New York: Oxford University Press.

The World Bank. 1999. *World Development Indicators.* Washington, DC: Communications Development.

PART III

TACKLING ROOT CAUSES

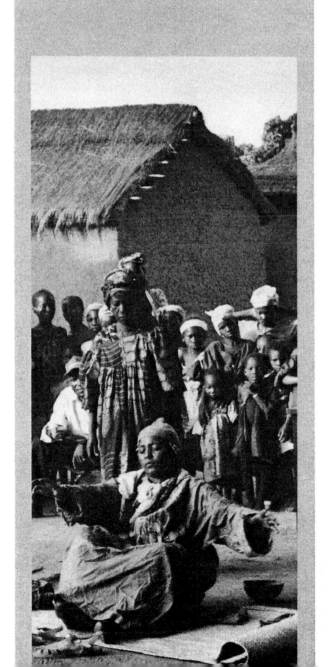

The identification and mapping of health disparities must be complemented by well-conceived policies designed to prevent and mitigate inequity. The development of sound policy to redress inequity in health is an undertaking made all the more complex, however, by the often obscured social and biological pathways along which inequities arise. Factors contributing to health inequities may cut across a range of sectors, such as labor, transport, and welfare, and levels of society—from nation to region to community. In addition, more subtle but pervasive issues like endemic corruption, institutionalized racism, and gender discrimination may underlie cultural norms that generate and perpetuate inequities in health. Untangling the root causes of disparities in health is central to the analyses undertaken in this section of the book.

The first chapter considers the issues of gender, equity, and health. The authors point out that gender bias is one of the fundamental causes of inequity in health and emphasize the need for more equitable gender relations. Through a gender lens they examine inequalities in mortality, morbidity, health care, and health research. A policy analysis describes recent progress in bringing gender issues to the global health agenda and suggests mechanisms for moving toward greater gender equity both in process and in outcomes.

The authors of the South Africa chapter trace the legacy of the apartheid system, pointing out draconian social and economic policies and their ramifications for the health of different groups in the population. The high infant mortality level and the nearly fivefold disparity in infant mortality rates between richer and poorer ethnic groups in the population are but two of the more obvious health impacts. South Africa is now trying to deal with this legacy of apartheid by developing policies with explicit equity objectives. The authors take a critical stance as to whether the government's policies are sufficient to redress the inequities of the past.

In the Kenyan analysis of road traffic accidents, the authors take a creative approach to analyzing policy issues in the transport and road safety sectors. The authors debunk the myth of purely behavioral explanations for the growing burden of road traffic accidents in Kenya, pointing instead to systemic corruption, inadequate labor protections, and lack of alternatives for low-income passengers as root causes of the problem. Rather than fall back on punitive and ineffective efforts to influence driver behavior through crippling fines, the study recommends a variety of policies aimed at engaging stakeholders and tackling the structural antecedents of the problem.

A case study on Bangladesh describes the separate and joint health benefits arising from a rural development program, designed to promote the rights and status of poor women, and a maternal child health program in rural Bangladesh. The case study is remarkable in that the interventions have been accompanied by reductions in inequities in health—differentials between socioeconomic and gender groups in child mortality have narrowed dramatically in the past decade. Not only have mortality rates declined across all social groups, but the greatest absolute and relative gains in child mortality were experienced by girls from the poorest households. This example of intervention research provides a valuable model with which to gather further empirical evidence on the ways to reduce socioeconomic and gender inequities in health.

In a comparison between two Western European countries, Sweden and the United Kingdom, the authors demonstrate a methodology for distinguishing empirically between causal pathways in order to explain the way that macropolicies affect health. The authors examine the hypothesis that the effect of poverty on health may be weaker in Sweden than in Britain—that being poor in Sweden may be less damaging to health than being poor in Britain. They question which aspects of the social and policy context in Britain add to and reinforce the negative experience of being poor—the synergistic effect between social context and poverty and, conversely, which aspects of living in Swedish society are more supportive for poor people, possibly making the experience of poverty less stressful and damaging to health. The two countries serve as a "natural experiment" for a comparative analysis of policy and make the case for more robust health equity impact assessments.

CHAPTER
1 3

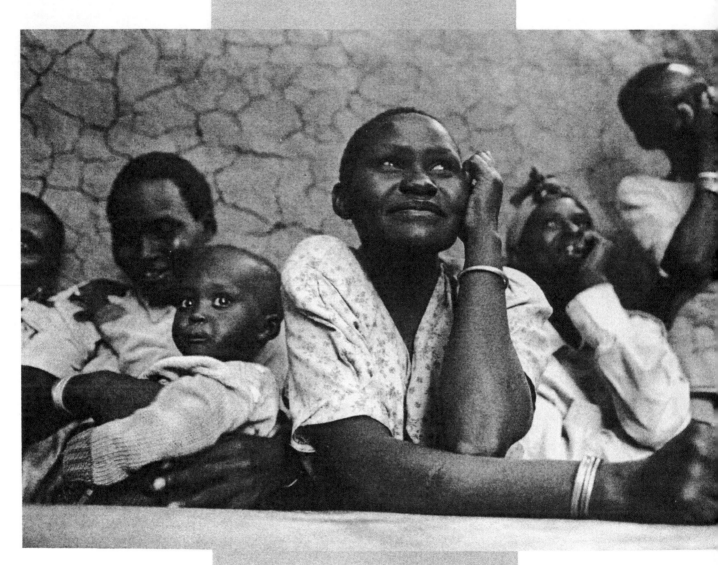

A Kenyan women's group, Tirken Village: "If one of us is ill, the others will help her—fetching wood, or whatever—our unity is really important."
Source: Crispin Hughes/Panos.

Gender, Health, and Equity: The Intersections

PIROSKA ÖSTLIN, ASHA GEORGE, AND GITA SEN

As a fundamental basis for grouping people, gender is a social stratifier that both influences and is influenced by multiple forms of discrimination. The resulting inequalities in health between women and men have not only stimulated medical and social science research during the last decade but also become one of the major public health concerns in policy debates in many countries. Research aimed at a deeper understanding of the social and biological determinants of gender inequalities in health and how such inequalities reflect and sustain social discrimination is an important prerequisite to enabling policy makers to address the health gap between women and men more effectively.

The purpose of this chapter is to illustrate the ways in which gender influences health inequalities. A more detailed discussion is found in our forthcoming review of the subject (G. Sen et al. 2002). This chapter is divided into three parts. In the first part, we describe what we mean by gender and how it informs a health equity perspective. In the second part, we focus on gender influences in four key areas of health: (1) mortality and longevity in general and maternal mortality in particular, (2) morbidity, (3) health care, and (4) medical research. The final section draws on selected examples of policies from both developing and developed countries that have a strong bearing on gender inequalities in health.

Conceptual Intersections: Gender, Health, and Equity

The terms *sex* and *gender* are often used synonymously, but in gender research the two concepts have fundamentally different meanings. Sex refers to the biologically recognized differences between men and women—chromosomes, internal and external sex organs, hormonal makeup and secondary sex characteristics. In contrast, the concept of gender "is related to how we are perceived and expected to think and act as women and men because of the way society is organized, not because of our biological differences" (World Health Organization 1998a). In this way, what is considered "appropriate" female and male behavior can vary across cultures.

However, gender is much more than the socialized relations between individuals. It is a key form of social stratification, which also determines unequal access to resources, biased public representation, and discriminatory institutional policies. Gender is distinct from but *interactive* with other social features like social class or race/ethnicity. All these social factors combine to determine power relations in society that lead not only to inequalities *between* women and men, but also to inequalities *within* different groups of women and different groups of men.

Lastly, although gender and sex are conceptually distinct, in practice, variations of interaction between the two exist. Biological differences between the sexes may be in part socially determined, while social differences arising from gender relations may also have a biological element (Hammarström et al. 2001; Krieger and Zierler 1995).

There are systematic gender differences in income, resources, and benefits. These include, for example, the division of labor both within the household and outside of it, levels of education or medical care received, and liberties that different members of society are permitted to enjoy (A. Sen 1992a). Gender equity, including equity in health, is contingent on fairness in the distribution of resources, benefits, and responsibilities between women and men. This idea of equity envisions health as being located within the larger realm of societal well-being (see chapter 3) and within overarching social and political contexts (see chapter 2).

The gender, health, and inequity interface can initially be broken down into two conceptually distinct dimensions: (1) biologically specific health needs of men and women that are not fairly accommodated and (2) inequalities in health and health care arising from unfair gender relations and not from biological differences between the sexes.

The failure to recognize the biologically specific health needs of women and men is most obviously related, but not limited to, the reproductive system. Perhaps the clearest and most appalling expression of this type of gender inequity is the persistence of extremely high rates of maternal death in childbirth in many developing countries despite the widespread public health know how to prevent such catastrophes (Fig. 1 and further discussion below).

Despite the need to recognize and address such differences, care must be taken to note that such specific needs do not lead to "naturally" different social roles or fewer social opportunities for women or men. Another example of this type of gender and health inequity is the tendency to interpret women's biological reproductive capacity as a basis to justify exclusive responsibility for reproduction to women. Instead, occupational regulations should protect both male and female reproductive health from exposure to toxic chemicals and radiation, and employment policies should support both male and female parenting.

Once these specific needs are addressed fairly, all other differences in health between women and men must be hypothesized as being caused by unequal social relations of gender. For example, although both females and males have similar biological risks for trachoma infection, males at all ages have a lower prevalence of the disease (West et al. 1991a,b). This reflects not only the higher exposure of females through their domestic roles as caregivers to young children who carry the infection, but also a gender bias in access to trachoma treatment favoring males (Congdon et al. 1993; Lane and Inhorn 1987).

Gendered patterns of employment also underlie differentials in occupational health. Women are also disproportionately hired in export factories notorious for their lack of occupational health standards and labor policies that respect their needs. At the same time, rigid gender roles are also dangerous to men's health. The pervasive expectation of men as the family breadwin-

Figure 1 Maternal mortality ratios in selected countries, 1990

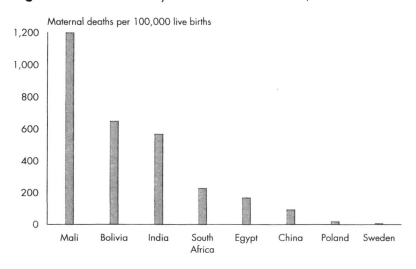

Source: United Nations Development Program 1999.

ner forces many poor men to take jobs that expose them to excessive health risks. If they are unable to meet expectations, they may also resort to health-damaging behaviors such as alcohol abuse and smoking (Sabo and Gordon 1993; see chapter 11). Hence gender roles and the extent to which health care provision is skewed along gender lines underlie male–female differences in health outcomes (Okojie 1994; Doyal 1995).

Women are also disproportionately affected by harmful traditional practices, such as female genital mutilation, which causes health problems and suffering in millions of girls and women (Santow 1995; Craft 1997b; World Health Organization 1997). Although female genital mutilation has recently attracted much public attention, it is only one part of the larger problem of violence against women implicitly and explicitly sanctioned by gender discrimination (Heise et al. 1994). Another disturbing form of social discrimination against women is the health and economic destitution of female-headed households and widows in many developing countries (Chen and Drèze 1995).

Evidence of Gender Inequality in Health

Mortality

Globally, the observed higher rates of male mortality are assumed to be based in biological fact. Women's survival advantage at all ages has been demonstrated in a wide range of countries (Waldron 1983; Hemström 1998). The degree of gender difference in life ex-

pectancy, however, varies across the age spectrum and across time periods (Hemström 1998). In an 11 country study, Hemström identified a range in the mortality rate ratio of men to women from a low of 1.25 at either end of the age spectrum to a high of 2.4 in the early adult years (Fig. 2). As demonstrated in Sweden, the pattern of excess male mortality has varied considerably over the last 50 years (Fig. 3). The variations across age, time, and place suggest that social factors have a significant influence on the biological difference in survival between the sexes.

Where social discrimination against women is less pervasive, women tend to increase their life expectancy beyond that of men (Waldron 1983). In countries where women's mortality rate is higher or equal to that of men, differential female deprivation of extraordinary proportions exists (A. Sen 1992a). Extremes in the range of gaps in life expectancy at birth between males and females are expressed as ratios in Table 1. At the low end are countries such as Nepal and India where women's survival advantage is suppressed, and at the other extreme are former socialist countries where men's survival has decreased even more than women's. In 1994, Russian women could expect to live 13.5 years longer than men, a gender gap in life expectancy that had widened significantly since 1989. In this volume, examples of the variation of this gender difference in survival are abundant (see chapters 7, 10, 11, and 16).

In comparing survival between sexes, one has to be careful not to confuse equality with equity. Amartya Sen argues that a "shortfall" from the optimal value

Figure 2 Average life-course pattern of male-female mortality rate ratios

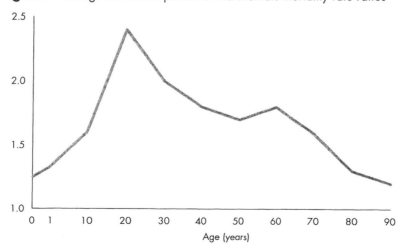

Age (years)

Note: The figure is based on data from Ecuador, Egypt, Finland, Hungary, Israel, Japan, the Netherlands, Portugal, Sri Lanka, Sweden, and the United States. There are two observations for each country (three for Sweden), the first for a year in the 1970s and the second for a year in the 1990s (or the most recent year available). For Sweden, data for 1945 are also used.
Source: Adapted from Hemström 1998.

Figure 3 Male-female mortality rate ratio in Sweden, selected years, 1945–94

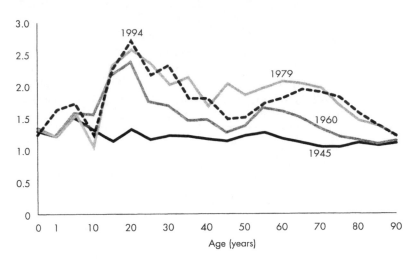

Source: Adapted from Hemström 1998, p. 19.

each sex could ideally achieve would be more useful in measuring gender differences in survival (A. Sen 1992a). A shortfall measure controls for biological differences between men and women and reveals the extent of social discrimination faced by both men and women across different countries. Such an approach raises the important issue of how an optimal value of life expectancy for each sex is agreed upon (see chapter 5).

Table 1 Ratio of female to male life expectancy at birth in selected countries, 1997

Country	Ratio
Maldives	0.96
Nepal	0.99
Bangladesh	1.00
India	1.01
Afghanistan	1.02
Belarus	1.16
Estonia	1.17
Lithuania	1.17
Latvia	1.19
Russia	1.23

Source: United Nations Development Program 1999.

In some countries where female survival is inferior or equal to that of males, sex ratios at birth provide another indication of gender inequity. Under normal circumstances, the male to female ratio at birth is expected to be 1.05 (105 males for every 100 females). In a number of countries, such as China, South Korea, and India, attention has been drawn to sex ratios that are significantly higher than the expected ratio of 1.05. These countries are facing a phenomenon of "missing" girls and women, reflecting differential treatment of women and men, and particularly of girls vis-à-vis boys (A. Sen 1992b; Das Gupta 1998). In China, gender discrimination against females before birth is particularly worrisome: 116.3 males (instead of an expected 105) were born for every 100 females in 1994 (State Statistical Bureau 1995). This unusually high ratio arises from sex-selective abortions, informal adoption of girl babies and concealment or nonregistration of female birth, and female infanticide—reflecting both China's one child per family policy and the culturally rooted preference for sons (Dalsimer and Nisonoff 1997; see chapter 7).

Within countries, average differentials in survival between men and women may mask significant variation across specific causes of death. For example, despite greater overall survival probabilities, women in China (and perhaps in many other countries of South and Southeast Asia) have markedly higher death rates from suicide than men, contradicting the pervasive global trend of greater suicide mortality among males (see chapter 10; World Health Organization 2000).

Gender also interacts with occupational class and race to differentially influence survival. Between 1987 and 1991 British male life expectancy at birth in the upper two occupational classes was 75 years while for the lower two classes it was 70 years. For women, life expectancy at birth was considerably longer, and the differences between the occupational classes were narrower (80 years in the upper two occupational classes and 77 years in the lower occupational classes; Hattersley 1997). In the United States in 1996, mean life expectancy for white women was 6 years longer than for black women, and white men lived an average of 8 years longer than black men (U.S. Department of Health and Human Services 1993).

A third example suggests differences in male–female survival gaps according to level of wealth (Fig. 4). Within a given country, as expected, nonpoor (rich) adult men have a significantly higher probability of dying between the ages of 15 and 59 years than do nonpoor (rich) women. Among the poor, beyond the markedly higher probability of deaths, we also observe that the female advantage in survival has virtually disappeared: from minimal female survival advantage in India and South Africa; to equal survival chances in Egypt, Niger, and Nicaragua; to a situation in which poor women have inferior survival in Sri Lanka, China, Poland, and the Czech Republic.

Although poor women and men in developing countries suffer primarily and disproportionately from infectious diseases, malnutrition, and lack of quality primary health care services, persistently high rates of maternal mortality in the developing world are symptomatic of more profound global gender inequities (see Fig. 1). Of the 585,000 annual deaths among young women in pregnancy or childbirth, 99% occur in developing countries (World Health Organization, 1998b). In Africa the risk of dying is 1 in 16 pregnancies compared with 1 in 65 in Asia and 1 in 1400 in Europe (World Health Organization 1998b). For the most part, maternal deaths are entirely preventable, yet remain unchecked due to lack of emergency health services for the poor and to historical neglect of women's broader reproductive health needs in developing countries. Such societal discrimination has restricted women's health issues to a narrow focus on the control of their fertility rather than on their rights to societal well being.

The social and economic costs of maternal mortality are enormous not only for the women themselves but also for their children's survival and well-being, their households, and society as a whole. When a mother dies or is disabled, household income for children's food, education, and health care is reduced. In such circumstances, daughters are at particular risk in soci-

Figure 4 Probability of dying between the ages of 15 and 59, by poverty status and sex, in selected countries, around 1990

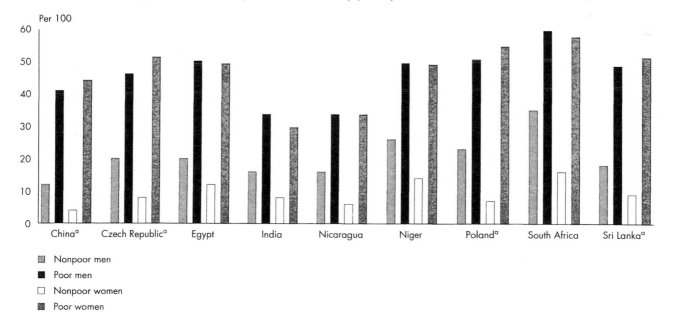

a. Poor women have higher mortality rates than poor men.
Source: World Health Organization 1999a.

eties in which sons are more valued than girls. For example, in Bangladesh one study found that a mother's death sharply increased the chances that surviving children, predominantly girls, up to the age of 10 years would die within 2 years (World Health Organization 1998c).

Morbidity

Because death is frequently preceded by illness, we might expect that those with higher mortality rates would similarly suffer from higher rates of morbidity. In other words, we might expect men, who are more likely to die prematurely, to be more affected by illness. Paradoxically, most research on gender differences in health shows higher rates of illness among women. Studies on morbidity, which are almost exclusively conducted in developed countries, indicate that women, more than men, perceive their health as worse and suffer greater disability. Thus, women's potential for greater longevity rarely results in them feeling healthier than men during their lifetimes. Furthermore, excess female morbidity can be observed in all socioeconomic groups, as illustrated in the Anglo-Swedish study (see chapter 17).

Although literature on morbidity in developing countries is scarce, several community surveys conducted in developing countries show similar patterns of higher female morbidity across the life cycle. A number of studies indicate that women are more likely than men to report feelings of anxiety and depression (Paltiel 1986). In China, a remarkably high disability rate for girls relative to boys under the age of 4 years is reflected in a female to male disability rate ratio of 1.89 (see chapter 7). It is important to note, however, that in poor or rural communities the workload of women is so heavy that societal thresholds for female illness are correspondingly very high (Okojie 1994). As a result, women in these societies endure a great deal of pain before they "admit" or "recognize" that they are ill or before they stop working (Zurayk et al. 1993). Hence, actual levels of female morbidity may be even higher than what is reported.

In this section we discuss several alternative hypotheses that attempt to explain the patterning of excess female morbidity. First, the weaker association between mortality and morbidity among men may suggest that many of the excess deaths among men are not preceded by prolonged related illness. For example, deaths from external causes such as violent deaths due to accidents, suicide, homicide, and war, and perhaps some deaths from heart attack as well, often occur without a preceding period of illness (Hemström 1998). Correspondingly, women's greater longevity in and of itself could be a cause of their higher rates of recorded morbidity. Longer life spans increase both biological and social risks associated with common disabling conditions among elderly women such as rheumatoid arthritis, osteoporosis, and Alzheimer's disease (World Health Organization 1998a; Verbrugge 1985). Even when controlling for differential life span, however, research has also found consistently poorer self-reported health for women in developing countries (Rahman et al. 1994).

Second, it has been hypothesized that women's reproductive ill health may account for their greater morbidity. In many parts of the world, pregnancy-related complications account for between 25% and 33% of all deaths of women of reproductive age and 18% of the global burden of disease for women of this age group (World Health Organization 1996). The true range of morbidity actually suffered is hard to quantify, however, and is potentially much larger than what is currently measured. Many argue that maternal mortality figures only represent the tip of the iceberg—for every maternal death, there are over 100 acute morbidity episodes (Koblinsky et al. 1993).

Although women are more likely to suffer health problems connected to their reproductive functions, one should not conflate all women's health issues with reproduction. This is especially important given the historical antecedents of attributing many female health problems, including mental disorders, to gynecological dysfunction—so-called "globus hystericus"—(Johannisson 1995; Laqueur 1994). A Dutch study has shown that 60% of women's health problems were unrelated to reproductive morbidity (Gijsbers van Wijk et al. 1995). Furthermore, women who do not report reproductive health problems still report worse health than men (Popay et al. 1993).

Third, cultural norms governing gender roles may determine the likelihood of reporting illness and therefore affect the apparent degree of morbidity differentials between the sexes. Some have interpreted excess female morbidity in developed countries as a sign that women may be more observant and more conscious of their bodies and consequently find it easier to report health problems and/or seek medical care. The traditional masculine ideal of remaining impervious to infirmities, on the other hand, may also contribute to gender differences in self-reported illness. Men may underreport morbidity, in keeping with their perceived gender roles (Sabo and Gordon 1993). Thus, it is hypothesized that women exaggerate real morbidity while men underreport it. The few studies in developed countries that compare reporting of morbidity with clinical examination, however, fail to support this hypothesis (Gijsbers van Wijk et al. 1995; Stenberg and Wall 1995).

An important corollary to mortality studies that document greater female longevity is the assessment of female morbidity, as longevity does not seem to translate into greater health and well-being during women's lives. The multidimensionality of morbidity makes gender equity assessments in this area a thorny issue. None of the aforementioned hypotheses provides a wholly convincing explanation of higher female morbidity relative to men. From an equity perspective, this argues against a reliance on single measures of mortality or morbidity when comparing the ill health of women and men. Rather, on a case by case basis, the social and biological antecedents of specific gender inequalities in health must be assessed in order to make an equity judgment.

Health Care

Gender inequities are endemic in health care systems globally. In part, this reflects a lack of gender analysis in the planning and provision of health care systems. It also reflects more general gender inequalities in society that impact on the equitable utilization or consumption of health care. Here we describe some manifestations of these inequities in the planning, provision, and utilization of health care.

In many health care systems there is often insufficient attention to the differential needs of men and women in planning health services. As a result, health services for women often focus on only reproductive functions. The widespread priority of maternal child health has focused primarily on children to the relative neglect of the mothers. Important women's health issues, unrelated to their reproductive role, tend to be shortchanged (Paolisso and Leslie 1995; Vlassoff 1994). In Tanzania, the gender bias in adolescent health policies has led to a disproportionate focus on female reproductive health to the virtual exclusion of policies addressing both male adolescents and young women with nonreproductive health needs (see chapter 12).

Gender inequality may also be manifest in the ways men and women are treated by the health care system. Mounting evidence suggests that male and female health providers may be gender biased in their perception of patient preferences and problems (Pittman and Hartigan 1996). Patient–physician differences in age, class, sex, race, or ethnicity are found to accentuate gender bias in quality of care. Studies from rural communities in West Africa (Prevention of Maternal Mortality Network 1992) and from Chile (Vera 1993) have shown that women are not always treated with respect by health providers. In many societies women complain about lack of privacy, confidentiality, and information about treatment options (Vlassoff 1994). Underpaid, overworked, and gender-insensitive health care workers will be unlikely to communicate with, examine, and prescribe appropriately for women (or men). Not surprisingly, women in some cultures prefer traditional providers (healers), who take the time to listen and explain ailments in easily understood terms. Given that many women are reluctant to be examined by male doctors, the lack of female medical personnel—itself a reflection of gender bias in educational opportunity—is an important barrier to utilization for many women (Zaidi 1996).

Studies in the Netherlands, Sweden, and United States highlight gender inequalities in the provision of certain technologies or treatment services for the same disease. Women with heart disease are less likely than men to receive coronary bypass surgery, and women are less likely to receive organ transplants such as kidney transplants (Kutner and Brogan 1990; Held et al. 1988). In the case of lung cancer, it has been found that women are less likely than men to have cytological tests of sputum ordered by their doctors (Wells and Feinstein 1988).

A wide variety of sociodemographic factors such as employment status and age interact with gender relations to generate inequalities in accessing health care (Puentes-Markides 1992). Although health care services may be available, girls and women may be unable to access them due to discrimination within the household, granting preferential allocation of resources to male needs. Girls are likely to receive less expensive and more home-based care than boys (Lane and Inhorn 1987) and also more likely to suffer from outright neglect of their health needs than boys (Chen et al. 1981; Das Gupta 1987; Ahmed et al. 2000). In general, vulnerable sections of society, such as poor, illiterate, or less educated rural women, may not even be aware of their legal rights to adequate health care (Gijsbers van Wijk et al. 1996).

Clinical Research

Medical research and clinical trials for new drugs have been heavily criticized during the last decade for their general lack of a gender perspective (Freedman and Maine 1993). Health problems that specifically or predominantly affect women have received less attention and funding than research on health problems mainly prevalent among men. The lack of research is obvious in areas concerning menstruation and nonlethal chronic diseases that affect women disproportionately, such as rheumatism, fibromyalgia, and chronic fatigue syndrome (Doyal 1995). The only exception to this trend is contraceptive research, which has historically neglected male methods and focused on controlling fertility rather than on enhancing women's contraceptive and reproductive options.

In the field of occupational health and safety, women are overlooked in toxicological studies. Even when women are considered, their biological specificity is seldom noted. For example, the effects of occupational exposures on lactating women have received little study despite research results indicating the adverse health effects of their exposure to certain chemicals (Messing et al. 1993). This is a particularly important issue for women, as their greater level of body fat means that they store more fat-soluble toxic material even when exposed to the same levels as men (Sims and Butter 2000).

An even more serious problem has been the exclusion of female subjects from study populations for medical and drug research. One rationale for excluding female subjects from research is that the menstrual cycle introduces a potentially confounding variable. Additional grounds for omitting women of childbearing age is the fear that experimental treatments or drugs may affect their fertility. Experimental use of treatment might, moreover, expose fetuses to unknown risk. Despite such concerns, the consequences for women of interpreting research results based on studies of male models and without convincing evidence of their applicability to women, continue to be harmful to women (Hammarström et al. 2001). Accumulating evidence shows that technology for diagnoses, treatment of diseases, and rehabilitation programs are not adapted to the specific characteristics and needs of women in general, let alone to women in various socioeconomic circumstances or cultural backgrounds.

Encouragingly, emerging research on gender differences in cardiovascular epidemiology has revealed the serious shortcomings of applying "male-based" diagnostic techniques and treatments to female patients (Gijsbers van Wijk et al. 1996). In part, this stems from increased recognition that symptoms of heart attack differ significantly between men and women (Loring and Powell 1988). Of particular concern, is recent evidence that life-threatening delays in diagnosis (via EKG) of women may occur because of lack of awareness of the unique nature of female symptomatology (Lerner and

Kannel 1986; Green and Raffin 1993; Heston and Lewis 1992).

There is an obvious need for further research to improve health care professionals' perception of, and response to, gender-specific needs and preferences. Greater gender sensitivity will minimize the risk of attitudinal biases in diagnostic and treatment decisions and help improve health outcomes. Formal medical education and training can be an excellent forum for sensitization to avoid gender bias by providers. Accordingly medical textbooks should reduce the stereotypic representation of the sexes (Mendelsohn et al. 1994). Apart from educational measures, funding guidelines, review boards, and the engagement of women's advocacy groups in research and policy also provide important institutional incentives for change.

Policies for Addressing Gender Inequities

The recognition by policy makers that something can be done about gender inequalities in health has long been obscured by the strong biological and individualistic orientation of medical research. Analysis of socioeconomic, cultural, and environmental influences has consequently been overshadowed by genetic and biomedical models. The resulting view that the determinants of gender inequalities in health are mainly of genetic and biological origin has led policy makers and practitioners to pay insufficient attention to which of these inequalities are genuinely unchangeable and fixed and which are in fact quite amenable to change (Hammarström et al. 2001).

Today there is a growing recognition that the most powerful determinants of health for both women and men are to be found in social, economic, and cultural circumstances. These include, among other things, economic growth, income distribution, sanitation, housing, nutrition, consumption, work environment, employment, social and family structures, education, community influences, and individual behaviors (Blane et al. 1996). All of these circumstances differentially affect women and men due to the positions they occupy in society, the different roles they perform, and the variety of social and cultural expectations and constraints placed on them.

Health promotion, disease prevention, and rehabilitation have until now been recognized as largely the responsibility of those working in the health sector. Health, however, does not arise from actions solely by the health sector, but as the result of all public policies and how they individually, or in interaction with each other, promote or damage health. A narrow focus on the health sector alone obscures the socially constructed gender roles and expectations that may exacerbate health inequalities.

The multisectoral responsibility for creating sustainable health has recently been recognized by the World Health Organization (1999b) policy document *Health 21: The Health for All Policy for the WHO European Region—21 Targets for the 21st Century*. The document emphasizes solidarity, equity, and gender sensitivity. It notes that "decision-makers in all sectors should take into consideration the benefits to be gained from investing for health in their particular sector and orient policies and actions accordingly." Furthermore, "Member States should have established mechanisms for health impact assessment and [ensure] that all sectors become accountable for the effects of their policies and actions on health." Accordingly, an evaluation of the health impacts of various policies on women or men occupying different positions in the social hierarchy is desirable.

In the following section we give examples of strategies that are important from a gender health equity perspective, ranging from macro to micro public policy levels. These strategies include interventions aimed at promoting gender equity in society in general and in health in particular by (*1*) ensuring a supportive macroeconomic and sectoral policy framework, (*2*) promoting gender equity in access to essential goods and services, and (*3*) reducing gender bias in communities and empowering women.

Gender and Macroeconomic Policies

Policies at the structural level include macroeconomic and social policies spanning sectors such as labor market, trade, environment, and more general efforts to improve women's status. Such major structural policies are seldom introduced for the specific purpose of altering the health status of the population, but they all have great potential to reduce or exacerbate gender inequality, including inequalities in health (Whitehead 1995).

The dramatic declines in mortality observed in *developing countries* during the last 50 years are due in part to advances in public health measures and in part to policies at the macroeconomic level. The most important policies leading to improved life expectancy were those aimed at poverty reduction and increased spending on public health measures (Anand 1996). Supportive macroeconomic and sectoral policies that increased income and educational levels allowed greater proportions of the population to obtain the pre-

requisites for good health—food, housing, clean water, and employment opportunities. Investments in schooling, particularly for girls, and policies that increased women's political and economic power have contributed to significant health improvements for women and for whole populations.

In Mauritius, the fertility rate of the population declined dramatically from 6.2 in 1963 to 3.2 in 1972. The rapid success is attributed to advances in girls' education, supportive policies that improved access to health and family planning services, and pension schemes providing for improved social security for all (Lutz et al. 1994). A striking feature of this change in Mauritius, as is also true for similar changes in Sri Lanka and the state of Kerala in India, is that it occurred in the absence of significant economic growth. Per capita income in Mauritius, for example, not only was relatively low but also actually fell during its period of rapid fertility decline in the 1960s before accelerating significantly during the subsequent decades. The ability of governments to retain and even strengthen supportive policies toward sectors such as health, education, and social security in an environment promoting gender equality made these advances possible (G. Sen 1992).

Equity-oriented policies in a social context in which women had traditional matrilineal rights to property and girls were valued as much as boys have resulted in laudable health gains in Kerala, India. Although state policies in Kerala during the twentieth century were not particularly focused on reducing gender inequalities, because the social and cultural environment was not strongly biased against women, it was possible for women to benefit from improvements in health care provision and to achieve high levels of literacy. Not surprisingly, Kerala is the only state in India where the population's sex ratio has been favorable to women throughout the twentieth century and is not plagued by the problem of "missing women."

Unfortunately there are many examples, particularly in the last two decades, of macroeconomic policies that have brought about increased gender inequalities in living conditions and health by worsening the position of women in absolute and/or relative terms. Many developing countries have, for example, introduced structural adjustment policies aimed at halting inflation, gaining economic efficiency, improving the balance of payments, promoting sustainable growth by switching resources to production of tradable goods and services, and allowing liberalization of imports. When, as in many cases, these policies have been implemented without adequate or effective safeguards for the social sectors, they have resulted in severe cuts in public expen-

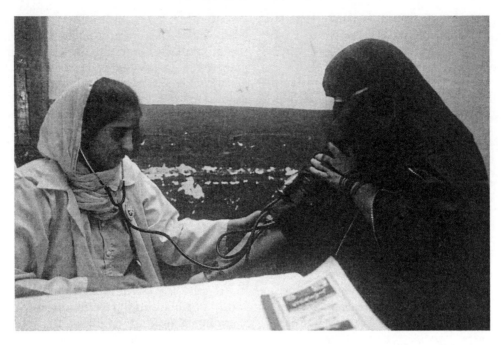

A woman service provider and woman client, Islamabad, Pakistan.
Source: Richard Lord/L & I.

diture on health, education, and other social programs. Privatization of many services including health care; tolerance of higher unemployment rates; promotion of more flexible and informal labor markets; removal of subsidies for food and other basic goods; and increased prices for drugs, foods, and health and educational services have been important parts of structural adjustment policy packages.

The impact of cuts in public expenditure tends to fall most heavily on the most disadvantaged sections of the population and especially on girls and women who have to shoulder the heaviest burden of poverty (Stewart 1992; Whiteford 1993). Econometric proof of causal associations between macroeconomic policies and health outcomes is quite challenging to obtain because of the complex web of associations inherent in such broad social and economic changes. The reallocation and cuts in public resources can, however, clearly lead to serious failures of access to health care, worsening of service delivery, and greater gender inequality as existing gender biases within communities and households interact with shrinking resource availability. A few examples below serve to illustrate the multidimensional impact of some macroeconomic policies on gender inequalities in developing countries.

Increased food prices and removal of food subsidies are major elements of adjustment programs at the macro level. These measures, together with declining earnings, translate into a steep fall in real household incomes and have a strong gender-differentiated impact on poor households (Stewart 1992). Available evidence indicates that decreases in household incomes result in significant malnutrition in girls and women—especially pregnant and lactating women. Many countries, including Brazil, Barbados, and Jamaica, have reported increases in the proportion of low-birth-weight babies during periods of structural adjustment (Dias et al. 1986).

Price reform has also involved the introduction of user charges for health and educational services. In Nigeria, enrollment was reduced by one-third when fees for primary and secondary schools were introduced, while in Sri Lanka several schools were shut down. The introduction of user charges for health care in Ghana was associated with lower attendance at clinics (Stewart 1992). Similar results were also found in Zambia. Cuts in public expenditure on health, drugs and educational services hit women harder than men. When these services are in short supply or increase costs for households, girls more often than boys are taken out of schools and deprived of health services such as immunizations (McPake 1993). Under the pressure of increased male unemployment and rising inflation, mothers are often forced to leave home in order to earn incomes. Girls are then withdrawn from school to care for younger siblings.

Evidence is just beginning to emerge from Southeast Asian countries on the health implications of the budget cuts and inflation following the late 1990s financial crisis. In Asia, International Monetary Fund–supported policies of budget deficit management without effective safeguards for social sector expenditures are, in part, blamed for the crisis. Relief organizations and nongovernmental organizations working at the community level report increasing incidences of hunger, school drop-outs, homelessness, and street children. Based on past experience it would not be far-fetched to anticipate rising gender inequalities from these macro policies. Few countries in the South have been able to protect the social sectors adequately in the face of structural adjustment programs. More recently however, there have been calls for ensuring adequate resources for the social sectors through such measures as the 20–20 compact (the proposition that both governments and international aid donors should allocate 20% of their resources to social sectors) and taxes on financial transactions.

In *industrialized countries* where evidence suggests that the magnitude of income differences is strongly linked to population health status (Wilkinson 1996), policies at the structural level aimed at reducing poverty and social disadvantage are just as important from a public health perspective as in developing countries. The strong association between more inequitable income distribution and lower life expectancy suggests that economic policies that increase income inequalities can therefore be characterized as "unhealthy."

Examples of "healthy" economic policies, on the other hand, aim at compensating those who for different reasons (e.g., unemployment, early retirement, parental leave) experience loss of income (Dahlgren 1997). High rates of universal family benefits are usually found to be linked to low rates of infant mortality (Wennemo 1993). It is likely that "healthy" economic policies influence not only the overall health profile of a population but also the health status of the most disadvantaged sections of the populations, such as single parents, early retirees, and people with very low incomes, many of whom are women.

Sweden, for example, has focused on full employment by developing a parent-worker model through extensive public child care provision and family-friendly employment policies. With gender equity already a national goal, this full employment policy has led to increased job opportunities for women in the public sector. As discussed in chapter 17, expanded provision of social services not only directly enabled more women to find employment but also indirectly enabled other women to pursue careers in other sectors. A cohort study by Vågerö and Lahelma (1998) has followed up and compared the mortality of women who took advantage of these employment policies with that of women who did not. The findings show significantly greater decreases in mortality among those employed. Positive health selection could not alone account for this mortality differential. Other than improving the health of employed women, the provision of social services in Sweden has also mitigated the negative effects of poverty for more disadvantaged women. As a result, poor Swedish women are no more likely than women who are not poor to report fair or poor health (see chapter 17).

Promoting Gender Equity in Access to Essential Goods and Services

Many developing countries continue to suffer from weak or deteriorating health services, infrastructures, and unaffordable services, a situation that disproportionately affects women. The inadequacy and lack of affordability of health services is compounded by physical and psychological barriers to care. At the national level, there have been some attempts to tackle the cost and affordability barriers to health services for women. For example, both South Africa and Sri Lanka provide free maternal and infant health services. Flat fee structures that cover not only regular antenatal and postnatal care but also delivery care, including complications, may be one way to ensure that cost barriers do not prevent families from bringing women in for such services, especially during obstetric emergencies (World Health Organization 1998c). When health insurance schemes are introduced, care should be taken to ensure that poor women are adequately covered (Carrin and Politi 1997).

Even such services as are available or affordable to the poor in general may still be out of the reach for girls and women. In some settings, this is a matter of distance or transport access, which may make it impossible for girls or women to visit health centers, particularly where gender taboos limit women's mobility. Upgrading local (village-level) health centers, setting up systems for reliable emergency transport, and making it possible for women and their attendants to stay near a health facility can help to bridge this gap (World Health Organization 1998c). Such measures have yielded good results in countries such as Cuba, Sri Lanka, Uganda, and, in the Matlab project, in Bangladesh.

Poor quality in patient–provider interactions can also make women unwilling to use health services. There is now substantial evidence showing that improving the quality of care in reproductive health services can significantly increase women's willingness to use such services (Jain et al. 1992). This requires, among other measures, improvement in the attitudes of providers toward women clients through effective training and gender sensitization.

Particularly nefarious are the health systems that exacerbate health inequalities through lack of gender sensitivity. All too often health policy makers tend to view women primarily as "reproducers" and narrowly focus their attention on women in the reproductive ages. In 1994, the International Conference on Population and Development attempted to correct this bias by including actions to meet the health needs of girls, adolescents, and older women.

Perhaps the most comprehensive attempt to design a more holistic policy has been the Comprehensive Program for Women's Health Care, which was created in Brazil in 1983. This program includes a range of reproductive and sexual health services, as well as occupational and mental health services. It includes not only women in the reproductive ages but also postmenopausal women and preadolescents, and it emphasizes that women need access to both preventive and curative care as well as information about their bodies and health (Garcia-Moreno and Claro 1994).

Another positive example of an integrated and gender-sensitive health policy is the "Health for Women, Women for Health" policy enunciated by the Ministry of Health in Colombia in 1992, which explicitly aims to reduce gender inequalities through a comprehensive approach. Its five programs include the promotion of self-help, reproductive health and sexuality, violence prevention and care for victims of violence, mental health, and occupational health. The policy document states explicitly that a "woman has the right to treatment and care from the health services as a whole being, with specific needs—according to her age, activity, social class, race, and place of origin, and not to be treated exclusively as a biological reproducer. She has the right to respectful and dignified treatment by health workers of her body, her fears, and her needs for intimacy and privacy" (Colombia Ministry of Health 1992).

Thus, quality of care and attention to women's health needs throughout the life cycle are critical components in the health system—and as essential to ensuring utilization as physical access and affordability.

Reducing Gender Bias at the Community Level and Empowering Women

Promoting gender equality and equity also requires tackling gender biases in communities and households through community education, empowering women, and training boys and men to reduce gender biases by promoting gender-sensitive behavior and reducing violence. The International Conference on Population and Development initiated a broad-based policy discussion on this subject. There are also many examples from both developed and developing countries of person-based strategies aimed at strengthening individuals in disadvantaged positions (Whitehead 1995). From a gender equity perspective, such strategies have focused mainly on strengthening women to better respond to, and control determinants of, health in the physical or social environment. The most effective interventions have been those with an *empowerment* focus. They aim to help disadvantaged women to gain their rights, improve their access to essential facilities and services, address perceived deficiencies in their knowledge, acquire personal or social skills, and thereby improve their health (for more discussion of empowerment strategies, see Batliwala 1994; G. Sen and Batliwala 2000; Whitehead 1995; Hashemi and Schuler 1996).

Empowerment initiatives aim at encouraging both sexes to challenge gender stereotypes. One of these projects, described by Craft (1997a), is The Girl Child Project (see also International Planned Parenthood Federation 1995), established by the Family Planning Association of Pakistan. The project raises awareness among young girls and their families about unfair and unnecessary discrimination against girls and thereby promotes the status and the value of the girl child. For example, according to the girls involved, the project made them aware that unequal food allocation in the family is wrong. In fact, just a few years ago, Pakistan was one of the countries where the female life expectancy was inferior to male life expectancy. By 1997, this situation had reversed (World Health Organization 1998b), indicating a positive trend toward the greater gender equity in longevity.

In Bangladesh, one of the initiatives (BRAC) integrated into a poverty alleviation project focused on the empowerment of poor rural women by provision of women's microcredit and female education. Gender equity in health was improved considerably via increased economic independence and improved social status relative to men in both public and personal spheres (Bhuiya and Ansary 1998). Positive changes were also reported in food allocation and educational attainment that led to decreasing male bias in a society where preference for sons is deeply rooted. The BRAC initiative, designed to increase gender equity, has also successfully contributed to the sharp decline in the socioeconomic gap in child mortality but has not significantly altered the gender gap in child mortality (see chapter 16).

Conclusion

This chapter has explored the ways in which gender acts as an important determinant of health inequalities and inequity in both high- and low-income countries. The analysis of mortality, morbidity, health care, and clinical health research suggests that gender biases are important and pervasive stratifiers of health outcomes for women and men. These outcomes not only arise from sociocultural beliefs and behaviors but may be sustained and accentuated by policies that are insensitive to the multiple manifestations of gender bias.

The chapter has also provided a range of examples of more gender-sensitive approaches to policy at the macro, sectoral, community, and individual levels. As stated at the outset, gender equity in health depends on fairness in the distribution of health-promoting resources, benefits, and responsibilities between girls and boys and women and men. It also requires policy assurance that men and women will be treated equally where they share common needs, as well as recognition that where their needs are different, these differences will be addressed in an equitable manner. The chapter illustrates that when policies are framed in this manner, they can go a fair way toward closing the health gaps between women and men.

References

Ahmed S.M., Adams A.M., Chowdhury A.M.R., Bhuiya A. 2000. Gender, socioeconomic development and health seeking behavior in Bangladesh. *Social Science and Medicine.* 51:361–372.

Anand S. 1996. Global Health Equity: Some Issues. Paper prepared for Workshop on Global Health Equity, September 20, Harvard Center for Population and Development Studies.

Batliwala S. 1994. The meaning of women's empowerment: new concepts from action. In: Sen G., Germain A., Chen L.C. (eds), *Population Policies Reconsidered: Health, Empowerment and Rights.* Cambridge, MA: Harvard University Press, pp. 127–138.

Bhuiya A., Ansary S. 1998. Status of Health and Health Equity in Bangladesh. Report prepared for the Global Health Equity Initiative (GHEI) Meeting in Dhaka, Bangladesh, December 11–17, 1998.

Blane D., Brunner E., Wilkinson R. 1996. *Health and Social Organization: Towards a Health Policy for the 21st Century.* London: Routledge.

Carrin G., Politi C. 1997. *Poverty and Health: An Overview of Basic Linkages and Public Policy Measures.* World Health Organization Task Force on Health Economics. Geneva: World Health Organization.

Chen L., Huq E., D'Souza S. 1981. Sex bias in the family allocation of food and health care in rural Bangladesh. *Population and Development Review.* 7:147–183.

Chen M., Drèze J. 1995. Widowhood and well-being in rural North India. *In:* Das Gupta M., Chen L.C., Krishnan T.N. (eds), *Women's Health in India: Risk and Vulnerability.* Delhi: Oxford University Press, pp. 245–288.

Colombia Ministry of Health. 1992. *Salud para las mujeres, mujeres para la salud.* Santafe de Bogota: Ministry of Health.

Congdon N., West S., Vitale S., Katala S., Mmbaga B.B. 1993. Exposure to children and risk of active trachoma in Tanzanian women. *American Journal of Epidemiology* 137(3):366–372.

Craft N. 1997a. Women's health is a global issue. *British Medical Journal* 315:1154–1157.

Craft N. 1997b. Life span: conception to adolescence. *British Medical Journal* 315:1227–1230.

Dahlgren G. 1997. Strategies for reducing social inequalities in health—visions and reality. In: Ollila E., Koivusalo M., Partonen T. (eds), *Equity in Health Through Public Policy.* Helsinki: STAKES, pp. 25–53.

Dalsimer M., Nisonoff L. 1997. Abuses against women and girls under the one-child family plan of the People's Republic of China. In: Visvanathan N., et al. (eds), *The Women, Gender and Development Reader.* London: Zed Books, pp. 227–283.

Das Gupta M. 1987. Selective discrimination against female children in rural Punjab, India. *Population and Development Review* 13:77–100.

Das Gupta M. 1998. "Missing Girls" in China, South Korea and India: Causes and Policy Implications. Working Paper Series, No. 98-03, Harvard Center for Population and Development Studies, Harvard School of Public Health, Cambridge.

Dias L.R., Camarano R., Lechtig A. 1986. Drought, recession and prevalence of low birth babies in poor urban populations of the North-East of Brazil. Letter to the editor. *Journal of Tropical Pediatrics.*

Doyal L. 1995. *What Makes Women Sick? Gender and the Political Economy of Health.* London: Macmillan Press.

Freedman L., Maine D. 1993. Women's mortality: a legacy of neglect. In: Koblinsky M., Timyan J., Gay J. (eds), *The Health of Women: A Global Perspective.* Boulder, CO: Westview Press, pp. 147–170.

Garcia-Moreno C., Claro A. 1994. Challenges from the women's health movement: women's rights versus population control. In: Sen G., Germain A., Chen L.C. (eds), *Population Policies Reconsidered: Health, Empowerment and Rights.* Cambridge, MA: Harvard University Press, pp. 47–62.

Gijsbers van Wijk C.M., Kolk A.M., van den Bosch W.J., van den Hoogen H.J. 1995. Male and female health problems in general practice: the differential impact of social position and social roles. *Social Science and Medicine* 40(5):597–611.

Gijsbers van Wijk C.M., van Vliet K.P., Kolk A.M. 1996. Gender perspectives and quality of care: towards appropriate and adequate health care for women. *Social Science and Medicine* 43:707–720.

Green L.A., Raffin M.T. 1993. Differences in management of suspected myocardial infarction in men and women. *Journal of Family Practice* 36(4):389–393.

Hammarström A., Härenstam A., Östlin P. 2001. Gender and health—Concepts and explanatory models. In: Östlin P., et al. (eds), *Gender Inequalities in Health: A Swedish Perspective.* Boston, MA: Harvard School of Public Health.

Hashemi S.M., Schuler S.R. 1996. Rural credit programs and women's empowerment in Bangladesh. *World Development* 24(4):635–653.

Hattersley L. 1997. Expectation of life by social class. In: Drever F., Whitehead M. (eds), *Health Inequalities.* Office for National Statistics, Series DS No. 15. London: The Stationery Office, pp. 73–82.

Heise L., Pitanguy J., Germain A. 1994. *Violence Against Women: The Hidden Health Burden.* Washington, DC: World Bank.

Held P.J., Pauly M.V., Bovbjerg R.R., Newmann J., Salvatierra O. 1988. Access to kidney transplantation, has the United states eliminated income and racial differences? *Archives of Internal Medicine* 148(12):2594–2600.

Hemström Ö. 1998. *Male Susceptibility and Female Emancipation. Studies on the Gender Difference in Mortality.* Doctoral thesis, University of Stockholm. Stockholm: Almqvist & Wiksell International.

Heston T.F., Lewis L.M. 1992. Gender bias in the evaluation and management of acute nontraumatic chest pain. The St. Louis Emergency Physicians' Association Research Group. *Family Practice Research Journal* 12(4):383–389.

Jain A.K., Bruce J., Kumar S. 1992. Quality of services, program efforts and fertility reduction. In: Phillips J.F., Ross J.A. (eds), *Family Planning Programs and Fertility.* Oxford: Clarendon Press.

Johannisson K. 1995. *Den mörka kontinenten. Kvinnan, Medicinen och fin-de-siècle.* Stockholm: Norstedt.

Koblinsky M., Campbell O., Harlow S. 1993. Mother and more: a broader perspective on women's health. In: Koblinsky M., Timyan J., Gay J. (eds), *The Health of Women: A Global Perspective.* Boulder, CO: Westview Press, pp. 33–62.

Krieger N., Zierler S. 1995. Accounting for health of women. *Current Issues in Public Health* 1:251–256.

Kutner N.G., Brogan D. 1990. Sex stereotypes and health care: the case of treatment for kidney failure. *Sex Roles* 24:279.

Lane S.D., Inhorn M. 1987. The "hierarchy of resort" examined: status and class differentials as determinants of therapy for eye disease in the Egyptian delta. *Urban Anthropology* 16(2):151–182.

Laqueur T. 1994. *Making Sex.* Cambridge, MA: Harvard University Press.

Lerner D.J., Kannel W.B. 1986. Patterns of coronary heart disease morbidity and mortality in the sexes: a 26 year follow-up of the Framingham population. *American Heart Journal* 111(2):383–390.

Loring M., Powell B. 1988. Gender, race and DSM III: a study of the objectivity of psychiatric diagnostic behavior. *Journal of Health and Social Behavior* 29:1–22.

Lutz W., Beguant J., Toth F.L., Wils A.B. 1994. *Population–Development–Environment: Understanding Their Interactions in Mauritius.* Berlin: Springer-Verlag.

McPake B. 1993. User charges for health services in developing countries: a review of the economic literature. *Social Science and Medicine* 36:1397–1405.

Mendelsohn K.D., Nieman L.Z., Isaacs C., Lee S., Levison S.P. 1994. Sex and gender bias in anatomy and physical diagnosis text illustrations. *Journal of the American Medical Association* 272:1267–1270.

Messing K., Dumais L., Romito P. 1993. Prostitutes and chimney sweeps both have problems: towards full integration of both sexes in the study of occupational health. *Social Science and Medicine* 36:47–55.

Okojie C.E.E. 1994. Gender inequalities of health in the third world. *Social Science and Medicine* 39:1237–1247.

Paltiel F. 1987. Women and mental health: a post Nairobi perspective. *World Health Statistics Quarterly* 40:233–266.

Paolissio M., Leslie J. 1995. Meeting the changing needs of women in developing countries. *Social Science and Medicine* 40:55–65.

Pittman P., Hartigan P. 1996. Gender inequity: an issue for quality assessment researchers and managers. *Health Care for Women International* 17(5):469–486.

Popay J., Bartley M., Owen C. 1993. Gender inequalities in health: social position, affective disorders and minor physical morbidity. *Social Science and Medicine* 36(1):21–32.

Prevention of Maternal Mortality Network. 1992. Barriers to treatment of obstetric emergencies in rural communities of West Africa. *Studies in Family Planning* 23:279.

Puentes-Markides C. 1992. Women and access to health care. *Social Science and Medicine* 35:619–626.

Rahman O., Strauss J., Gertler P., Ashley D., Fox K. 1994. Gender differences in adult health: an international comparison. *Gerontological Society of America* 34(4):463–469.

Sabo D., Gordon G. 1993. *Men's Health and Illness: Gender, Power and the Body.* London: Sage Publications.

Santow G. 1995. Social roles and physical health: the case of female disadvantage in poor countries. *Social Science and Medicine* 40:147–161.

Sen A. 1992a. *Inequality Reexamined.* Cambridge, MA: Harvard University Press.

Sen A. 1992b. Missing women: social inequality outweighs women's survival advantage in Asia and north Africa. *British Medical Journal* 304:587–588.

Sen G. 1992. Social needs and public accountability—the case of Kerala. In: Wuyts M., et al. (eds), *Development Policy and Public Action.* Oxford: Oxford University Press, pp. 253–278.

Sen G., Batliwala S. 2000. Empowering women for reproductive rights. In: Presser H., Sen G. (eds), *Women's Empowerment and Reproductive Rights: Moving Beyond Cairo.* Oxford: Oxford University Press.

Sen G., George A., Östlin P. 2002. Engendering health equity: a review of research and policy. In: Sen G., George A., Östlin P. (eds), *Engendering International Health: The Challenge of Equity.* Cambridge, MA: MIT Press.

Sims J., Butter M. 2000. Gender Equity and Environmental Health. Working Paper Series, Vol. 10, No. 6. Cambridge, MA: Harvard Center for Population and Development Studies.

State Statistical Bureau. 1995. *Social Statistic Information of China.* Beijing: State Statistical Bureau.

Stenberg B., Wall S. 1995. Why do women report "sick building symptoms" more often than men? *Social Science and Medicine* 40(4):491–502.

Stewart F. 1992. Can adjustment programs incorporate the interest of women? In: Asfhar H., Dennis C. (eds), *Women and Adjustment Policies in the Third World.* London: Macmillan.

U.S. Department of Health and Human Services. 1993. *Health in United States 1992.* Hyattsville, MD: Department of Health and Human Services.

Vågerö D., Lahelma E. 1998. Women, work and mortality: an analysis of the relation between female mortality rates. In: Orth-Gomér K., Chesney M., Wenger N.K. (eds), *Women, Stress and Heart Disease.* Mahwah, NJ: Erlbaum, pp. 73–85.

Vera H. 1993. The client's view of high quality care in Santiago, Chile. *Studies in Family Planning* 24:40.

Verbrugge L.M. 1985. Gender and health: an update on hypotheses and evidence. *Journal of Health and Social Behavior* 26(3):156–182.

Vlassoff C. 1994. Gender inequalities in health in the third world: uncharted ground. *Social Science and Medicine* 39:1249–1259.

Waldron I. 1983. Sex differences in human mortality: the role of genetic factors. *Social Science and Medicine* 17:321–333.

Wells C.K., Feinstein A.R. 1988. Detection bias in diagnostic pursuit of lung cancer. *American Journal of Epidemiology* 128(5):1016–1026.

Wennemo I. 1993. Infant mortality, public policy and inequality—a comparison of 18 industrialized countries. *Sociology of Health and Illness* 15:429–446.

West S.K., Munoz B., Turner V.M., Mmbaga B.B., Taylor H.R. 1991a. The epidemiology of trachoma in central Tanzania. *International Journal of Epidemiology* 20(4):1088–1092.

West S.K., Rapoza P., Munoz B., Katala S., Taylor H.R. 1991b. Epidemiology of ocular chlamydial infection in a trachoma-hyperendemic area. *Journal of Infectious Diseases* 163(4):752–756.

Whiteford L. 1993. Child and maternal health and international economic policies. *Social Science and Medicine* 37(11):1391–1400.

Whitehead M. 1995. Tackling inequalities: a review of policy initiatives. In: Benzeval M., Judge K., Whitehead M. (eds), *Tackling Inequalities in Health. An Agenda for Action*. London: King's Fund.

Wilkinson R.G. 1996. *Unhealthy Societies. The Afflictions of Inequality*. London: Routledge.

World Health Organization. 1996. *Safe Motherhood Progress Report 1993–1995*. Geneva: World Health Organization.

World Health Organization. 1997. *Female Genital Mutilation—A Joint WHO/UNICEF/UNFPA statement*. Geneva: World Health Organization.

World Health Organization. 1998a. *Gender and Health: Technical Paper*. Women's Health and Development, Family and Reproductive Health. Geneva: World Health Organization.

World Health Organization. 1998b. *The World Health Report 1998. Life in the 21st Century. A Vision for All*. Geneva: World Health Organization.

World Health Organization. 1998c. *Report of the Technical Consultation on Safe Motherhood*. October 19–23, 1997, Sri Lanka. Geneva: World Health Organization.

World Health Organization. 1999a. *World Health Report 1999*. Geneva: World Health Organization.

World Health Organization. 1999b. *Health 21: The Health for All Policy for the WHO European Region—21 Targets for the 21st Century*. Copenhagen: World Health Organization Regional Office for Europe.

World Health Organization. 2000. *World Health Report 2000*. Geneva: World Health Organization.

Zaidi A.S. 1996. Gender perspectives and quality of care in underdeveloped countries: disease, gender and contextuality. *Social Science and Medicine* 43:721–730.

Zurayk H., Khattab H., Younnis N., El-Mouelhy M., Fadle M. 1993. Concepts and measures of reproductive morbidity. *Health Transition Review* 3(1):17–40.

CHAPTER

14

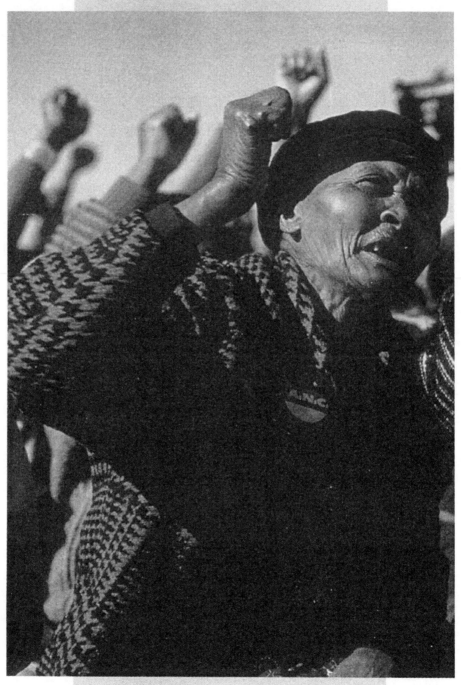

African National Congress rally, Freedom Charter Day, Freedom Square, Kliptown, South Africa.
Source: Joao Silva/Black Star Publishing/ Picture Quest.

South Africa: Addressing the Legacy of Apartheid

LUCY GILSON AND DI McINTYRE

The first post-apartheid government in South Africa came into office in 1994 with a clear mandate: redress inequity. Through the Reconstruction and Development Program (African National Congress 1994a), the dominant partner of the new Government of National Unity, the African National Congress (ANC), committed itself to tackling the huge disparities in the distribution of income and social services it inherited and to reducing poverty. The ANC also emphasized equity as the priority goal of its health policy, rooting the achievement of health gains in broader equitable social and economic development (African National Congress 1994b). Such an approach reflects the largely preventable burden of disease in the country (Health Systems Trust 1997) and the country's relatively poor health performance in comparison with countries of similar or lower income levels (McIntyre and Gilson 2001).

There is growing concern, however, about the government's ability to achieve its socioeconomic goals. There is, in particular, debate and disagreement about the potential influence of the government's current macroeconomic framework—the Growth, Employment and Redistribution strategy (GEAR)—on economic and social change. Given international debate about the potentially negative health effects of other orthodox macroeconomic policies (e.g., Loewenson 1993; Pinstrup-Andersen 1993), as well as the specific potential

of macroeconomic policy to influence health equity (Wilkinson 1996), this chapter has two aims. The first is to understand how macroeconomic policies such as GEAR might have an impact on health equity in South Africa, and the second to consider how to monitor the health equity impact of such policies.

As GEAR was only introduced in 1996, it is not yet possible to undertake a full analysis of its impact. Instead, this chapter explores the policy's potential longer term impact on health equity. It reviews first the pattern of poverty inherited from the apartheid era and then the policy framework underlying it. Following consideration of the weaknesses of available data, it then provides an overview of the pattern of inherited health inequity and an exploration of the influence of socioeconomic factors over this pattern. This analysis demonstrates the broad impact of the apartheid policies on health and health system inequity. It also provides a foundation for an initial assessment of the potential impact of GEAR on this apartheid health legacy. Finally, on the basis of these analyses, future policy, advocacy, and monitoring requirements are considered.

The overall analytical approach of this chapter places inequities, rather than inequalities, at its heart and unashamedly lays responsibility for promoting equity at the government's door. This approach is in line with the South African government's own approach to social policy development, as well as with the broader

South Africa

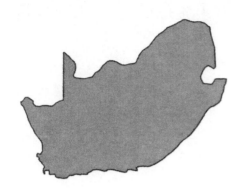

Total population (millions), 1997	38.8
Human development index, 1999	0.695
Human development index rank, 1999	101
Infant mortality rate (per 1,000 live births), 1997	49
Real GDP per capita (PPP$), 1997	7,380
Public spending on health as percentage of GDP, 1995	—

— Not available.
Source: UNDP 1999. [Human Development Report]

trend of reaccepting the importance of the state in development (World Bank 1997). Although health inequality may be biologically or genetically determined, health inequity results from differences in health outcomes between groups that are unnecessary, avoidable, and unfair (Whitehead 1992). Health inequities can be seen explicitly in the differences between groups in their achievement of health potential. These inequities are the result of, or have been exacerbated by, past government actions such as those of the apartheid era in South Africa.

Household Poverty: The Apartheid Legacy Shaping Health Inequity in South Africa

Who Are the Poor and Health Vulnerable?

The first post-apartheid census, taken in 1996, estimates the total population of the country as 40.6 million people. The black population (referring to black African in this chapter) represents 77% of this total, with whites (around 11%), coloreds (around 9%) and Indians (3%) making up the balance. The terms *black*,

white, *colored* and *Indian* indicate a statutory stratification of the South African population in terms of the former Population Registration Act. In South Africa the term "colored" refers to those of mixed race. The use of these terms here does not imply the legitimacy of this racist terminology.

South Africa is categorized as an upper middle income country by the World Bank, with an average per capita gross national product of US$3160 in 1995 (World Bank 1997). Yet the 1998 *Poverty and Inequality Report* (May 1998), prepared for the South African government, indicates that just over 50% of the population is "poor" and 27% is "ultra-poor," assessed against consumption-based income poverty lines. It identifies the most significant indicators of poverty as

- *Race*, with 61% of the black, 38% of the colored, 5% of the Indian, and only 1% of the white population categories being poor
- *The household head's gender*, with 60% of female-headed households being poor compared with 31% of male-headed households
- *Household members' educational levels*, in that those household members who have at least fully completed secondary education tend to assist the household to escape poverty
- *Unemployment*, with the probability of poverty increasing with additional unemployed household members and decreasing with increasing numbers of employed household members
- *Rural residence*, in that 71% of the rural population is poor compared with 29% of the urban population; urban households are, however, significantly poorer than those in metropolitan areas (the term *metropolitan* refers to major urban conglomerations of the country, such as Cape Town), and households in the former "independent homeland" states (see later explanation) face especially high probabilities of being poor
- *Provincial residence*, with three of the nine new provinces having poverty rates of 60% to 70% and accounting for 51% of the total "poverty gap" in the country despite being home to only 36% of the total population. The concept of *poverty gap* is used here to give a sense of the depth of poverty; it is "the aggregate poverty deficit of the poor relative to the poverty line. In other words, it is the [annual] amount needed to lift the poor to the poverty line through a perfectly targeted transfer to the poor" (May 1998: 27).

The provinces, listed in descending order according to poverty rates, are Eastern Cape (71% of residents are poor), Free State (63%), North West (62%), Northern Province (59%), Mpumalanga (57%), Northern Cape (55%), KwaZulu-Natal (52%), Western Cape (28%), and Gauteng (17%) (May 1998).

What Has Made Them Poor and Health Vulnerable?

Apartheid policies essentially served to further the economic privileges and interests of the white minority at the expense of the so-called nonwhite majority population, using a variety of economic and social policy instruments. Of particular importance was the creation and maintenance of a cheap labor system to secure industrial profits. This was achieved by forcing the majority of the black population to live in specified rural areas and then limiting their access to urban areas as part of the broader control over the employment opportunities offered to black, colored, and Indian people.

As early as 1913, the Native Land Act had designated 13% of the available land as the only areas that the black population could purchase and reside in. The apartheid government built on this act by developing the "homelands" as the place of permanent residence for the majority of the black population. Between 1960 and 1982, 3.5 million people were forcibly removed by the state to these areas, and a further 700,000 people were removed from urban areas declared as exclusively for white residence. As these overpopulated homelands were among the most unproductive areas in the country, young and able-bodied men were forced to seek work elsewhere to supplement household income and welfare levels (women were less likely to become migrant workers). These "internal migrants" were then controlled through a diverse set of policies that included requiring them to register with labor bureaus, reserving certain jobs for whites only, and enacting measures, such as the infamous "pass laws," which restricted the movements of the black population within the country. Marais (1998: 22) has consequently called apartheid "an exclusionary regime of accumulation" in which the labor surplus was barricaded "on a periphery which took economic, social, political and geographic forms."

The promotion of a cheap labor supply combined with capital-intensive modes of production had three particularly important consequences for poverty: the development of a heavily segmented labor market, high levels of unemployment, and huge income inequalities between population categories.

In South Africa the labor market is divided by job type, race, gender, and location, and movement between segments is almost impossible (Heintz and Jardine 1998). Highly paid professional and managerial jobs, in which unemployment was low and security high, have largely been the preserve of white men. Production workers and service employees face higher levels of unemployment, less job security, lower wages, and few benefits. Finally, workers in the informal economy suffer very unsteady employment and little legal protection or regulation of employment conditions. A disproportionate number of women and members of the black population work within the lower paid and less secure labor market segments, facing much greater risk of unemployment. Rural residents have particular difficulties in gaining access to the labor market, and even in the informal economy they have lower incomes. The poor employed include domestic workers and rural farm workers whose wage levels fall well below the "minimum living level." This level is derived from the World Bank's definition of poverty, the inability to attain a minimal standard of living, and is determined as the income level an individual requires to satisfy basic consumption needs. It is in effect a "poverty line," and those below it are defined as living in poverty. Rural farm workers are also heavily dependent on their employers for additional services like schools, housing, electricity, medical care, water, and transport.

Overall, "astronomically high unemployment rates prevail" (Heintz and Jardine 1998: 25). Total unemployment in 1995 was around 29%, but over half the black women looking for work could not find jobs, and the rural rates of unemployment for both men and women were nearly twice those in urban areas. Sixty-nine percent of the unemployed have never worked. These conditions have translated into huge income inequalities. The degree of income inequality in South Africa is exceeded only by that in Brazil and Guatemala (World Bank 1997). The poorest 40% of households account for only 11% of total income, while the richest 10% capture 40% of total income (May 1998). Income distribution is unequal across many dimensions. In 1995, the average household income of whites was over four times that of the black population, urban households had double the average income of rural households, and average household income varied by a factor of three across provinces. These income distribution patterns are consolidated and exacerbated by highly concentrated asset (land, capital, financial holdings, real estate) ownership patterns (Heintz and Jardine 1998).

Social policy broadly supported the thrust of economic policy. Housing policy, for example, specifically reinforced influx control by preventing the majority of the black urban labor force from owning or buying houses in urban areas. Instead, hostel accommodation was built for migrant workers in urban areas, while some housing developments in the homelands sought to dampen unwanted rural/urban migration (Hindson 1987). One analyst also argues that health policy in the

Figure 1 Policy influences on health and individual and household welfare

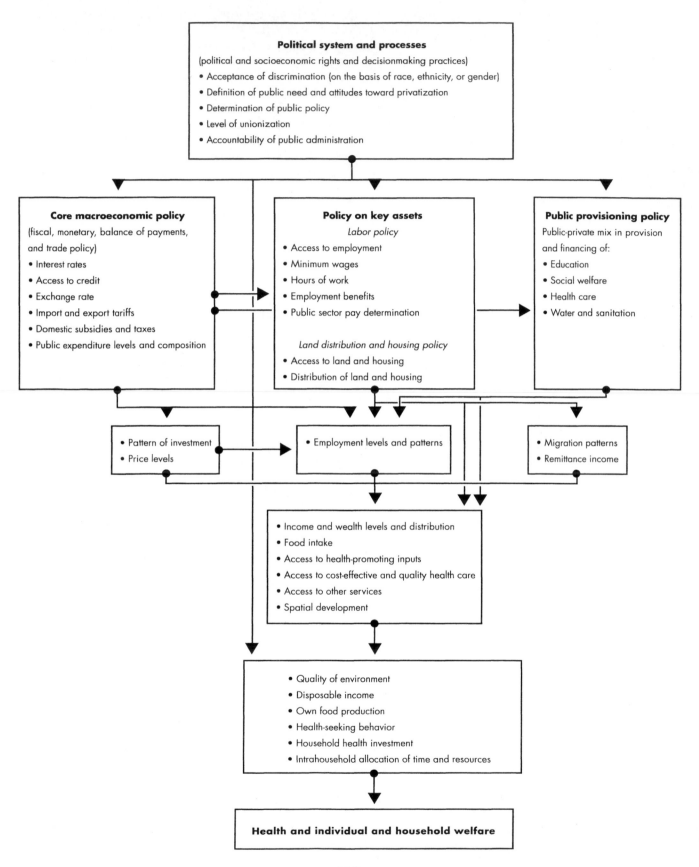

1980s was specifically used as an instrument to support the broader government policy of "co-opting" the increasingly skilled, urban black labor force in the face of economic and political turbulence (Price 1986). He argues that the government spent more on health care in urban than in rural areas in order to limit the loss of working time due to sickness among the black labor force as well as to improve their standards of living. At the same time, the policy supported the maintenance of a good, cheap health care service for the poorer white community, which owed political allegiance to the ruling National Party. In 1985, only 13% of total public health expenditure was spent on health care in the homeland areas, where 32% of the total population (and 40% of blacks) resided (de Beer et al. 1988). Spending patterns generally supported the apartheid bias in favor of the white population. In 1980–1981, the government spent, on average, five to six times more on education (Jinabhai and Coovadia 1984) and in 1985 nearly four times more per head on health care for the white than for the black population (Savage and Benatar 1990). The lack of basic mortality and morbidity statistics for the black population is a clear sign that their needs were simply not considered in health policy development (Jinabhai and Coovadia 1984).

The consequences of apartheid policies for the health system include inequitable resource allocation patterns (biased toward the more wealthy and more urban of the new provinces) and health care provision patterns biased toward less cost-effective, higher level curative care demanded by the more wealthy white population (McIntyre et al. 1995; McIntyre and Gilson 2001).

A further legacy of the apartheid era is the dominance within the health system of the private sector. Although serving only 23% of the population on a regular basis, it accounted for nearly 60% of total health care spending in 1992–1993 (McIntyre et al. 1995). Nearly 39% of the respondents in a large, national 1995 household survey who sought care used private sector services, including 23% of those in the lowest income quintile (McIntyre et al. 1998a).

The political system and processes clearly shaped the overall nature of the economic policies and economic exclusion in the apartheid era, as well as the definitions of public need and approaches to public provisioning. Thus, the denial of political rights to the "nonwhite" population underpinned the apartheid policy package. Not only were the "nonwhite" prohibited from voting, but strict controls also restricted levels of unionization. Political reforms were, however, among the first to be implemented in response to the apartheid crisis of the 1970s. Government first sought to restructure labor relations (Marais 1998) and then, through the 1984 constitution, to extend political rights marginally. It established a "tricameral parliament" with three different sets of political representatives—one for each of the white, colored, and Indian populations. The white population, however, remained dominant while blacks remained excluded from even this small degree of political power. Not surprisingly, these reforms were "too little, too late" to redress several decades of unremitting political and economic exclusion. Powerlessness remains "almost a defining characteristic of the poor" in South Africa (May 1998: 41).

Figure 1 provides a schematic overview of these policy influences over household and personal health and welfare in the apartheid era and highlights key mediating factors. Reflecting wider international evidence and thinking on these issues, it also illustrates that South Africa provides one of the clearest examples of how government policy can directly influence household health and welfare.

It also highlights key issues that must be considered by policy makers seeking to offset the apartheid legacy. The post-apartheid democratic processes and structures represent a political foundation for more inclusive practices. Their overall equity impact will, however, depend on their broader influence. The impact of government policies is, at one level, mediated through household and community factors. For example, an individual's access to income or other resources is often a function of intrahousehold decision making practices that commonly discriminate against certain age groups and women. Political change must be translated into the practice of policy making and public administration and into broader equity-supporting socioeconomic policy change. Although international experience emphasizes the particular influence of core macroeconomic policies (see Fig. 1) over health and welfare, South African experience points rather to the critical influence of the overall labor policy. Future policy must also take into account the internal migration promoted by apartheid, and the subsequent creation of fragile households primarily dependent on the remittance income received from these workers.

Data and Methods Used in Analyzing Health Inequity

Data Sources and Weaknesses

Routine health data are largely unavailable, and what exist are both limited and weak. There are, for example, few morbidity data other than those reported from health facilities for notifiable diseases such as tuberculosis. Currently available mortality data undercount deaths in black and rural populations as a result of the past government's failure to include data from the former homeland areas, as well as severe inadequacies in birth and death notification systems, particularly in rural areas. In addition, few data are available to monitor trends over time, and few data or analyses disaggregated by factors other than race (or area) are available.

Given these problems, the analyses presented here draw on data from the two available national household surveys with relevant information at the time of analysis, representing the best available data at this time. Both the 1993–1994 *Living Standards and Development Survey* (LSDS) and the 1995 *October Household Survey* (OHS) provide data on various socioeconomic indicators (income, employment, education, and so forth) as well as some limited health status and health care utilization data (see Box 1).

Approaches Used in Analyzing Health Inequity

Two health status indicators are used in these analyses: the self-reported diarrhea rate and the infant mortality rate (IMR). The diarrhea rate was selected as an indicator of a type of disease burden in the population that is both preventable and greatly influenced by access to basic public health amenities, such as clean water, safe food supply, and sanitation. It is also a relatively straightforward symptom for self-reporting purposes, less open to the problem of differential perception of general ill health among different income groups described by Amartya Sen in chapter 6. Unlike other cause-specific reported illness rates, this measure offers sufficiently large sample sizes to allow relevant analyses (McIntyre et al. 1998b). A utilization level was also determined for different population categories to allow consideration of health system inequity (see Box 1).

Infant mortality rates calculated from household survey data are often underestimated, as infant deaths tend to be underreported compared with the reporting of surviving children (Nannan et al. 1998: 1585). In contrast, there is concern that the LSDS data used to determine IMRs here may overestimate mortality levels (I. Timaeus, personal communication). The current analyses are, therefore, intended only to illuminate broad patterns of inequity as well as to allow identification of useful analyses to undertake with the more reliable data sets soon to be available (such as the 1996 population census and the 1998 Demographic and Health Survey).

The population categories used in this analysis are summarized in Table 1, and information about how they were determined and how they were used as socioeconomic proxies is provided. They were selected after consideration of the apartheid poverty and policy legacy and were chosen to allow both reflection of the consequences for health of particular aspects of government policy and consideration of the differences in health and health care utilization between socioeconomic groups. Such analysis was, however, constrained by the data available within the available household surveys and the analytical approaches of the past. For example, few gender-specific data of sufficiently large sample size (when cross-tabulated by socioeconomic categories) were available, and there is no commonly

---

BOX 1: DATA SOURCES

Living Standards and Development Survey, 1993

- National household survey
- Small sample size of 8848 households, but with regional stratification to ensure geographic and racial representativeness
- Conducted by the South African Labour and Development Research Unit

Indicators

- Infant mortality rate—deaths among children under 1 year of age per 1000 live births
- Self-reported diarrhea rate—diarrhea as a percentage of all self-reported illnesses

October Household Survey, 1995

- National household survey
- Sample size of 29,700 households
- Conducted by the Central Statistical Service (recently renamed Statistics South Africa)
- Most recent and comprehensive survey available

Indicator

- Utilization level—consultations with formal health care providers per person per year, based on reported contacts during a 1 month period; calculated as number of contacts per person times 12 months

Table 1 Population categories used in analyses in tables 2–10

Criterion for category, by policy area	Categories	Variable used for indicator
Race	Standard definitions: black, colored, Indian, white	Race of dead or sick person
Macroeconomic policy		
Household income level	Quintiles based on per capita household income	Quintile of dead or sick person's household
Employment status	Not economically active, unemployed, employed in formal sector, employed in informal sector	For infant mortality rate, mother's employment status; for diarrhea rate, employment status of sick person
Social policy		
Education level	No education, primary, secondary, postmatriculation qualifications (obtained after leaving school), currently studying	For infant mortality rate, mother's education level; for diarrhea rate, education level of sick person
	For data from the October Household Survey, two categories, certificate or diploma and degree, are used rather than post-matriculation qualifications	
Environmental health index	Determined from household survey data on water supply, type of sanitation, and energy source used for cooking (with each element scored 0 or 1 using criteria reflecting standards appropriate to South Africa). Index ranges from 0 (worst) to 3 (best)	Household environmental health index
Government resource allocation (based on geographical area)		
Area of household residence	Rural, informal urban (informal settlements in urban areas), other urban (formal settlements), homeland, nonhomeland	Household residence
Province of household residence	The nine new provinces: Eastern Cape, Free State, Gauteng, KwaZulu-Natal, Mpumalanga, Northern Cape, Northern Province, North West, Western Cape	Household residence

accepted definition of "social class" currently in use in South Africa.

The explicit use of a racial categorization in this analysis does not imply any acceptance of the idea that health status differences between racial groups in South Africa are primarily biologically or genetically determined. It is, instead, used as a reflection of the apartheid policy framework and is intended to contribute to the current and important debate about the use of race in health analyses (e.g., Ellison et al. 1996).

The rate ratio has been determined for each health status indicator and for each population group, using the group with the highest socioeconomic status as the reference group (Mackenbach and Kunst 1997). The significance of the difference within each population grouping was tested using the z-test and a 1% level. To allow a closer examination of the influence of income on health, IMR variation across income quintiles is also presented for the black and colored populations (sample sizes being too small to allow presentation of these data for the Indian and white groups). Two alternative ways of calculating rate ratios, using different reference groups, are then presented for the income quintiles within the black and colored populations.

Further analyses explored patterns of health system inequity on the basis of utilization data. The correlation between utilization levels and health status indicators is assessed using data for population groups categorized by race and income combined. A mean annual per capita formal care utilization level is then determined for each population category, and variations between population categories are explored. This is based on utilization of nurses, doctors, dentists, specialists, and pharmacists working in the public or private health sectors.

Table 2 Health status indicators by racial group in South Africa, 1993

Group	Infant mortality rate (per 1,000 live births)	Diarrhea rate (percentage of all self-reported illnesses)
Black	72	7.2
Colored	22	4.1
Indian	32	3.9
White	13	3.0
Rate ratio: black to white	5.5*	2.4*

* Significant at the 1 percent level.
Source: 1993 South African Living Standards and Development Survey.

The Apartheid Legacy of Health Inequity

Tables 2 through 8 show health inequity using 1993 data on IMR and reported diarrhea rates for the range of population categories used in this analysis. They suggest that there is a relationship between indicators of health status and socioeconomic status and point to the range of socioeconomic factors underlying the inherited distributions of ill health. This range, in turn, clearly reflects the intertwined economic and social policy package of the apartheid era as outlined above, with its specific racial bias.

Race was clearly important within the range of factors considered. The black population suffered greater levels of ill health than the white population for the two indicators presented. From Table 2, for example, there was a five-fold difference in IMR between the black and white populations and a more than twofold difference in reported diarrhea.

Table 3 illustrates the fact that households in the lowest income quintile suffered greater levels of ill health than those in the highest quintile. In relation to infant mortality, there was a three-fold differential between the poorest and the richest groups.

The lowest income households within the black and colored groups also suffered higher levels of ill health than the highest income quintile, but the differences were only significant for IMR within the black population (Table 4). It was not possible to look at this pattern within the Indian and white population groups because there were no reports of infant deaths or diarrhea cases in some of the low-income categories.

The small differences in levels of ill health across employment status levels, using the "unemployed" category as the low socioeconomic status group, were not significant (Table 5). This may suggest that there is no relationship between employment and health. However, as Table 5 also indicates, the levels of both health

Table 3 Health status indicators by household income quintile in South Africa, 1993

Income quintile	Infant mortality rate (per 1,000 live births)	Diarrhea rate (percentage of all self-reported illnesses)
Poorest	86	11.0
Second	75	7.3
Third	60	7.5
Fourth	49	4.6
Richest	30	3.3
Rate ratio: poorest to richest quintile	2.9*	3.3*

* Significant at the 1 percent level.
Note: Households were assigned to quintiles by per capita household income.
Source: 1993 South African Living Standards and Development Survey.

Table 4 Health status indicators by race and household income quintile in South Africa, 1993

Race and income quintile	Infant mortality rate (per 1,000 live births)	Diarrhea rate (percentage of all self-reported illnesses)
Black		
Poorest	87	11.2
Second	78	7.1
Third	66	8.0
Fourth	60	4.9
Richest	54	4.1
Rate ratio: poorest to richest quintile	1.6*	2.7*
Colored		
Poorest	55	n.a.ᵃ
Second	33	5.1
Third	13	4.8
Fourth	19	3.7
Richest	23	4.6
Rate ratio: poorest to richest quintile	2.4	n.a.

* Significant at the 1 percent level.
n.a. Not applicable.
Note: Households were assigned to quintiles by per capita household income.
a. No reported cases.
Source: 1993 South African Living Standards and Development Survey.

status indicators were worse for the "not economically active" category than for the "unemployed" category. Further consideration of the subcategories used in this analysis would, therefore, be useful in clarifying the nature of any relationship between employment status and health.

In relation to social policy, there were significant differences for both health indicators across education groups and across households categorized by the environmental health index (Tables 6 and 7). Among these indicators, the greatest difference was in IMR between the children of mothers with no education and those

Table 5 Health status indicators by employment status in South Africa, 1993

Employment status	Infant mortality rate (per 1,000 live births)	Diarrhea rate (percentage of all self-reported illnesses)
Not economically active	70	5.7
Unemployed	51	5.6
Employed in informal sector	55	3.6
Employed in formal sector	51	4.7
Rate ratio: unemployed to employed in formal sector	1.0	1.2

Note: For the infant mortality rate, the employment status is that of the mother; for the diarrhea rate, it is that of the sick person.
Source: 1993 South African Living Standards and Development Survey.

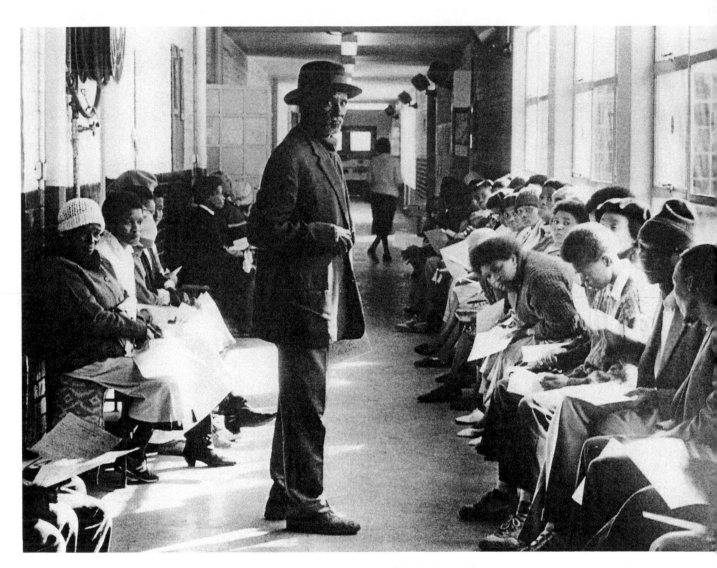

Alexandra Clinic, Alexandra township, Johannesburg.
Source: Gisele Wulfsohn/Panos.

Table 6 Health status indicators by level of maternal education in South Africa, 1993

Maternal education level	Infant mortality rate (per 1,000 live births)	Diarrhea rate (percentage of all self-reported illnesses)
No education	83	8.3
Primary	81	3.8
Secondary	39	3.5
Currently studying	43	6.4
Postmatriculation qualifications[a]	21	3.0
Rate ratio: no education to postmatriculation qualifications	3.9*	2.8*

* Significant at the 1 percent level.
Note: For the infant mortality rate, the education level is that of the mother; for the diarrhea rate, it is that of the sick person.
a. Qualifications obtained after leaving school.
Source: 1993 South African Living Standards and Development Survey.

with the highest levels of education—a fourfold difference in rates (still not as large as the more than fivefold difference observed across racial groups).

Finally, Table 8 shows that people living in rural, informal urban, and homeland areas (the more disadvantaged areas) suffered worse levels of ill health than those living in urban and nonhomeland areas (the wealthier geographic areas). The differences were significant in most cases, except for that of reported diarrhea between informal urban and other urban areas. Relatively high, and significant, levels of variation in health status were also identified in the comparison of the two indicators across all provinces (Table 8). Although sample sizes preclude detailed analysis, geographic inequities were also seen within provinces between rural/urban and homeland/nonhomeland areas.

Interrelationships between geographic and socioeconomic inequities are difficult to interpret, however, and cannot be inferred from these data.

Figure 2 provides further evidence to explore the mediating factor of income over the observed relationship between race and health status. It shows that IMR improves quite clearly across income levels for the black group and across quintiles 1 to 3 for the colored group—and the improvement is greatest at the lowest income levels for these groups.

We used three alternative norms to measure inequity within the black and colored groups, determining rate ratios using data on IMR (Table 9). The use of the IMR of the richest white group (quintile 5) as the reference rate generates larger rate ratios than the use of each group's own quintile 5 rate (comparison of column 3

Table 7 Health status indicators by household environmental health index in South Africa, 1993

Environmental health index[a]	Infant mortality rate (per 1,000 live births)	Diarrhea rate (percentage of all self-reported illnesses)
0 (worst conditions)	89	8.5
1	69	6.1
2	54	4.2
3 (best conditions)	31	3.2
Rate ratio: category 0 to category 3	2.9*	2.7*

* Significant at the 1 percent level.
a. The index is determined from household survey data on water supply, type of sanitation, and energy source for cooking, with each element scored 0 or 1 based on criteria reflecting standards appropriate to South Africa.
Source: 1993 South African Living Standards and Development Survey.

Table 8 Health status indicators by geographical area of residence
in South Africa, 1993

Geographical area of residence	Infant mortality rate (per 1,000 live births)	Diarrhea rate (percentage of all self-reported illnesses)
Rural	78	7.3
Informal urban	64	6.0
Other urban	37	3.5
Rate ratio: rural to other urban	2.1*	2.1*
Rate ratio: informal urban to other urban[a]	1.7*	1.7
Homeland	76	7.3
Nonhomeland	46	3.8
Rate ratio: homeland to nonhomeland	1.7*	1.9*
Province with highest rate	103[b]	8.6[c]
Province with lowest rate	22[d]	3.0[e]
Rate ratio: highest to lowest province	4.7*	2.9*

* Significant at the 1 percent level.
a. Informal urban means informal settlement areas which tend to be poorer than other urban areas.
b. Free State.
c. Eastern Cape.
d. Northern Cape.
e. Western Cape.
Source: 1993 South African Living Standards and Development Survey.

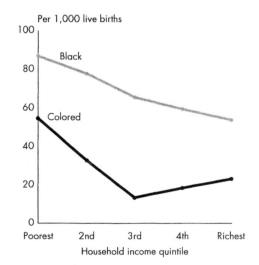

Figure 2 Infant mortality rate for black and colored population groups by income quintile in South Africa, 1993

Source: 1993 South African Living Standards and Development Survey.

with column 2). This might be seen as an inappropriate reference rate, however, because the health status of this group is exceptionally good even for countries of a similar income level. The white quintile 5 estimated IMR of around 14 per 1000 is less than half the average rate for all upper-middle-income countries (36 per 1000, according to World Bank 1995). The fourth column, thus, uses the average IMR of all upper-middle-income countries as the reference rate. Although the rate ratios in this column are considerably lower than those of the third column for both races, they still measure greater levels of inequity than when the black quintile 5 rate is used as the reference rate. For the colored population, the lower rate ratios of the fourth column in comparison with the second indicate that the IMRs of this group are relatively good by international "standards."

A final aspect of the apartheid legacy is that of health system inequity. As noted, public expenditure patterns systematically discriminated against the black, colored, and Indian populations and against less wealthy geographical areas. In addition, nonparametric correlation analysis (using Spearman's rho) indicates that higher levels of utilization are associated with better health status across groups categorized by the combination of race and income quintile, although the significance of

Table 9 Infant mortality rate ratios using different norms in South Africa, 1993

Race and household income quintile	Richest quintile for racial group[a]	Richest quintile for white population[a]	Average for all upper-middle-income countries[a]
Black			
Poorest	1.6	6.1	2.4
Second	1.4	5.5	2.2
Third	1.2	4.6	1.8
Fourth	1.1	4.1	1.7
Richest	1.0	3.8	1.5
Colored			
Poorest	2.4	3.8	1.5
Second	1.4	2.3	0.9
Third	0.6	0.9	0.4
Fourth	0.8	1.3	0.5
Richest	1.0	1.6	0.7

a. Reference rate.
Source: Based on data from the 1993 South African Living Standards and Development Survey.

the association varied. The association is not significant for reported diarrhea, but is significant at the 5% level for IMR (analysis not shown).

This finding is broadly supported by Table 10, which presents data on utilization levels for a range of population categories. They suggest that lower socioeconomic groups tend to use health care less than high socioeconomic groups, despite their generally worse levels of health status. The exceptions are the low-income group within the white population, who appear to use health care significantly more than the white high-income group, and the lower income group within

the medically insured population (although this difference is not significant). These findings are also generally supported by further multivariate analyses.

Overall, these data suggest that utilization is particularly sensitive to race, household income level, employment status, education status, household environmental health status, geographical area, and insurance status. The influence of these factors confirms the impact of the broad apartheid policy package on the health system.

Finally, Box 2 highlights the key issues that this analysis suggests should be considered when policies are

---

BOX 2: ISSUES TO CONSIDER IN THE DEVELOPMENT OF NEW POLICIES TO TACKLE THE APARTHEID LEGACY OF HEALTH INEQUITY

- The lowest income black and colored groups may benefit proportionately more in health terms than other groups from actions to raise household income (although income levels may only partially offset the disadvantage associated with the racial differentials of the past).
- Health status gains for low-income groups are likely to be supported by social policy action at both individual (e.g., education) and household (e.g., environmental conditions) levels.
- Geographical health inequities might be partially tackled through public sector resource re-allocations across and within sectors (which indirectly target the black and col-

ored populations who live in poor rural and informal urban areas).
- Utilization inequity between population groups is likely to require broad socioeconomic policy action, as well as specific action concerning access to health insurance.
- Financial inequities within the public health system can be addressed through health sector resource reallocations.

Note: Two important policy issues that could not be considered are the influence of pension income over health and the impact of migration on household health and welfare.

Table 10 Health care utilization level by socioeconomic status in South Africa, 1995

Groups with high socioeconomic status	Utilization level	Groups with low socioeconomic status	Utilization level	Rate ratio
All whites	3.5	All blacks	1.7	2.1
Richest quintile		Poorest quintile		
All racial groups	3.0	All racial groups	1.1	2.7
Black	2.3	Black	1.3	1.8
Colored	2.7	Colored	1.4	1.9
White	3.5	White	4.2	0.8
Indian	3.5	Indian	2.8	1.3**
Employed	2.0	Unemployed	1.4	1.4
Degree-holders	3.6	No education	2.2	1.6
EHI3 (best)[a]	2.7	EHI0 (worst)[a]	1.6	1.7
Medically insured (richest quintile)	3.4	Medically insured (poorest quintile)	3.5	1.0**
Medically uninsured (richest quintile)	2.6	Medically uninsured (poorest quintile)	1.4	1.9
Other urban	2.6	Rural	1.7	1.5
Other urban	2.6	Informal urban	1.6	1.6

** Not significant at the 1 percent level.
Note: Utilization level refers to the number of consultations with formal health care providers per person per year.
a. EHI is environmental health index. See notes to Table 7.
Source: 1995 October Household Survey.

developed to tackle the apartheid legacy of health and health system inequity. Are these issues being tackled by GEAR, the current macroeconomic policy framework?

Exploring the Potential Impact of Postapartheid Macroeconomic Policy on Health Equity

Key Components

GEAR establishes economic growth as its preeminent goal, to be achieved primarily through greater private, particularly foreign, investment, greater export competitiveness, and productivity improvements (Department of Finance 1996; Heintz and Jardine 1998; Marais 1997; May 1998).

Reducing the government deficit, from 5.7% of the gross domestic product in 1996 to 3% in 2000 (in late 1998, this target figure was revised to 3.9%), is a central strategy for improving business confidence and encouraging private investment. This deficit reduction in turn requires that public spending is rationalized and

controlled, as GEAR argues that taxes should not be increased above current levels and that government spending should increase at a slower rate than any growth in the overall economy. Other policies to promote investment include tight monetary policy (using high interest rates to keep inflation low, maintain the value of the currency, and discourage increases in credit availability), as well as the removal of import tariffs and exchange controls in order to encourage foreign investment. Trade policy is then directed at ensuring export-led growth, with more labor-intensive patterns of production to be promoted through tax incentives for businesses.

Productivity increases are also encouraged through a three-fold strategy. First, labor market flexibility is to be regulated so that even though labor market outcomes will be negotiated through collective bargaining, there will be flexibility in relation to employment standards and wage moderation. In addition, there will be education and training for the labor force while public asset restructuring will improve the operation of existing public enterprises (through privatization or the development of public–private partnerships).

Overall, however, GEAR represents a policy package that gives preeminent emphasis to the policy levers highlighted in the box on "core macroeconomic policy" in Figure 1 as mechanisms through which to generate economic growth and, ultimately, redistribution. It identifies job creation resulting from economic growth as the main route to redistribution, supported by the public provisioning made possible through economic growth. As Heintz and Jardine (1998: 17) note

The logic of GEAR is straightforward: as unemployment drops, poverty will gradually disappear. In addition, economic growth, once it happens, will also generate additional public resources which can then be used to provide public services and poverty relief. The document argues that reducing government spending in order to bring down the deficit will actually pave the way for increased spending in the future, made possible by rapid economic growth.

How Might GEAR Affect Household Health and Health Inequity?

The analysis presented earlier clearly suggests that, like broader redistribution, GEAR's influence over the apartheid legacy of health inequity will be strongly mediated by its impact on the income levels of the unemployed and poor employed and on job creation for these groups (see also Box 2). International experience (e.g., Wilkinson 1996) suggests that these and other policies with an impact on income distribution patterns may have particular importance in tackling health inequity.

Data on economic growth and job creation within South Africa since 1994, however, are not encouraging. The initial projection of 3% economic growth for the 1998–99 fiscal year was reduced in late 1998 to 0.2%, and the 1999–2000 fiscal year projection was halved from 4% to 2% (Ensor and Steyn 1998). At the same time, the unemployment rate has risen since GEAR was introduced—from 32% (or 20% under a narrower definition of "unemployed") in 1994 to 38% in 1997 (23% under the narrower definition) (*The Star: Business Report*, August 15, 1998: 5; see also Heintz and Jardine 1998; Marais 1997). These data suggest that the low income levels and the poverty associated with employment patterns from the pre-1994 government are hardly being touched, and macroeconomic policy post-1994 is unlikely to have begun to offset inherited patterns of health inequity.

As GEAR was only introduced in 1996, however, these problems are clearly not only a function of GEAR. Indeed, as is common in such debates, some suggest that GEAR has not been fully implemented and thus cannot be judged on the basis of these figures (*Business Report on Sunday*, November 8, 1998). The South African economy was also strongly affected in 1998 by the consequences of the Asian economic crises. Critics, however, argue that GEAR is likely to fail in its intentions, as it ignores the fundamental need to transform the economic structures, particularly the segmented labor market, inherited from the apartheid era (Heintz and Jardine 1998). This criticism receives support from a review of Figure 1. GEAR is primarily reflected in the "core macroeconomic policies" box in Figure 1 and so does not explicitly address the wider range of apartheid legacies influencing health and welfare, even while affecting policies designed to tackle them.

Critics identify the promotion of wage restraint and a flexible job market as the most important constraints on GEAR's potential to create jobs and raise the income levels of the poor (Adelzadeh 1996; Maganya 1996; Marais 1997). Job creation in the low-wage sector, spurred by market flexibility and international competition, will do little to reduce poverty and inequality, while wage moderation will have limited impact on the huge income differentials among the formally employed. Those likely to be hardest hit by labor market flexibility are women, and thus GEAR is said to have the potential to exacerbate gender inequality within the household (Budlender 1997; Heintz and Jardine 1998). Some analysts even suggest that current macroeconomic policies will create a strong division between a core pool of organized labor able to demand improved working conditions and an increasingly disorganized segment of the labor force unable to negotiate improved wage levels, working conditions, or social benefits (Nattrass and Seekings 1996). Overall, the International Labor Organization (1996: 18) suggests that although job creation is one way of reducing inequalities, "one would be a little skeptical that it would do so quickly or substantially."

Other aspects of GEAR may also be counterproductive to the goals of creating jobs for, and raising income levels among, the poorest. Critically, the pursuit of low inflation through high interest rates may actually contract job opportunities by discouraging investment. The potential of public investment to attract other investment is being ignored, and policy development reveals how little understanding the government has of job creation within the informal economy. Finally, public sector restructuring involving public sector employment cuts is likely to hit both the poorest provinces and women hardest (Adelzadeh 1996; Budlender 1997; Maganya 1996; May 1998).

The wide range of other policies being implemented might, however, offset these negative impacts. The package of new labor laws is particularly important. It seeks to address problems such as low wage levels and poor conditions of service (Basic Conditions of Employment Act of 1998); skills development policies; poor employment security and limited organizational rights (Labor Relations Act of 1995); and historical recruitment and promotion practices biased in favor of white employees (Employment Equity Act of 1998). Again, some critics suggest that these policies may only promote greater unemployment. Moreover, because the casually and informally employed are largely excluded from the regulatory safety net introduced by these policies, they offer only limited relief for the lowest income groups, which are also ignored by GEAR (May 1998; Murphy 1995). It also remains unclear how the implicit tension between the labor flexibility promoted by GEAR and the restrictions on that flexibility encouraged by new labor laws will affect implementation of either set of policy actions. To date, GEAR is being given greater weight in terms of policy rhetoric.

Other important redistributive policies include land reform, housing provisions, public works employment programs, and the transformation of public provisioning by reprioritizing public expenditure policies. These may also, however, be constrained by GEAR. For example, the high interest rates and limited access to credit and productive capital that GEAR promotes are likely to raise the cost of financing land redistribution and housing development (Heintz and Jardine 1998). Policy implementation in these areas has also been criticized for being slow (May 1998; Eveleth 1998).

GEAR also has the potential to undermine public provisioning, including public works and skills development programs, through three mechanisms: its deficit target (which critics suggest need be neither so low nor so speedy; Lewis 1998), its refusal to allow higher taxation levels, and its determination to reduce the public debt through orthodox measures that maintain investor confidence. As the second largest government expenditure after education, interest payments effectively reduce the availability of resources for social and other spending. Many commentators in South Africa suggest that because the debt is largely held internally and is primarily a function of the nature of the civil service pension scheme, the debt burden could be relieved by restructuring this scheme or even by measures such as a "1 year interest holiday" (Duffy 1998; May 1998). In the health sector, for example, public expenditure ceilings mean that it is likely to be more difficult to shift resources away from higher level hospital care towards primary care and to redirect resources to the most disadvantaged of the rural areas (McIntyre and Gilson 2001). Indeed, there is already

some evidence to suggest that the pace of resource reallocations in favor of previously deprived provinces has slowed, and in some provinces, the redistribution process has been reversed since the 1997–1998 financial year (McIntyre et al. 1998b). Although this problem is partly a result of provincial administrations being given responsibility for allocating resources between sectors, GEAR's critics argue that the national deficit target contributes to provincial budgeting failures by unfairly penalizing relatively underresourced provinces (van Zyl 1998). Moreover, provincial deficits are not counted as part of the national deficit, and this allocation approach allows the central government to move toward national deficit targets despite social service failings within provinces (May 1998; van Zyl 1998). Overall, while GEAR's supporters claim that constrained public sector expenditure levels will only encourage retargeting of public expenditures in favor of the poorest (Donaldson 1997), critics emphasize that redistribution is always "more difficult when it goes hand in hand with cost containment" (Budlender 1997: 20; see also May 1998).

The debates over GEAR will continue, but there are already warning signals about its potential to have a negative impact on households. In failing to enable actions such as those outlined in Box 2, its policies may do little to tackle the underlying causes of health inequity within South Africa and may also undermine efforts to strengthen public provisioning.

Policy and Monitoring Conclusions

Strong political foundations for redressing the exclusionary policies of apartheid have clearly been established in South Africa, including a Constitution based on the idea of substantive, rather than formal, equality. This is rooted in the understanding that "it is not enough to ensure that all people are treated the same if starting points are unequal. Instead, one might need to treat different groups and individuals differently in order to ensure that their finishing points are equal" (de Bruyn and Budlender 1998: 56). As Figure 1 illustrates, however, these political foundations are not enough by themselves to redress the inherited health and socioeconomic inequities, a goal that must be secured by wide-ranging action to tackle the pervasive and inimical apartheid legacy.

Inevitably, South Africa reflects international experience in its continuing debate over what range of broader policy actions is feasible and appropriate in the drive to redress inequity. In some senses, the debates over GEAR are largely rhetorical. Policy, as implemented, generally diverges from written or spoken intentions of the policy so that focusing criticism on the GEAR document may lead to the implementation issues simply being ignored. The debates are important, however, because they illuminate the need to build socioeconomic policy on the specific features of the South African context. For example, to address the peculiar nature of the labor market inherited from the apartheid era, one might begin by giving particular attention to the needs of women in better-funded public works and skills development programs and by supporting microcredit facilities for the poor (Budlender 1998; Heintz and Jardine 1998; Ndungane 1998).

What is the role for health policy makers in relation to these debates and policy interventions? Almost inevitably, health policy makers have focused primarily on the public medical care system since 1994, introducing a wide range of changes designed to orient the system more closely to the needs of the poorest and most vulnerable (McIntyre and Gilson 2001). Although important, these actions are not enough by themselves to redress apartheid's health inequities. The removal of primary care fees, for example, may signal the government's commitment to the poorest, but the impact of this action is inevitably constrained by the geographical and cultural barriers that are often the more important deterrents of utilization by such groups. Although new primary care facilities are being built to improve access, these actions are in turn constrained by financial limits (exacerbated by GEAR's deficit targets) and a bias toward more organized and less disadvantaged communities (McIntryre and Gilson 2001; see also Friedman 1997; Marais 1997). Moreover, despite relevant policy development (Department of Health 1995), none of the government's implemented policies has given clear direction on how to tackle the inherited division between public and private health care (although action has been taken to improve regulation of the insurance industry). The influence of insurance status on utilization patterns clearly highlights the importance of the issue in redressing health system inequity.

Outside the health sector, health policy makers also have a legitimate role to play in developing an understanding of the broad policy framework necessary to redress health inequity, as it is a key element of past socioeconomic exclusion. Such a framework needs to address both questions of content and institutional design—most importantly, the arrangements required to allow the multisectoral action necessary to promote health. Health policy makers also have a vital role in signaling when other policies may undermine efforts to promote health equity. For example, the early signs that inequities in interprovincial health resource allocations may grow over time has spurred national and provincial action seeking to protect health sector resource allocations.

To enter into broader policy debates, however, it is vital to develop an effective and appropriate monitoring system that allows consideration of the impact on *health* inequity of the changing range of economic and social policies. The past influence of race strongly suggests that it should continue to be used to monitor the impact of new policy strategies on health inequity. Its use will allow changes in inequity over time to be identified and thus will permit close review of whether and how the apartheid legacy is being tackled. On both moral and practical grounds, however, it must no longer be the only category used. As identified in this chapter, socioeconomic differentiation within the population also influences health status, and its influence might be expected to grow with time. Future monitoring must, therefore, allow detailed and careful analysis of the socioeconomic determinants of health inequity and trends over time.

Critical steps toward developing an effective health equity monitoring system include

- Changes in the attitudes of policy makers, given Budlender's comment (1997: 25) that "sometimes categories such as women, rural, or even race, are being used to avoid less comfortable categories such as class, income and employment inequalities"
- Routine scanning of the macroeconomic and sociopolitical policy environment and its changes that are likely to have a bearing on health (such as the extent, range, and nature of job creation; wage level changes in different segments of the labor market; price changes and their relative impact on households of different income levels; asset redistribution; and broader changes in the pattern of sociopolitical exclusion/inclusion)
- Improved data collection to support and strengthen the existing efforts to address the weaknesses of the birth and death registration and to develop a national health information system, giving specific attention to ways of tackling the problems that may affect the collection and use of data (such as migration)
- Identifying the health status indicators that can best reflect health inequities, such as cause-specific mortality and morbidity (giving particular attention to preventable causes), and indicators such as the perinatal mortality rate or immunization rates that directly reflect health system performance
- Collecting individual and household socioeconomic data that will allow appropriate social categorization, including specific review of employment/occupational categorizations, and moving toward the creation of a nationally acceptable index of social position (Krieger and Moss 1996)

- Collecting data at the level of small geographical areas to allow more detailed analysis of the influence of factors better measured at the areal level (such as income distribution) over health equity (Krieger and Moss 1996) and to inform geographical resource allocation patterns
- Conducting multivariate analyses of the determinants of health inequalities, using trend data wherever possible; and investigating, through cross-sectional qualitative inquiry and/or longitudinal investigation, factors such as life cycle issues, influencing the health and economic situation of specific vulnerable groups (such as women, rural farm workers, and groups living within urban informal settlement areas), and the influence of migration over household socioeconomic and health status.

Finally, an effective health equity monitoring system must also promote broad engagement in understanding and interpreting patterns of health inequity and the influence of policy over them. The process of monitoring must be open and transparent, engaging all sectors of society. On the one hand, South Africa boasts an active civil society that can implement and support aspects of the monitoring process, as well as disseminate information to communities and their organizations. On the other hand, a diverse range of political and government bodies could be drawn into the process—from the South African Human Rights Commission (whose mandate includes monitoring socioeconomic rights) to the parliamentary committees specifically charged with responsibility for overseeing policy development at national and provincial levels. Wide-ranging ownership is as important as government leadership and action in developing an effective health equity monitoring strategy.

We are very grateful to Eyob Asbu, Debby Muirhead, Neil Soderlund, Nicole Valentine, and Haroon Wadee for their analytical and research support. In addition, Debbie Bradshaw, Debby Budlender, Lesley London, Francie Lund, and Ian Timeaus provided helpful comments on an earlier version of the paper, as did the editors and reviewers involved in this volume. However, the authors accept final responsibility for the paper. Funding for the study was provided by the Swedish International Development Agency (SIDA). The Centre for Health Policy has been accorded the status of Research Group on Health Policy by the South African Medical Research Council (MRC), and receives MRC funding in terms of that status. Lucy Gilson is a part-time member of the London School of Hygiene and Tropical Medicine's Health Economics and Financing Programme, which receives support from the UK's Department for International Development.

References

Adelzadeh A. 1996. *GEAR: Neo-Liberalism in RDP Clothing*. Johannesburg: National Institute of Economic Policy.

African National Congress. 1994a. *The Reconstruction and Development Program: A Policy Framework*. Johannesburg: Umanyano Publications.

African National Congress. 1994b. *A National Health Plan for South Africa*. Johannesburg: African National Congress.

Budlender D. 1997. Introduction. In: Budlender D. (ed), *The Second Women's Budget*. Cape Town: Institute for Democracy in South Africa, pp. 9–39.

Budlender D. 1998. Policy priorities through gender lens. *Budget Watch* 4(3):7.

de Beer C., Buch E., Mavradonis J. 1988. *A National Health Service for South Africa Part 1: A Case for Change*. Johannesburg: Center for Study of Health Policy, Department of Community Health, University of Witwatersrand.

de Bruyn J., Budlender D. 1998. Intergovernmental fiscal relations. In: Budlender D. (ed), *The Third Women's Budget*. Johannesburg: Institute for Democracy in South Africa, pp. 50–88.

Department of Finance, Republic of South Africa. 1996. *Growth, Employment and Redistribution: A Macroeconomic Framework*. Pretoria: Department of Finance.

Department of Health, Republic of South Africa. 1995. *Report of the Commission of Inquiry into Social Health Insurance*. Pretoria: Department of Health.

Donaldson A.R. 1997. Social development and macroeconomic policy. *Development Southern Africa* 14(3):447–463.

Duffy G. 1998. *The Economics of South Africa's Public Debt Problem*. Report prepared for South African Non-Governmental Organization Coalition and Alternative Information Development Center, Johannesburg/Cape Town.

Editorial. 1998. *Business Report on Sunday*, November 8, 1998, p.4.

Ellison G., de Wet T., Ijselmuiden C., Richter L. 1996. Desegregating health statistics and health research in South Africa. *South African Medical Journal* 86(10):1257–1262.

Ensor L., Steyn G. 1998. Budget deficit up to 3.9% of GDP. *Business Day*, November 3, 1998, p.2.

Eveleth A. 1998. Land reform targets are far, far away. *Weekly Mail and Guardian*, June 5–11, 1998, p. 41.

Friedman S. 1997. Delivery and its discontents: delivery targets and the development challenge. *Development Southern Africa* 14(3):463–470.

Health Systems Trust. 1997. *South African Health Review 1997*. Durban: Health Systems Trust.

Heintz J., Jardine C. 1998. *Poverty and Economics in South Africa*. SANGOCO Occasional Paper Series, prepared for the South African NGO Coalition, The South African Human Rights Commission and the Commission for Gender Equality, Johannesburg.

Hindson D. 1987. *Pass Controls and the Urban African Proletariat in South Africa*. Johannesburg: Ravan Press.

International Labor Organization. 1996. *Restructuring the Labor Market: The South African Challenge*. Geneva: International Labor Organization.

Jinabhai C.C., Coovadia H.M. 1984. Socio-Medical Indicators for Monitoring Progress Towards Health-for-All in South Africa. Paper presented at the Second Carnegie Inquiry into Poverty and Development in Southern Africa, Cape Town.

Krieger N., Moss N. 1996. Accounting for the public's health: an introduction to selected papers from a U.S. conference on "Measuring Social Inequalities in Health." *International Journal of Health Services* 26(3):383–390.

Lewis D. 1998. Exploding the myths about job creation. *Sunday Independent*, July 26, 1998, p. 11.

Loewenson R. 1993. Structural adjustment and health policy in Africa. *International Journal of Health Services* 23(4):717–730.

Mackenbach J., Kunst A. 1997. Measuring the magnitude of socioeconomic inequalities in health: an overview of available measures illustrated with two examples from Europe. *Social Science and Medicine* 44(6):757–771.

Maganya E. 1996. The contemporary development paradigm and South African policy-making in the 1990s. In: Maganya E., Houghton R. (eds), *Transformation in South Africa? Policy Debates in the 1990s*. Johannesburg: Institute for African Alternatives, pp. 2–13.

Marais H. 1997. The RDP: is there life after GEAR? *Development Update* 1(1):1–20.

Marais H. 1998. *South Africa: Limits to Change: The Political Economy of Transformation*. London: Zed Press.

May J. (ed). 1998. *Poverty and Inequality in South Africa*. Report prepared for the Office of the Executive Deputy President and Inter-Ministerial Committee for Poverty and Inequality. Durban: Praxis Publishing.

McIntyre D., Baba L., Makan B. 1998b. Equity in Public Sector Health Care Financing and Expenditure in South Africa. Input paper for the 1998 Annual Health Review, Health Economics Unit, University of Cape Town, Cape Town.

McIntyre D., Bloom G., Doherty J., Brijlal P. 1995. *Health Expenditure and Finance in South Africa*. Durban: Health Systems Trust and World Bank.

McIntyre D., Gilson L. 2001. Putting equity in health back onto the social policy agenda: experience from South Africa. *Social Science and Medicine*. In press.

McIntyre D., Gilson L., Valentine N., Soderlund N. 1998a. *Equity of Health Sector Revenue Generation and Allocation: A South African Case Study*. Cape Town: Health Economics Unit, University of Cape Town and Johannesburg: Center for Health Policy, University of Witwatersrand.

Murphy M. 1995. South African farm workers: is trade union organization possible? *South African Labor Bulletin* 19(3):20–26.

Nannan N., Bradshaw D., Mazur R., Maphumulo S. 1998. What is the mortality rate in South Africa? The need for improved data. *South African Medical Journal* 88(12):1583–1587.

Nattrass N., Seekings J. 1996. The challenge ahead: unemployment and inequality in South Africa. *South African Labor Bulletin* 20(1):66–72.

Ndungane N. 1998. The challenge to transform. *Budget Watch* 4(3):1–3.

Pinstrup-Andersen P. 1993. Economics crises and policy reforms during the 1980s and their impact on the poor. In: Jancloes M., Carrin G. (eds.) *Macroeconomic Environment and Health*. Geneva: WHO, pp. 85–115.

Price M. 1986. Health care as an instrument of apartheid. *Health Policy and Planning* 1(2):158–170.

Savage M., Benatar S.R. 1990. Analysis of health and health services. In: Schirre R.A. (ed), *Critical Choices for South Africa: An Agenda for the 1990s*. Cape Town: Oxford University Press.

The Star: Business Report. August 15, 1998.

United Nations Development Programme (UNDP). 1999. *Human Development Report 1999*. New York: UNDP.

van Zyl A. 1998. Can provinces stick to budgets? *Budget Watch* 4(1):3.

Whitehead M. 1992. The concepts and principles of equity and health. *International Journal of Health Services* 22(3):429–445.

Wilkinson R. 1996. *Unhealthy Societies*. London: Routledge.

World Bank. 1995. *World Development Report 1995*. Washington, DC: World Bank.

World Bank. 1997. *World Development Report 1997*. Washington, DC: World Bank.

CHAPTER
1 5

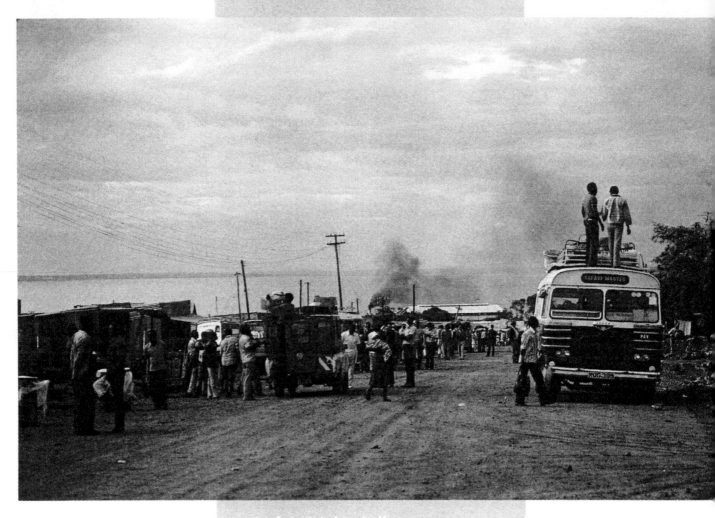

A *matatu* bus in Kenya.
Source: Dominic Dibson/Panos.

Kenya: Uncovering the Social Determinants of Road Traffic Accidents

VINAND M. NANTULYA AND FLORENCE MULI-MUSIIME

An Emerging Health Problem

Road traffic accidents (RTAs) are a burgeoning public health problem worldwide, with a 1990 estimate of over 500,000 deaths and 10 million people injured or crippled per year. Globally, the problem of road traffic accidents is ranked ninth among the major causes of mortality and disability (Murray and Lopez 1996). The forecast for the year 2020 raises it to third position, just behind heart disease and clinical depression, and ahead of respiratory infections, tuberculosis, war, and human immunodeficiency virus and the acquired immunodeficiency syndrome (HIV/AIDS).

In developing countries, although underreported for a variety of reasons (Razzak and Luby 1998; Tercero et al. 1998), RTAs are rapidly emerging as a leading cause of death and disability at rates far exceeding those in most developed countries. In the Asia–Pacific Region alone, over 2 million people died and approximately 17 million were crippled or injured in RTAs in the 1990s. During the next decade it is expected that over 6 million people will die and over 60 million will be crippled or injured in developing countries as a result of RTAs. Although developed countries have experienced a marked decline in RTA deaths, Africa has experienced a rapid growth in this cause of death over the last several decades.

Economic Costs

In economic terms, the cost of RTAs to the global economy is enormous, an estimated US$500 billion a year, of which about US$100 billion is lost in the developing and the transition countries of Eastern Europe. The annual losses in developing countries exceed the total annual development aid and loans received by these countries. It has been suggested that the cost to the economy due to RTAs is approximately 1% to 2% of a country's gross national product (GNP).

Equity Dimensions of Road Traffic Accidents

One striking aspect of the problem in both developed and developing countries alike is that the risk of traffic injury is disproportionately borne by the underprivileged. Laflamme (1998), in her review of the evidence in developed countries, concluded that traffic injury was one of the causes of mortality with the steepest social class gradient, especially for children and young people. Injuries are sustained above all by non-car users—pedestrians and cyclists. Research suggests that the main explanation for the social gradient is greater exposure to various hazards coupled with

211

Kenya

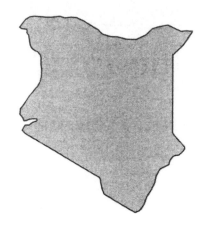

Total population (millions), 1997	28.4
Human development index, 1999	0.519
Human development index rank, 1999	136
Infant mortality rate (per 1,000 live births), 1997	57
Real GDP per capita (PPP$), 1997	1,190
Public spending on health as percentage of GDP, 1995	—

— Not available.

Source: UNDP 1999. [Human Development Report]

young males and pedestrians—often children, adolescents, and poorer segments of the population (Mohan and Tiwari 1998; Ayuthaya 1997; Laflamme 1998; Andrews et al. 1999; Odero et al. 1997).

In a review of 38 studies on road traffic injuries in developing countries, it was found that pedestrian fatalities were higher than fatalities involving drivers, cyclists, and other victims in 75% of the studies (Odero et al. 1997). The gender dimensions of RTAs have not been widely explored, although a number of studies suggest that men are at greater risk for injury and death than are women (Barss et al. 1998; Odero et al. 1997). Other types of studies examine the inequitable medical, social, and economic consequences of RTAs (Rahman et al. 1998b; 1999). Critical factors such as availability of medical care, trauma services, rehabiliation, insurance, ability to pay for care, and foregone income due to death of a breadwinner disproportionately burden the poor and vulnerable once they have suffered an RTA.

Although the social gradient in RTAs may persist in developed and developing countries alike, their causes are likely to be quite disparate across countries. Mohan and Tiwari (1988) argue that the mix of vehicles—high-speed high-technology, low-technology, and foot traffic—in the context of less advanced roadways and enforcement systems sets the scene for an unprecedented confluence of risks on the roadways of developing countries. The unreliability of official statistics and the nontransferability of lessons from developed countries' road safety efforts necessitate new methods for research on RTAs in developing countries. Although the epidemiological literature on RTAs in developing

poorer access to health services following accidents in deprived areas rather than a behavioral explanation (Laflamme 1998). The evidence in developing countries is more fragmentary, but points in a similar direction. The most vulnerable groups on the roads are

Figure 1 Public opinion of the trend of road traffic accidents in Kenya.
Source: The Nation Newspaper, Kenya.

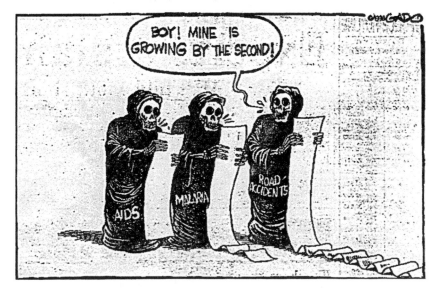

countries is sparse (Rahman 1998), analysis of the broader socioeconomic determinants of RTAs in a developing country setting is virtually nonexistent.

Kenyan Context

In Kenya, the rising number of RTAs in the country and the magnitude of associated deaths and injuries have raised public awareness and concern. This public concern is vividly captured by the cartoonist for Kenya's most popular daily, *The Nation*, which runs a serial count of the number of people killed instantly in RTAs and compares deaths due to malaria and HIV/AIDS (see Fig. 1). Beyond the human toll, RTAs exact a tremendous loss for the Kenyan economy (Economic Commission for Africa 1997). For example, in 1996 it was estimated that between 26% and 52% of Kenya's total earnings from the road transport sector were lost due to RTAs. Despite the increasing number of RTAs, the public outcry, and the socioeconomic losses associated with them, policy responses have been ineffective. Improvements of road and rail systems have been recommended, as have greater efforts to encourage road safety. As the cartoon in the *The Nation* suggests, however, much remains to be done.

This chapter, part of a larger study of RTAs in Kenya, attempts to shed light on the contextual determinants of unsafe roads with a specific focus on the *matatu* culture. *Matatus* are privately operated minibuses that stop anywhere to pick up or drop off passengers. Through a participatory design, it seeks to engage key stakeholders in developing a shared understanding and collective engagement in efforts to reduce RTAs.

Study Framework and Methods

Guiding the design of this study is a conceptual model of determinants of RTAs and their health outcomes (Fig. 2). In this model, a number of factors interact within the overarching socioeconomic environment to bring about RTAs and their adverse health outcomes. The major determinants of RTAs are human factors (behavior of motorists, pedestrians, passengers); vehicular factors (condition of the vehicle, presence of seatbelts); the physical environment (location—rural/urban—road conditions, weather conditions); and the socioeconomic environment (e.g., the organization of the transport industry, pervasiveness of corruption, informal labor markets, the policing system). Although not a specific focus of this study, the model also encompasses the consequences of RTAs that are a function of evacuation services, care-seeking behavior, medical care, and rehabilitation. Given that limited data preclude elaborate quantitative analysis, a range of qualitative methods including stakeholder participation, group discussions, interview surveys, and policy analysis are employed to construct an understanding of the main causes of RTAs.

Figure 2 Road traffic accidents and related health outcomes in the context of the socioeconomic environment in Kenya

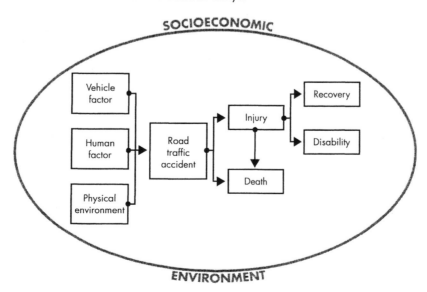

Stakeholder Involvement

Engaging public sector stakeholders (the police, Ministry of Health, and Ministry of Transport) from the outset of the study was undertaken to create a sense of ownership of both the study process and the results. Discussions as to the nature of the problem and availability of information were undertaken at this early stage. Formal and informal consultations were the main methods used such that by the time the other study activities were begun, we had established a common understanding of the RTA problem, the aims of the study, and formal contact points and responsibility arrangements at the key offices and departments.

As a result, the police, a distinct stakeholder group, became an integral component of the study team. The police participation included senior officers from Kenya police headquarters and traffic police headquarters, provincial police officers, and staff at police stations. The key involvement of the police in the research team was a primary facilitator of the subsequent study. Moreover, their positive involvement strengthened public confidence and participation, especially during interviews and group discussions.

Existing Records on Road Traffic Accidents

The routine statistics collected by governmental agencies are neither complete nor harmonized. For example, records kept by the Registrar of Motor Vehicles do not include RTAs. Furthermore, the Ministry of Health does not disaggregate accidents into separate categories—all accidents whether domestic or industrial are reported in composite statistics. Moreover, in the police statistics, records related to RTA health outcomes after evacuation (death or disability) are incomplete due to deficiencies in follow up, although the law does mandate full reporting. It was suggested that a considerable number of accidents were not reported to the police in order to avoid punitive action and loss of time. At the National Bureau of Statistics the story is the same, as the Bureau has no mechanism for analysis and data validation. The tendency, therefore, is to reproduce the data from their original sources, without subjecting them to any critical appraisal.

Despite these drawbacks, some quantitative assessment of trends in RTAs is necessary. Contacts with public sector stakeholders permitted access to traffic police records to analyze routine data on accident occurrences and their immediate outcomes (injuries and deaths). Forty-nine police stations were selected through a sampling frame designed to be nationally representative. Traffic police records from a 20 year period (1977–1996) were reviewed to gain information on the number of deaths and injuries and on the causes of the RTAs.

Surveys of Road Users and Accident Victims

To investigate perceptions of the causes of the RTA problem in Kenya, three distinct categories of road users—motorists of private vehicles and privately owned Public Service Vehicles, nonmotorists (passengers/pedestrians, *matatu* owners), and traffic police officers—were interviewed via questionnaires. Interviewees in this "road users" survey included 259 nonmotorists, 200 motorists and, 39 traffic police officers. To ensure adequate involvement of different socioeconomic groups, nonmotorists were randomly selected by using a stratified sampling frame. Relative levels of deprivation or affluence were determined by place of residence: The nonmotorists were selected from 17 sites, including affluent estates, medium socioeconomic level estates, relatively deprived estates, slum dwellings, and the central business district in Nairobi.

We also carried out a "hospital survey" in which similar questionnaires on causes of RTAs were administered to 213 inpatient RTA victims. A random sample of 53 hospitals was selected by systematic sampling using a sampling frame that consisted of all hospitals, stratified by whether they were public or private.

Group Discussions

In settings with limited quantitative data, group discussions provide a valuable means of "generating ideas about why events and behaviors happen" (Otten 1994). Based on a review of the literature and knowledge of the local context, diverse institutions were identified as critical players in the prevention or perpetuation of RTAs. The participants included senior managers of the Road Safety Network and St. John's Ambulance, traffic officers from Nairobi City Council, instructors from major driving schools, traffic police officers, *matatu* drivers, officers and engineers from the Ministry of Transport, and lecturers from Nairobi University. The group discussions covered issues pertinent to RTAs, such as perceived causes of RTAs, the road safety behavior and knowledge of the various categories of road users in the context of road safety, and perceptions of existing policy and legislation. The discussions took place in the offices of the selected institutions. Sessions involving groups of eight lasted an average of 2 hours and were facilitated by one principal investigator and at least two research assistants. Confidentiality was ensured by undertaking the discussions in private, by not allowing police officers to participate in nonpolice groups, and by

Figure 3 Trends in road traffic accident deaths and injuries by severity in Kenya, 1977–96

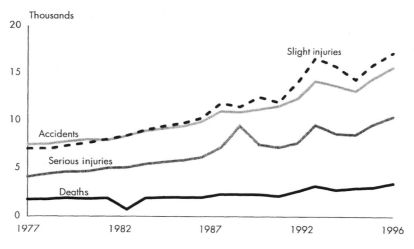

Source: Police records, 1977–96.

separating junior police officers from senior officers for the discussions.

Insights From the Study Findings

Trends in Road Traffic Accidents

From 1977 to 1996 there was a substantial upward trend in the numbers of RTAs in Kenya together with the associated fatalities and injuries (Fig. 3). Based on police records, the total number of road traffic accidents for the 10 year period (1987–1996) was 114,741. These accidents resulted in 23,124 deaths and 125,907 injuries. Thirty-nine percent of injuries were reported to have been severe. Information from follow ups of the injuries to determine eventual health outcomes was not readily available. In the 10 year interval from 1987 to 1996, the number of RTAs had risen by 65% while fatalities had increased by 69%. The routine police statistics from 1992 to 1996 identify two major causes of RTAs—driver error and pedestrians—with passengers, pedal cyclists, and vehicle defects accounting for a small number of RTAs (Fig. 4).

Human Factors

Young, reckless drivers

The routine police statistics record that driver error was the most common cause of RTAs, accounting for 41% of the accidents on record. The other causes recorded by police include passengers, pedestrians, motor cyclists, and pedal cyclists (see Fig. 4). In line with the police records, which highlighted human factors as primary causes of RTAs, 77% of traffic police respondents apportioned the blame for accidents to drivers, especially young men. The perceived driver error could be due to a number of factors. It is of particular note that 1% of the accidents involved vehicles that were being driven by underage drivers, and of these one-third were ferrying passengers. In addition, 39% of vehicles involved in accidents were driven by young men aged 18 to 24 years.

Interviews with road users and accident victims in hospitals revealed common perceptions of causes of the RTA problem. Data obtained reinforce the view that *matatus* were particularly vulnerable to accidents: 44% of the patients had been traveling in *matatus* at the time of the accident. In our road-user survey, 69% of the traffic police respondents asserted that drivers aged 20 to 30 years generally behaved in a manner that threatened road safety. The nonmotorists argued that most drivers of public transport vehicles, especially *matatus*, were fairly young, and those interviewed considered the drivers irresponsible; 90% of nonmotorists and 74% of the police argued that the drivers had risk-taking characteristics. The commuters who used public transport perceived the conventional buses as the safest mode of transport, driven by more competent drivers.

Drunk drivers

Although the general assumption in Kenya is that substance abuse, especially alcohol, has a high correlation with RTAs, evidence to support this is not available, as the police do not routinely check drivers for their

Figure 4 Road traffic accidents by cause, as recorded by police, in Kenya, 1992–96

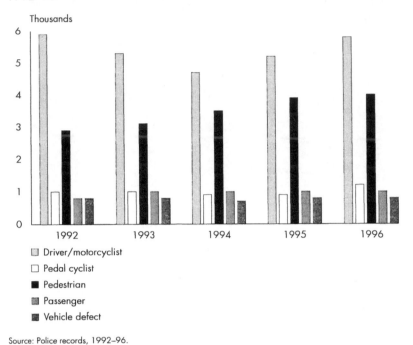

Source: Police records, 1992–96.

Figure 5 Road traffic accident deaths by casualty category in Kenya, 1992–96

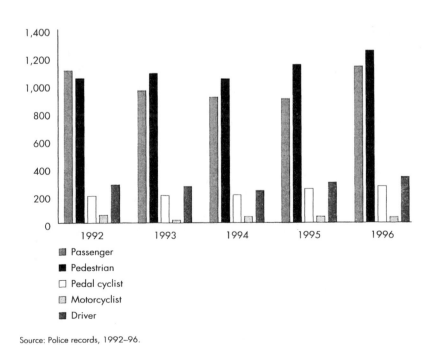

Source: Police records, 1992–96.

blood alcohol levels after an accident. The main reasons for not doing so are the lack of equipment and the lack of a systematic surveillance system for drunk driving.

To obtain some data on substance abuse we included this issue in the road-user survey. When asked about the factors contributing to RTAs, 75% of the respondents said that drunk driving was responsible for most RTAs; 92% of the police agreed. Interestingly, restricting the response to those road users previously involved in accidents (160 of 459 road users) yields a different picture—speeding was a far more prevalent perceived cause of the accident than substance abuse (106 of 160 cases). In contrast, overloading was involved in 38 of 160 cases and drunk driving in only 22 of 160 cases. The accident victims interviewed in the hospital survey corroborated this assessment of the relative role of alcohol in RTAs—of 213 victims interviewed, 10% said that the driver was under the influence of alcohol (32% stated that the driver was not under the influence and over 50% were not sure or did not know).

Pedestrians and passengers

The differential impact of RTAs on road users—pedestrians, passengers, cyclists, and drivers—provides some indication as to those who are at greatest risk for accidents or fatalities. The literature on RTAs in developing countries substantiates the extraordinarily high risk to pedestrians (Egan and Tesha 1999; World Disaster Report 1998; Mohan and Tiwari 1988; Barss et al. 1998). Our analysis of the data on more than 13,000 recorded deaths from road traffic accidents for the period 1992–1996 showed that pedestrians (42%) and passengers (38%) accounted for the majority of deaths from RTAs nationwide (Fig. 5). These proportions did not vary significantly over the 5-year period. In the urban province (Nairobi), pedestrians constituted by far the highest category of road users killed in road accidents every year over the 5-year period (1992–1996), with drivers and pedal cyclists following, in that order. In the more rural province of Nyanza, however, there were roughly equal numbers of pedestrians and passengers involved in accidents. The use of pedal cycles is higher in the rural areas.

The vulnerability of pedestrians to RTAs may be related to a lack of awareness of important road safety procedures and practices among this group. Most pedestrians are poor people who have been born and brought up in the rural areas where the volume of vehicles and density of road networks are low. Because road safety has not been part of the school curriculum, most pedestrians other than those who drive, lack

awareness of road safety practices and behavior. In our road-user survey, 92% of police respondents cited lack of awareness of the highway code by pedestrians as one of the important predisposing factors to their involvement in accidents. Equally important, environmental factors may be coming into play. The pedestrians in urban areas, for example, are particularly at risk because of poor traffic management with regard to the lack of pedestrian walkways along roads running through the city and residential areas, speeding on roads in residential areas, and poor street lighting.

Matatu Passengers' Views: "Taking Our Lives into Our Own Hands"

Despite the obvious risks, nonmotorists still prefer to travel by *matatu*. The reasons given in the group discussions were that the services provided by *matatus* were flexible, affordable, convenient, and, in some cases, the only transport available; *matatus* stop anywhere at the request of a passenger, whereas buses stop only at designated bus stops. In addition, *matatu* drivers can speed and overtake other vehicles, giving them a competitive edge over the conventional buses. The result, however, is a dangerous driving culture—a situation about which passengers in the discussion groups expressed feelings of apathy and powerlessness to influence. Riders described the experience of traveling on a *matatu* as a strange feeling of incapacity to express or verbalize any opinion, especially regarding the conduct of the driver and his assistants. Some said that traveling up country in an overloaded and fast-driven *matatu* was a chilling experience, which made them feel numb and incapable of any reaction. Others said each time they have attempted to talk the driver into some sensible driving, other passengers had told them they were wasting their time—hence the culture of silence. Asked why they still traveled by *matatu* under such circumstances, most said that there was no alternative transport to their destination. This phenomenon is becoming very common even in Nairobi, where the conventional bus service has pulled out of many routes mainly due to the poor condition of the roads.

Physical Environment

The distribution of road accidents in Kenya by province is shown in Figure 6. A third (35%) of the accidents occurred in Nairobi Province. Rift Valley Province, the largest and with several medium-sized urban centers and highways, recorded 12% of the accidents. North-Eastern province had the least accidents (the most common mode of transport in this area is the camel). Analy-

Figure 6 Road traffic accidents by province in Kenya, 1992–96

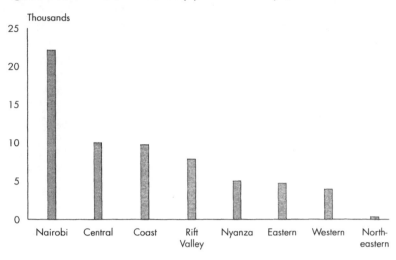

Source: Police records, 1992–96.

sis of the data according to day of the week and by month did not reveal any statistically significant differences. From the police data, the condition of the roads due to bad weather as well as defective roads was blamed for only 1% of the accidents. This contrasted with the views of participants drawn from outside police ranks in the discussion groups, who commented on the deplorable condition of Kenyan roads.

Vehicle Factors

The only factor related to vehicle safety explored in this study is seatbelts, a highly controversial issue in Kenya. The government has issued policy statements about the use of seatbelts, but have provided inadequate follow-up or implementation strategies. Data about the use of safety belts are not recorded in the police records or in routine statistics on RTAs. Of 213 RTA victims in our hospital survey, only 1% said they were wearing a safety belt; 32% said they were not, while 67% said it was not applicable. Those stating that seatbelt use was "not applicable" may have been passengers in *matatus*, virtually none of which have safety belts. The indication from these data is that demand for seatbelts has yet to become part of the culture in Kenya.

Socioeconomic Context

Internal migration

Urbanization in Kenya has been dictated by the main rail and road links, along which economic hubs have developed. Populations migrate from the less-developed peripheral areas to these hubs, leading to tremendous growth of the urban centers—currently estimated at 7% per annum. Most of the population has rural roots, and those who work and reside in urban areas seek to maintain social and economic ties with families and relatives living in the rural areas by making regular visits and sending them money. The poor rural dwellers also send some form of farm produce to the urban areas to overcome food shortages. This reciprocal relationship between the urban and rural populations has introduced another form of transient or recurrent migration, which in turn has translated into growth in the transport industry. In addition, most of the Kenyan African population tend to have two homes, a rural and an urban one, a carryover from the colonial system when Kenyans of African decent did not legally qualify to have permanent urban residency. Dual home ownership also feeds into the transport industry and explains the high level of personal vehicles on the major roadways into the rural areas.

Roads in the Kenyan economy

To improve communication and transportation to, from, and within the rural areas, the 1974 Rural Access Road Program and later the Minor Roads Program were established, roads were graveled, bridges were improved, and culverts were built. These programs resulted in tremendous improvement and expansion of the road transport network. Revenue generated from passengers and goods transported by road has increased from 19 million Kenya pounds in 1972 to 1030 million in 1992, an annual growth rate estimated at 22%

per annum according to the Economic Survey of 1997 and the Development Plan, 1994–1996 (Ministry of Planning and National Development 1997; Republic of Kenya 1994). Due to the underdevelopment of the rail transport system for both goods and passengers, the road transport network, with its attendant corollary of road traffic accidents and related implications, will continue to play a greater economic role for both freight and passenger traffic in the foreseeable future.

Informal public transport

Above all, the key to understanding the determinants of RTAs in Kenya may be in recognizing the dynamics of the *matatu* industry and culture. The original nature of the matatu industry has changed considerably, while the requisite regulations and policies have not kept pace. In Kenya, there is no *public* transport system equivalent to that found in most developed economies. The system for transport service to the public is by means of privately owned vehicles of various types, including conventional buses, minibuses, covered pick-up trucks, and midibuses. The private means of transport include saloon cars, bicycles, and motorcycles, while freight is carried by trucks and trailers.

The other form of public transport, private conventional buses (privately operated public service vehicles), is better regulated and is considered a safer mode of transport. Privately owned saloon cars are the main means of transport for the affluent. In a 1982 study, Kapila and colleagues found that Nairobi residents who had not attended school were far more likely to walk (27%) or use public transport (55%) rather than to use a private car (9%), while those with more than a secondary school education traveled in private cars (81%) and none walked. Now, as then, the poorer populations walk or ride *matatus*, the most dangerous forms of transportation.

The *matatu* is equivalent to the light buses of Hong Kong, the minibuses of Singapore, the jeepneys of Manila, the colt of Jakarta, and the dolmus-minibus of Istanbul. This mode of transport falls between the private car and the conventional bus transport system, described by Rao (1978) as an "intermediate transport mode," the main features being the convenience of stopping anywhere to pick up or drop off passengers, unfixed time schedules, and lower fares. Worldwide, the informal, unregulated nature of these forms of transport connotes greater risks to the passengers.

In Kenya, the midibuses, minibuses, and converted pick-ups constitute what is locally known as the *matatus*. The word *matatu* originates from the phrase in a local language "*mang'otore matatu*," meaning "thirty cents." In 1960, when the *matatus* were first intro-duced, the standard fare for commuting from one end of the city to another in Nairobi was 30 cents. The total number of *matatus* in Nairobi was then under 400, and they operated illegally as a means of public transport, provoking the watchful eye and wrath of the police, who would religiously pursue them for operating as "pirate taxis." It was not until 1973 that, as a result of intense lobbying by the owners, *matatus* were authorized by presidential decree to operate legally. At this time, total ridership on *matatus* constituted only 16% of the total volume of commuters using public transport. Today, the proportion of ridership on *matatus* may represent upward of 70% of the public transport users, and these vehicles criss-cross the whole country.

Originally, *matatus* were operated by relatively low-income people mainly to carry fare-paying passengers as a means of livelihood for the owner. By the 1970s, therefore, the government provided certain incentives to the owners as an encouragement to a less privileged segment of the population. These incentives included exemption from control and regulation by the Transport Licensing Board (TLB) and from income taxation. The *matatus* are licensed by the Registrar of Motor Vehicles, while other public service vehicles are licensed by the TLB, which is the regulating body for road transport (both public and goods transport). Thus the TLB has no record of the *matatu* industry or its safety record, allowing the *matatu* to avoid adherence to the stringent TLB regulations. The profile of ownership has evolved such that *matatus* are now a major form of investment for business people, farmers, professionals, senior civil servants, policy makers, law makers, law enforcers, and others who see in the business a lucrative source of supplemental income. With this shift in ownership came the practice of hiring drivers, conductors, and "turnboys" to operate the *matatus*.

Pervasive corruption

The group discussions with traffic police officers helped uncover the underlying determinants of the transport problems in the country. Both senior and junior officers mentioned the problem of bribery, about which (not surprisingly) we found no official statistics. Nevertheless, the issue was raised spontaneously in several of the groups and was considered to be a contributory factor in the gravity of the RTA situation in Kenya. Several police officers, for example, said that in their opinion bribery allowed the operation of unsafe vehicles as well as the use of underage drivers with little or no driving instruction. Likewise, penalties for road traffic offences such as speeding were not enforced in some cases because members of the police force took

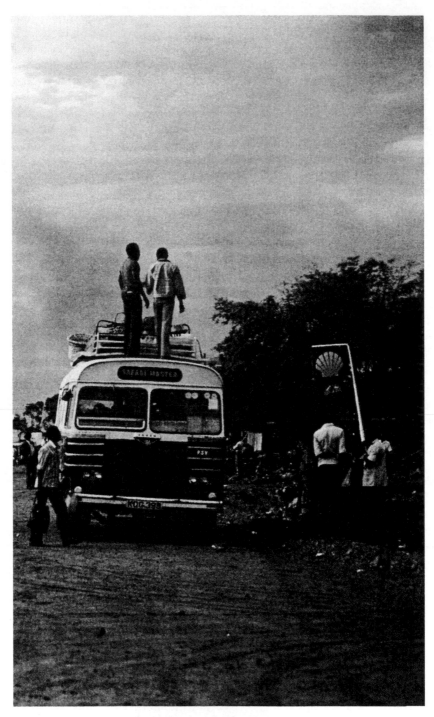

A *matatu* bus in Kenya.
Source: Dominic Dibson/Panos.

bribes. Existing road safety measures and fines were perceived as "toothless" as long as this endemic practice continues—a theme that was repeated in the group discussions with members of the general public and transport industry as reported below.

Both the motorists and *matatu* owners mentioned bribery as a regrettable, but widespread feature of traveling on Kenyan roads. During the group discussions, both *matatu* drivers and *matatu* owners said that TKK ("*Toa Kitu kidogo*"), meaning "*give something small*" is necessary if the *matatu* is to operate. Others used phrases like "*you have to shake hands, man*," a common practice between *matatu* touts and drivers devised to pass money to police discreetly, or the necessity of "*toa chai*" ("*bring tea*"), slang for kickbacks or bribes. The general consensus was that one has to pay to survive as a *matatu* operative. Unlike the powerlessness exhibited by *matatu* passengers, the attitude of owners, drivers, and touts was one of innovation and creativity. They said they had to keep on inventing new methods of paying the TKK rather than feel intimidated by it.

Lack of labor protections

The *matatu* industry is now a major employment sector for boys and young men who have dropped out of school. A 1982 study showed that the educational level of *matatu* drivers, conductors, and "turnboys" was less than 8 years of basic education and that it is an industry serving many in the informal and formal sector. On average a *matatu* driver worked 7 days a week and 14 hours a day (Kapila et al. 1982). Currently, the *matatu* drivers must meet all their contractual agreements with the owners before they can keep any revenue for themselves. Returns above the set target are kept by the driver and his co-workers once fuel and incidental costs such as "tips" to traffic police officers are netted out. This system provides powerful incentives for reckless driving, speeding, and overloading as the drivers try to maximize their daily earnings. The drivers themselves recount the pressures in "The Life of a *Matatu* Driver" (see Box 1). As the *matatu* industry evolved, worker protections for this new group of drivers and "turnboys" fell between the cracks of an unregulated informal industry.

BOX 1: THE LIFE OF A *MATATU* DRIVER

The group discussions with the *matatu* drivers revealed the reasons for reckless operation of vehicles. In the discussion groups, *matatu* drivers revealed that it was not unusual for them to work 17 hours per day, often starting as early as 5 o'clock in the morning and continuing until 10 o'clock at night. A *matatu* driver could cover well over 200 km per day on a town run. Some of the *matatu* drivers in the groups described what it was like to work day after day under such conditions. Most admitted that it was not good for them to be on the road for long hours, but they said that they had to do it to survive. "To survive, one had to be first on the road and last to leave," which meant no sleep and no time to attend to other needs, like going to the hospital when sick.

Others, especially the teenagers, said that the only time they had to spend with their girlfriends was during the evening working hours, when the girls could ride and chat with them in the *matatu* (a practice that has often been cited in city schools as a major factor of truancy among girls). In some cases drivers said it was useless to rent a house as they have so little time to use it, and there were some who slept in their vehicles, especially the long-haul drivers who arrived in the city late at night and were scheduled to depart very early in the morning.

To fight fatigue, some of the touts and drivers admitted using stimulants that often led to substance abuse. The heavy demand for long hours sometimes led to the use of amphetamines in the form of a local herb called *Miraa*, which is chewed continuously to stimulate improved alertness. *Miraa* chewing was reported to be common among the drivers of conventional buses. Drivers were also exposed to health hazards, especially sexually transmitted infections including HIV/AIDS, as sex is perceived as a convenient and easy to obtain form of stress relief.

The other issue of major concern was that *matatu* drivers complained of constant harassment by traffic police. Asked to describe the harassment, the drivers said that at most traffic check points they are expected to "handshake" or be grounded. Anything from the color of the vehicle to the playing of loud music or one faulty indicator light was reason for grounding unless they handed over TKK ("*Toa Kitu kidogo*," a payment).

These drivers and their touts lived an impoverished existence in a continual struggle for survival. Violence is an increasing problem in the *matatu* culture. As this chapter was being written, a *matatu* owner was stoned to death by touts who were protesting that the owners had colluded with city officials to run them out of business by sacking them and replacing them with Masai guards. The Masai in Kenya were chosen because their lack of education and organized structure renders them more vulnerable to exploitation. In up country bus and *matatu* stations, similar fights necessitating police intervention had also erupted with the touts accusing the police of colluding with the *matatu* owners to run them out of business.

Summary of the Main Determinants of Road Traffic Accidents

From the above evidence, it is clear that RTAs in Kenya are a serious and complex public health problem. The full range of factors associated with RTAs include the following: vehicle factors such as seatbelts; human factors such as speeding, overloading, reckless driving, drunk driving, fatigue, pedestrian/passengers' lack of knowledge of road safety procedures and their rights to road safety; and the physical environment such as rural/urban migration, road conditions, absence of pedestrian walkways, poor road surfaces, poor road signs and weather conditions. The interplay among all these determinants takes place within the overarching socioeconomic environment whose most significant causal mechanisms include lack of labor rights; corruption; insufficient and fragmented regulation of the *matatu* industry; absence of a traffic management and road safety system; poor law enforcement (lack of motivation in the police force, lack of regulation by the licensing and motor registration authorities); and minimal participation of critical stakeholders—the *matatu* industry (owner, driver, tout, and so forth), the local authorities, and the public.

Toward a New Approach to Road Traffic Accident Policy

Drawing on these findings, we offer a critique of the current policies of the Kenyan government and make some further recommendations.

Assessing the Current Policy Proposals

On November 6, 1998, the Traffic (Amendment) Bill 1998 was published by the government and sent out for consultation and debate before being passed into law. The most noticeable aspect of the Traffic Bill is that it proposes to increase the penalties for traffic offences as a deterrent to the breaking of existing traffic laws and regulations (see Table 1). The strategy of increasing penalties is focused almost exclusively on the irresponsible behavior of individual drivers and passengers. In light of our findings, the Traffic Bill is impressive in its failure to address the underlying socioeconomic inequities that give rise to these irresponsible behaviors. This assessment echoes and confirms previous assessments (JICA 1984; Ogonda 1984; Khayesi 1996, 1997, 1998).

This oversight is well illustrated by two sections of the Traffic Act (Sections 66A and 100), which are to be amended. Section 66A of the 1993 Traffic Act requires that the working hours for drivers of public service and commercial vehicles not exceed 8 hours in any 24 hour period, yet *matatu* drivers continue to work 14 to 17 hours a day. The only change proposed in the 1998 Traffic Bill is an increase in the penalties charged. The proposed increase in penalties, however, does not address the fundamental circumstances that propel the drivers to work beyond the maximum legislated working hours—they must work such long hours in order to survive.

Section 100 of the 1993 Traffic Act relates to overloading of public service vehicles with passengers. Despite this legislation having been in existence since 1993, passenger overloading is still a routine practice

Table 1 Penalties for traffic offenses in Kenyan law, 1993–98

Offense	Penalty imposed by Traffic Act, 1993	Penalty proposed by Traffic (Amendment) Bill, 1998
Improper condition of vehicle	Ksh 20,000 and/or 9 months in prison	Ksh 75,000 and/or 9 months in prison
Drunken driving	Ksh 10,000 and/or 18 months in prison	Ksh 50,000 and/or 2 years in prison
Careless driving	First conviction: Ksh 5,000 Subsequent conviction: Ksh 5,000 or 3 months in prison	First conviction: Ksh 10,000 Subsequent conviction: Ksh 20,000 and/or 6 months in prison
Reckless driving	Ksh 5,000 and/or 6 months in prison	First conviction: Ksh 50,000 and/or 6 months in prison Subsequent conviction: Ksh 75,000 and/or 12 months in prison
Causing death by driving	10 years in prison; withdrawal of driving license for 3 years	15 years in prison; withdrawal of driving license for 5 years

Note: Ksh is Kenyan shilling.

of the *matatus*. The proposed amendment to this section increases penalties for the owner, the driver, and the conductor of any overloaded vehicle that is apprehended by police. The section also provides for a fine of Ksh 200–500 to be charged to any passenger boarding a vehicle that is already carrying the maximum number of passengers. This is to be increased to Ksh 1000. Increasing the penalties is not a viable strategy in a context where bribery is rampant and alternative forms of transport are unavailable for the passengers.

Our data from both the road-user survey and the group discussions with stakeholders suggested that bribery to avoid the paying of penalties and prosecution is widespread. It is noteworthy that not only members of the general public expressed concern about bribery; vehicle drivers, owners, and the police, among whose ranks the bribery takes place, were concerned as well about the level of bribery. The proposed fines are so high that most of the poorer groups in the population will not be able to afford them and will have to go to prison. To avoid such penalties, it is likely that increased bribes will be given to police and other law enforcers so that offences are not recorded. In this scenario, the end result would be increased income for the bribe takers, but little or no change in individual road safety behavior.

A second aspect of the Traffic Bill is the proposed setting up of a Road Safety Authority. The Authority would formulate and implement national road safety policies and act as a regulatory body for setting safety standards. The Traffic Bill also proposes to establish a fund to be known as the Kenya Road Safety Fund. Money will be generated by way of a government levy on vehicle registration and licensing and on vehicle insurance premiums. This is one component of the Traffic Bill that holds promise for future development of a national road safety policy, but it appears to be given only minor emphasis so far.

What More Could Be Done?

In considering the way forward, we offer suggestions of what could be done to enhance road safety within existing legal provisions. From our study findings we contend that opportunities exist within the present regulations to address the concerns of different stakeholders (drivers, vehicle owners, the public, law enforcement agents, and policy makers).

Regulate the *matatu* industry
To deal with the pressures and exploitation of public service and commercial vehicle drivers, especially the *matatu* drivers, amendments need to be made in the employment act to give legal protection and all relevant labor rights to the driver. The terms of employment for the driver as well as the assistants (the conductors and touts) require legal recognition to protect them from exploitation and to enhance equity in job security, dignity, and health. In other words, the government would facilitate *matatu* drivers' shift from the informal to the formal economy. The benefits derived from regularized employment would go a long way toward reducing RTA risks associated with *matatus.*

In particular, the *matatu* owners need to see themselves as switching from informal to formal employers with responsibilities to their employees as governed by the labor laws. They need also to be recognized as major contributors to national development. This would allow them a say in policies affecting their sector, including access to affordable insurance, financing, and traffic management. Moreover, the *matatu* owners would benefit from capacity building in business management skills for their members, which would remove the investment insecurity and the risk-taking behavior rampant in the industry and thereby promote road safety. The *matatu* owners would need to be involved in the intervention to ensure success.

The importance of involving stakeholders in problem identification, intervention design, and implementation was underscored by the public furor that broke out between the Transport Licensing Board and the *matatu* owners while this chapter was being prepared. Matatu owners issued a strike threat on the grounds that they were not consulted before publication of the legal notice. The secretary to the Kenya Commuters Organization writes thus in a letter to the editor in another popular local daily, *The East African Standard* of Thursday, April 8, 1999: "We welcome the proposal by the government to regulate the matatu industry. The new regulations should be sorted out amicably. The government should listen to the matatu owners, touts and commuters to arrive at an agreement."

Increase surveillance
Despite the importance of engaging stakeholders in RTA policies, the lack of information on the dimensions of the problem is glaring. Policies should be based to a greater extent on statistics and data, and, ideally, public health surveillance should be used to drive public health programs (Graitcer 1992). Protection of vulnerable road users relies on accurate identification of "blackspot analysis" where incidence of fatalities is particularly high (Barss et al. 1998). The current Kenyan reporting system, however, suffers from the following shortcomings: no links between traffic accidents and hospital outcomes; high rates of underreporting, with

the poorest being the most likely not to report; and death and injuries not being disaggregated by cause (RTA vs. other causes). In Tanzania, the establishment of the Road Safety Program constituted a significant institutional change targeting injury control through a health management information system, standardization of health statistics, and emergency medical services (Egan and Tesha 1999). The wider literature on the subject indicates that population-based and community-based surveillance systems provide the most reliable alternatives for collecting data on RTAs and their outcomes in a developing country setting (Otten 1994; Tercero et al. 1998).

Increase public participation

One of the revelations of this study was the apparent powerlessness and fatalism expressed by the *matatu*-using public. The public not only uses transport that is perceived as dangerous, but also does not see itself as part of the solution to RTAs. How can the public be engaged in finding solutions to the problem of RTAs? Mechanisms for informing the public and enlightening them about their rights to safe transport and safe road use are needed.

Building confidence in public action is one key to broader change. In this regard, it is instructive to take note of a public mobilization effort occurring in Uganda. Around 1986, the Head of State mobilized the taxi (equivalent to *matatu*) users to take responsibility for their own safety and comfort. Public transport users were advised to organize themselves into a stakeholder group during the journey and appoint from among them a leader to take responsibility for ensuring that the vehicle does not become overloaded. The degree of empowerment was such that if a driver brought on board an extra passenger, the rest would walk out and wait for another vehicle. Thus, a problem was solved that law enforcement officers had failed to solve, and, furthermore, the impact has been self-sustaining. A similar initiative in Kenya holds great potential for changing this deep-seated problem.

Given that pedestrians constitute a large proportion of road traffic fatalities, efforts specifically designed to protect them must be developed. Improved road safety also needs to be approached from the traffic management angle. At present the system is not well coordinated. Traffic problems such as congestion, environmental hazards (e.g., poor street lighting and absence of pedestrian walkways) could be tackled within the existing legal provisions such as the proposed 1998 Traffic (Amendment) Bill. To address this in a sustainable manner, however, there is a need for a change of orientation of the bill from a penal approach to one

that would promote public road safety through stakeholder involvement and participation. To build public awareness and mobilize public action, the Road Safety Fund monies might be used toward a media campaign targeting pedestrians and passengers alike. Additional preventive measures must target prevention-oriented interventions to protect pedestrians—such as pedestrian crosswalks or pedestrian-only zones.

The strategy of looking at RTAs from an emerging health problem perspective within the broad framework of health equity unites both the offender and the offended as partners rather than adversaries. It also presents an entry point for positive and constructive engagement of important stakeholders such as policy makers and police in a context in which policy action has been at an impasse for years.

This research was funded by The Swedish International Development Agency. We are grateful for the valuable input to this study from William M. Macharia, Tom Omurwa, Paul Mbatia, and Erastus Njeru.

References

Ayuthya Rampai Suksawasdi Na and Danmar Böhning 1997. Risk factors for traffic accidents in Bangkok metropolis: a case-reference study. *Southeast Asian Journal of Tropical Medicine and Public Health.* 28(4):881–885.

Barrss P., Smith G.S., Baker S.P., Mohan D. 1998. *Injury Prevention: An International Perspective—Epidemiology, Surveillance, and Policy.* New York: Oxford University Press.

Economic Commission for Africa. 1997. *Study on Improvement of Pedestrian and Child Safety in Urban Areas.* Addis Ababa: Regional Cooperation & Integration Division.

Egan E., Tesha J. 1999. The changing profile of road trauma in Tanzania: an ecological perspective. In: *Trends in Health, Economics and Development: Challenges for the 21st Century.* Proceedings of the 8th Annual International Congress of the World Federation of Public Health Associations. Washington, DC: World Federation of Public Health Associations.

Graitcer P.L. 1992. Injury surveillance. In: Halperin W., Baker E.L., Monson R.R. (eds), *Public Health Surveillance.* New York: John Wiley & Sons, pp. 142–156.

International Federation of Red Cross and Red Crescent Societies. 1998. *The World Disaster Report.* London: Oxford University Press.

Japan International Cooperation Agency (JICA). 1984. Study on National Transport Plan in the Republic of Kenya. Draft Final Report, vol 1. Comprehensive Plan: Economy, Transport Demand and Investment. Nairobi: JICA.

Kapila S., Manundu M., Lamba D. 1982. *The Matatu Mode of Public Transport in Metropolitan Nairobi.* The Mazingira Institute Report. Nairobi: Mazingira Insitute.

Khayesi M. 1996. Road carnage in Kenya: a lamentor dialogues with the invisible hand. *Transafrica Journal of History.* 25:12–19.

Khayesi M. 1997. Livable streets for pedestrians in Nairobi: the challenge of RTAs. *World Transport Policy and Practice* 3(1):4–7.

Khayesi M. 1998. An Analysis of the Pattern of RTAs in Relation to Selected Socioeconomic Dynamics and Intervention Measures in Kenya. Unpublished PhD thesis, Kenyatta University.

Laflamme, L. 1998. *Social Inequality in Injury Risks: Knowledge Accumulated and Plans for the Future.* Stockholm: Sweden's National Institute of Public Health.

Ministry of Planning and National Development, Republic of Kenya. 1997. *The Republic of Kenya Economic Survey, 1997.* Nairobi: Government Printer.

Mohan D., Tiwari G. 1988. Traffic safety in low-income countries: issues and concerns regarding technology transfer from high-income countries. In: *Reflections of the Transfer of Traffic Safety Knowledge to Motorising Nations.* Melbourne: Global Traffic Safety Trust.

Murray C.J.L., Lopez A.D. (eds) 1996. *The Global Burden of Disease.* Cambridge, MA: Harvard School of Public Health on behalf of the World Health Organization and the World Bank.

Odero W., Garner P., Zwi A. 1997. Road traffic injuries in developing countires: a comprehensive review of epidemiological studies. *Tropical Medicine and International Health* 2(5):445–460.

Otten M.W. 1994. Surveillance issues in developing countries. In: *Principles and Practice of Public Health Surveillance.* Ed: Steven M. Teutsch and R. Elliott Churchill. New York: Oxford University Press.

Oucho J. 1979. The interrelationship of population with economic and social development: a macro-case study of Kenya. In: *Population and Economy of Kenya—Case Study Series 1.* New York: United Nations.

Rahman F., Andersson R., Svanström L. 1998. Health impact of injuries: A population-based epidemiological investigation in a local community of Bangladesh. *Journal of Safety Research.* 29:4, 213–222.

Rao M.S.V. 1978. The role of intermediate public transport in urban areas. *Urban and Rural Planning Thought* 21(1/2):27–54.

Razzak J.A., Luby S.P. 1998. Estimating deaths and injuries due to road traffic accidents in Karachi, Pakistan, through the capture-recapture method. *International Journal of Epidemiology.* 27: 866–870.

Republic of Kenya. 1994. *The Republic of Kenya Development Plan, 1994–1996.* Nairobi: Government Printer.

Tercero F., Anderrson R., Peña R., Svanström L. 1998. Can valid and prevention-oriented information on injury occurrence be obtained from existing data sources in developing countries? An example from Nicaragua. *International Journal for Consumer and Product Safety* 5(2):99–105.

United Nations Development Programme (UNDP). 1999. *Human Development Report 1999.* New York: UNDP.

CHAPTER 16

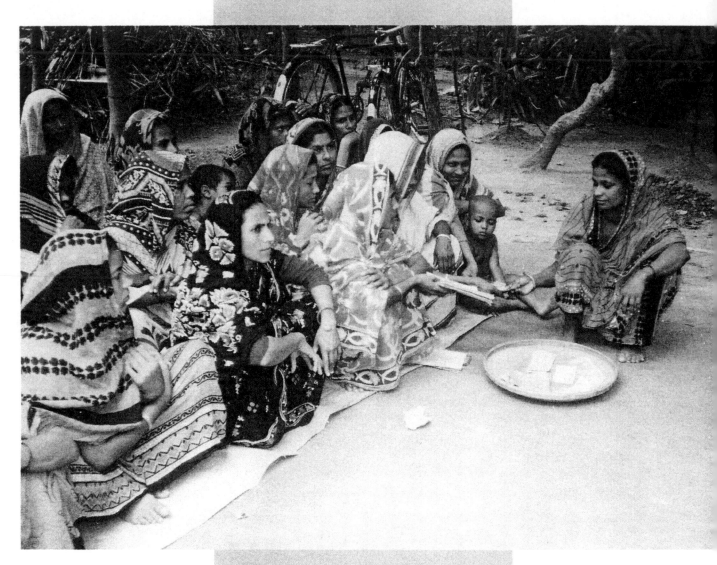

Microcredit meeting in Bangladesh.
Source: BRAC.

Bangladesh: An Intervention Study of Factors Underlying Increasing Equity in Child Survival

ABBAS BHUIYA, MUSHTAQUE CHOWDHURY, FARUQUE AHMED, AND ALAYNE M. ADAMS

Bangladesh has in the last two decades witnessed a large decline in infant and child mortality, a health gain that is particularly remarkable given its conditions of prevailing poverty and inadequate health services. Bangladesh ranks among the poorest and most densely populated countries in the developing world, with less than 45% of its population having access to primary health care services beyond childhood immunization and family planning (United Nations Development Program 1997). Malnutrition rates are among the highest in the world, with more than one-third of infants born annually classified as low birth weight (less than 2.5 kg). Approximately two-thirds of children under 6 years of age are underweight or stunted, and over 17% are moderately to severely wasted (Bangladesh Bureau of Statistics [BBS] 1997).

Bangladesh is also one of the few countries in the world where gender differentials in life expectancy and child survival contradict expected patterns that reflect women's biological advantage (D'Souza and Chen 1980; Bhuiya et al. 1986, 1989; Koenig and D'Souza 1986; Sen 1990). Numerous national and regional surveys have documented large differentials in child survival following the first 5 months of life, when the in-

fluence of social factors such as male preference in intrahousehold food distribution and sickness care become more apparent (Chen et al. 1981; Bhuiya et al. 1987). Indeed, gender bias in favor of males is so ingrained in the social consciousness that even mothers' education, the oft-cited panacea for improved child survival, appears to have no perceptible effect on male–female differentials in survival (Bhuiya and Streatfield 1991).

Given this context, the precipitous decline in child mortality from approximately 20 per 1000 mid-year population in 1981 to 7 per 1000 in 1996 (BBS 1990, 1996) raises two important questions. First, what factors underlie these remarkable improvements in child survival? Concomitant with observed trends in child mortality has been an exponential growth in large-scale public health and poverty alleviation programs, the overwhelming majority of which have been undertaken by the nongovernmental sector. To what extent do the benefits of these programs explain these trends? Second, have improvements in child survival been experienced equitably by all groups in the population? Specifically, are differentials between socioeconomic and gender groups narrowing, such that the disadvantaged

227

Bangladesh

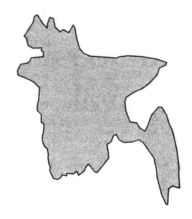

Total population (millions), 1997	122.7
Human development index, 1999	0.440
Human development index rank, 1999	150
Infant mortality rate (per 1,000 live births), 1997	81
Real GDP per capita (PPP$), 1997	1,050
Public spending on health as percentage of GDP, 1995	1.2

Source: UNDP 1999. [Human Development Report]

are experiencing disproportionately large improvements in survival?

This chapter examines these two questions using published and unpublished national and district-level data spanning the period 1982 to 1996. It considers the impact of health extension and poverty alleviation programs on trends in child mortality from socioeconomic and gender equity perspectives, with a view to informing equity-oriented policy in Bangladesh and elsewhere.

The Definition and Measurement of Socioeconomic and Gender Equity in Health

Health equity refers to a state in which good health is distributed optimally and fairly regardless of socioeconomic status or gender. For the purposes of this chapter, the examination of equity in health is confined to socioeconomic and gender differentials in the child mortality rate (CMR), expressed as the number of deaths among children aged 1 through 4 years per 10,000 mid-year population. This age group represents a stage in the life cycle that is particularly sensitive to socioeconomic context (weaning, vulnerability to environmen-

tal exposures, and so forth) and avails sufficient numbers of deaths to make robust intergroup comparisons.

Inequity in child mortality is measured in terms of socioeconomic status and gender using Sen's concepts (1992) of "shortfall" and "attainment" equality. Sen describes attainment equality as the comparison of absolute levels of achievement between groups. Attainment equality assumes that each group is capable of reaching the same absolute level of a particular health state. For the equity assessment of socioeconomic differentials in health, it could be argued that there are no unavoidable (e.g. biological) or justified reasons why expectations of health status or access to health care should differ according to income or education. Therefore, if the optimal life expectancy is 70 years, socioeconomic equity is attained when all socioeconomic groups have a life expectancy of 70 years. In other words, attainment equality is assessed by comparing the achievement of different socioeconomic groups against a common optimal norm.

In contrast, when assessing the fairness of gender differentials in health, the assumptions of a common norm for both men and women may not be justified. There is a large body of evidence that supports the idea of a biological advantage in survival of females over males (Waldron 1983; Anand 1993). As stated by Anand and Sen (1995: 4–5) "given symmetric treatment in nutrition, health care, and other conditions of living . . . women have systematically lower age-specific mortality rates than men, resulting in a life expectancy for women that is significantly higher than that for men—possibly by some five years or more." For this reason, Sen (1992) defines equality between gender groups in terms of shortfalls from the optimal value that each sex can respectively attain. If the maximal life expectancy of women and men is 85 and 80 years, respectively, yet a life expectancy of only 60 years is achieved, the "shortfall equality" for women (25 years) would be greater than for men (20 years).

Materials and Methods

Data Sources

The health and socioeconomic data used in this chapter come from Matlab, a rural subdistrict situated about 55 km southeast of Dhaka, the capital of Bangladesh. A low-lying deltaic area intersected with numerous rivers and canals, Matlab is subject to annual flooding of variable severity. Communication between the villages of Matlab is achieved mostly on foot and by rickshaw and small nonmotorized boats. Rice constitutes the staple food and is cultivated in two seasons. Given that a large proportion of the population is landless, agricultural labor, share-cropping, and fishing represent the main sources of livelihood in Matlab. Rates of illiteracy are high (40% in 1996) and increase with age. Differentials between male and female illiteracy rates are also more apparent in older age groups (Razzaque et al. 1998).

Since 1963, Matlab has served as the field station of the International Centre for Diarrhoeal Disease (ICDDR,B), an international research institution based in Bangladesh and renowned for its work on demographic surveillance and maternal and child health research and service delivery. In 1966, ICDDR,B established a demographic surveillance system (DSS) involving the monthly house to house registration of vital events such as births, deaths, migrations, and marriages in approximately 142 villages in Matlab (population, 211,306) (D'Souza 1984; Fauveau 1994; van Ginneken et al. 1998). Periodic cross-sectional censuses have also been conducted, with the inclusion of socioeconomic data in 1974, 1982, and 1996. In 1977, ICDDR,B initiated a Maternal and Child Health and Family Planning Program (MCH-FP) in one-half of the DSS area. The program currently includes family planning counseling, contraceptive provision, safe-delivery services, and illness treatment and referral for women and their children. These village-level services are provided by Community Health Workers and supported by midwives based in four health subcenters (Fauveau 1994).

Further data are furnished by the BRAC-ICDDR,B Joint Project, a collaborative research initiative that was forged in 1992 when BRAC introduced its Rural Development Program into Matlab. The largest nongovernmental organization in Bangladesh, BRAC operates in over 50,000 villages and has a total membership of over 2 million families (BRAC 1997). With the dual goals of poverty alleviation and women's development, BRAC undertakes a variety of development activities through its Rural Development Program, including group formation in Village Organizations, skill development training, essential health care, and the provision of nonformal education and collateral free loans for income-generating activities (Lovell 1992; Chowdhury and Alam 1997). The large majority of program activities are targeted to poor women and children. In 1992, a baseline survey of 12,000 households was conducted prior to the introduction of BRAC's rural development activities. A subsample was resurveyed 3 years later in 1995, and a post-test on the full sample was conducted in 1999.

The BRAC-ICDDR,B Joint Project aims to examine prospectively the joint and independent effects of health and socioeconomic development interventions on human well being (Bhuiya and Chowdhury 1995; Chowdhury et al. 1995). Linked to the DSS, the study design incorporates four distinct intervention cells where (1) only BRAC's socioeconomic development program is operating; (2) only intensive health extension activities (MCH-FP) are provided by ICDDR,B; (3) both socioeconomic development and health extension activities are undertaken; and (4) only government services are provided (comparison cell).

The analyses in this chapter are based on longitudinal DSS data collected between 1980 and 1996 and socioeconomic data from censuses carried out in 1982 and 1996. These data are linked with results from the BRAC-ICDDR,B Joint Project survey in 1995 to examine the impact of health extension and socioeconomic development on gender and socioeconomic inequality in child mortality.

Data Analysis

Mortality rates for children aged 1 to 4 years were calculated by dividing the total child deaths in the year by the mid-year population using DSS data. To calculate gender differentials in child mortality in 1982 and 1996 and to determine trends over time, measures of shortfall equality were derived using Japanese male and female child mortality rates from 1982 and 1994 as norms for comparison (World Health Organization 1984, 1996). Japan is selected as a normative standard given that its child mortality rate ranks among the lowest in the world and its female longevity is the highest.

To assess changes in socioeconomic differentials in child survival, census mortality data for 1982 and 1996 were compared according to household socioeconomic status. Area of the household dwelling (m²) was selected as the principle measure of socioeconomic status given its pertinence to the rural Bangladeshi context of acute land shortage and high population density. Further substantiating its selection is a study by Islam and Becker (1981) in Matlab indicating the comparative reliability and validity of dwelling size over other measures such as occupation, education, and income calculated on the basis of annual household land yield. Dwelling area was categorized into three groups that represent different levels of socioeconomic status: the "poor" (less than 15.7 m²), the "middle-income" (between 15.8 and 22.5 m²), and the "wealthier" group (greater than 22.6 m²). Using Sen's concept of attainment equality, child mortality is expressed in terms of "shortfall" from optimal Japanese norms to assess socioeconomic group differences and trends over time.

The impact of the socioeconomic development programs on child survival is assessed using data from the BRAC-ICDDR,B Joint Project. A cohort of children born during 1993–1997 were prospectively studied and life-table survival curves calculated for three groups of children identified on the basis of whether or not they came from poor households. In this analysis, socioeconomic status is defined according to BRAC's eligibility criteria that participating households own less than 0.5 hectares of land and rely on wage labor income for at least 100 days a year. The first group constitutes children from households participating in BRAC's Rural Development Program (BRAC member households), the second group are children from eligible households who did not join BRAC (poor nonmember), and the third group is comprised of children from noneligible, relatively better off, households (rich nonmember).

Finally, to assess the impact of ICDDR,B's MCH-FP health extension activities on childhood mortality and trends in gender and socioeconomic inequity, children were grouped based on whether their households were located in the catchment area receiving intensive health extension services (the MCH-FP group) or in the nonintervention area (the comparison group).

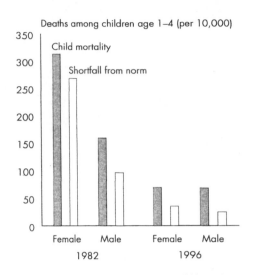

Figure 1 Child mortality rate and shortfall from norm by sex in Matlab, Bangladesh, 1982 and 1996

Note: The norm for 1982 is the 1982 Japanese child mortality rate (49 for females, 63 for males), and that for 1996 is the 1994 Japanese rate (35 for females, 44 for males).
Source: International Centre for Diarrhoeal Disease Research, Bangladesh, Demographic Surveillance System data.

Findings

Gender Inequity in Child Mortality

As described above, gender inequity in child mortality in Matlab is assessed using Sen's concept of shortfall equality, which measures achievement vis à vis gender-appropriate norms. Child mortality rate (CMR) is expressed per 10,000 mid-year population to make more apparent gender differences in optimal and actual attainment.

As shown in Figure 1, in 1982 the child mortality rate is strikingly higher among girls than boys (313 to 96 per 10,000, respectively). This disparity is even more vivid using measures of shortfall equality, whereby the levels of shortfall are almost three times

Table 1 Child mortality rate and shortfall from norm by socioeconomic status in Matlab, Bangladesh, 1982 and 1996
(per 10,000; age 1–4)

Socioeconomic status (by square meters of dwelling area)	1982 Child mortality rate	1982 Shortfall from norm[a]	1996 Child mortality rate	1996 Shortfall from norm[a]	Reduction in shortfall, 1982–96
Poor (less than 15.7)	322	266	70	30	236
Middle income (15.8–22.5)	278	222	104	64	158
Wealthy (22.6 or more)	163	107	46	6	101
All	233	177	68	28	149

a. The norm for 1982 is the 1982 Japanese child mortality rate (56), and that for 1996 is the 1994 Japanese rate (40).
Source: International Centre for Diarrhoeal Disease Research, Bangladesh, Demographic Surveillance System data.

greater for girls than for boys (280 vs. 96 per 10,000, respectively). By 1996, gender differentials in child mortality rate have all but disappeared (69 and 68 per 10,000 respectively). While the shortfall from Japanese norms also declines over this period, in 1996 it remains almost 50% higher for girls than for boys (34 vs. 24 per 10,000, respectively). The absolute reduction in shortfall between 1982 and 1996, however, indicates that substantially greater gains were experienced among girls (235 per 10,000) than among boys (72 per 10,000). Otherwise stated, over this 15 year period, there were 163 more deaths prevented among girls per 10,000 mid-year population than among boys.

Socioeconomic Inequity in Child Mortality

An assessment of the degree of socioeconomic inequity in child mortality over the interval 1982 to 1996, using household dwelling area as an indicator of socioeconomic status, is summarized in Table 1. In 1982, a marked socioeconomic gradient is apparent in absolute measures of child mortality and child mortality expressed as the degree of "shortfall" from optimal norms. Poor households experienced a child mortality rate of 322 per 10,000. This dropped to 278 per 10,000 in the middle-income group and further still to 163 per 10,000 among relatively wealthy households. In 1996, the steep decreases in CMR across all socioeconomic strata have flattened this gradient, although the lowest CMRs continue to be reported by households belonging to the wealthiest group. Trends in the reduction in shortfall also reveal similar dramatic improvements for all strata. Notably, the overall gain in socioeconomic equity is greatest among children from the poorest

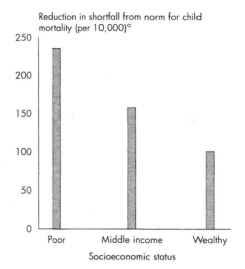

Figure 2 Gains in socioeconomic equity in child mortality rate in Matlab, Bangladesh, 1982–96

Note: Socioeconomic status is based on square meters of dwelling area; see table 1.
a. The norm for 1982 is the 1982 Japanese child mortality rate (56), and that for 1996 is the 1994 Japanese rate (40).
Source: International Centre for Diarrhoeal Disease Research, Bangladesh, Demographic Surveillance System data.

households, followed by those in the middle-income and wealthier households (Fig. 2).

To evaluate how socioeconomic status affects trends in gender equity in CMR, shortfall measures were applied (Table 2). In 1982, a striking survival disadvantage for females is evident across all socioeconomic strata. This disparity is particularly vivid when com-

Table 2 Child mortality rate and shortfall from norm by socioeconomic status and sex in Matlab, Bangladesh, 1982 and 1996
(per 10,000; age 1–4)

Socioeconomic status (by square meters of dwelling area)	1982				1996				Reduction in shortfall, 1982–96	
	Child mortality rate		Shortfall from norm[a]		Child mortality rate		Shortfall from norm[a]			
	Male	Female	Male	Female	Male	Female	Male	Female	Male	Female
Poor (less than 15.7)	247	404	184	355	70	71	26	36	158	319
Middle income (15.8–22.5)	210	357	147	308	110	98	54	63	93	245
Wealthy (22.6 or more)	87	244	24	195	42	51	7	16	17	179

a. The norm for 1982 is the 1982 Japanese child mortality rate (63 for males, 49 for females), and that for 1996 is the 1994 Japanese rate (44 for males, 35 for females).
Source: International Centre for Diarrhoeal Disease Research, Bangladesh, Demographic Surveillance System data.

Figure 3 Gains in gender equity in child mortality rate by socioeconomic status in Matlab, Bangladesh, 1982–96

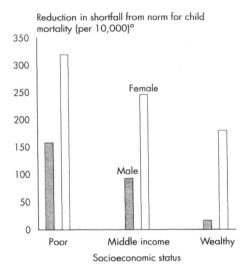

Reduction in shortfall from norm for child mortality (per 10,000)[a]

Note: Socioeconomic status is based on square meters of dwelling area; see table 1.
a. The norm for 1982 is the 1982 Japanese child mortality rate (63 for males, 49 for females), and that for 1996 is the 1994 Japanese rate (44 for males, 35 for females).
Source: International Centre for Diarrhoeal Disease Research, Bangladesh, Demographic Surveillance System data.

where the shortfall is eight times greater for girls than for boys.

In 1996, child mortality levels are dramatically lower and gender differentials are much less apparent between boys and girls. Calculation of shortfall equality reveals that the mortality rate for females is about one-tenth the level reported in 1982. Curiously, in 1996 the middle-income group had the highest shortfall for both boys and girls. In general, however, the trend in shortfall gender equality between 1982 and 1996 suggests massive improvements in female (relative to male) survival across all socioeconomic strata. The greatest absolute and relative gains in child survival are experienced by girls in the poorest socioeconomic circumstances. It is also interesting that the relative shortfall between girls and boys is greatest in the wealthier group in both 1982 and 1996.

The Effect of MCH-FP Health Extension Activities on Gender and Socioeconomic Inequity

Table 3 presents CMRs for boys and girls in 1982 and 1996 based on whether they have been exposed to the intensive MCH-FP health extension activities of ICDDR,B. Sharp declines in CMRs are observed among boys and girls in both groups during the period 1982 to 1996.

Table 4 presents data on socioeconomic differentials in CMRs as a function of exposure to the MCH-FP health extension activities of ICDDR,B. In 1982, a socioeconomic gradient in absolute levels of child mortality and measures of shortfall is evident in both MCH-

paring male and female shortfalls from norms (see Fig. 3). In poor and middle-income groups, the levels of shortfall are approximately two times greater for women than for men. The most pronounced gender differential in shortfall is apparent in the wealthier group,

Table 3 Child mortality rate by sex and participation in maternal and child health activities in Matlab, Bangladesh, 1982 and 1996

(per 10,000; age 1–4)

Participation in maternal and child health activities	1982				1996					
	Child mortality rate		Shortfall from norm[a]		Child mortality rate		Shortfall from norm[a]		Reduction in shortfall, 1982–96	
	Male	Female	Male	Female	Male	Female	Male	Female	Male	Female
Yes	120	264	57	215	57	64	13	29	44	186
No	193	365	130	316	76	84	32	49	98	267

a. The norm for 1982 is the 1982 Japanese child mortality rate (63 for males, 49 for females), and that for 1996 is the 1994 Japanese rate (44 for males, 35 for females).
Source: International Centre for Diarrhoeal Disease Research, Bangladesh, Demographic Surveillance System data.

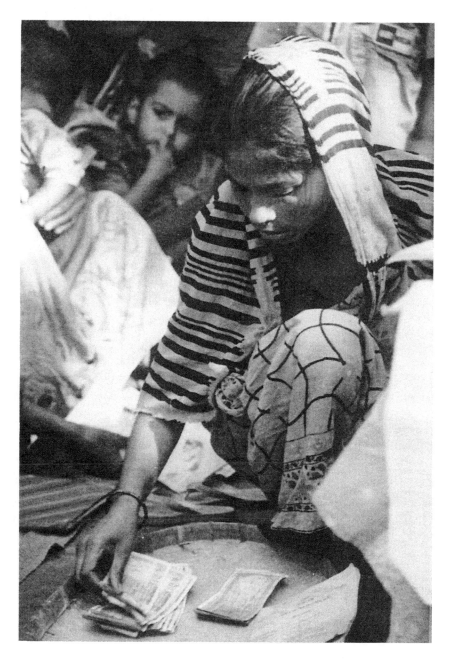

A payment for a family planning consultation,
Bangladesh. *Source:* Norman Daniels.

Table 4 Child mortality rate and shortfall from norm by socioeconomic status and participation in maternal and child health (MCH) activities in Matlab, Bangladesh, 1982 and 1996

(per 10,000; age 1–4)

Socioeconomic status (by square meters of dwelling area)	1982 Child mortality rate MCH	1982 Child mortality rate No MCH	1982 Shortfall from norm[a] MCH	1982 Shortfall from norm[a] No MCH	1996 Child mortality rate MCH	1996 Child mortality rate No MCH	1996 Shortfall from norm[a] MCH	1996 Shortfall from norm[a] No MCH	Reduction in shortfall, 1982–96 MCH	Reduction in shortfall, 1982–96 No MCH
Poor (less than 15.7)	147	173	97	117	60	81	20	41	77	76
Middle income (15.8–22.5)	124	151	68	95	71	126	31	86	37	9
Wealthy (22.6 or more)	64	98	8	42	52	41	12	1	7	41

a. The norm for 1982 is the 1982 Japanese child mortality rate (56), and that for 1996 is the 1994 Japanese rate (40).
Source: International Centre for Diarrhoeal Disease Research, Bangladesh, Demographic Surveillance System data.

FP and comparison areas. The magnitude of shortfall in each socioeconomic group, however, is greater in the comparison area than in the MCH-FP area. In 1996, the socioeconomic gradient is no longer evident due to the dramatic declines in CMR in the lowest socioeconomic group and similar improvements in the middle group. In both the MCH-FP and comparison areas the steepest declines in CMR in the period 1982 to 1992 are observed in the poorest group, with more marginal declines in the middle-income group. Between 1982 and 1996, the MCH-FP area registers greater absolute and relative shortfall reductions in the poorest and middle-income groups compared with the comparison area.

Rural Development and Socioeconomic Equity in Child Mortality

Figure 4 presents the cumulative life-table survival probability of three groups of children categorized on the basis of whether they lived in households that met the eligibility criteria for participation in BRAC's Rural Development Program, and/or whether their mothers were currently BRAC members. The curves suggest that the children of mothers who participate in BRAC's programs have a higher survival probability than poor nonmembers (p = 0.0002) and are statistically similar to "rich nonmembers" (p = 0.9171). If BRAC eligibility is considered a proxy measure for socioeconomic status, it appears that socioeconomic disparities in child mortality are decreasing between the rich and poor households that are beneficiaries of the women-focused socioeconomic development activities of BRAC. Socioeconomic differentials in CMR between

BRAC members and poor nonmembers who do not benefit from the program, however, appear to be widening.

Although the 1995 data set provides insufficient numbers to determine the effect of BRAC membership on gender differentials in survival, trends indicate that male advantage, although declining, persists among BRAC member households as well as in non-BRAC member households, both poor and rich.

Figure 4 Cumulative child survival probability by household membership in BRAC's Rural Development Program in Matlab, Bangladesh, 1993–97

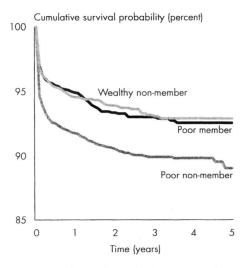

Source: International Centre for Diarrhoeal Disease Research, Bangladesh, Demographic Surveillance System data.

Figure 5 Cumulative child survival probability by participation in maternal and child health (MCH) activities and household membership in BRAC's Rural Development Program in Matlab, Bangladesh, 1993–97

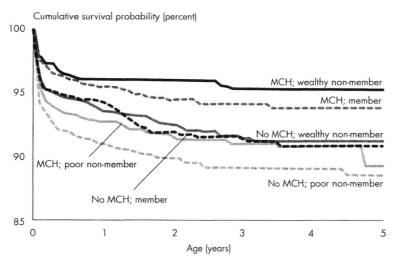

Source: International Centre for Diarrhoeal Disease Research, Bangladesh, Demographic Surveillance System data.

The Joint Impact of Rural Development and Health Extension Activities on Socioeconomic Disparities in Child Mortality

The joint impact of membership in BRAC's Rural Development Program and intensive MCH-FP health extension activities on socioeconomic equity in health is presented in Figure 5. It appears that children from economically better-off households (rich nonmembers) in the MCH-FP area have the highest survival probability. Children from BRAC member families in the MCH-FP area have the second highest survival prospects, which exceed those of children from economically better-off families in the comparison area where only government health and development programs are available. Of concern is the marginal improvement in child survival among poor nonmembers with access to MCH-FP in contrast to the very large survival improvement of the rich with access to MCH-FP. Finally, the survival improvement of BRAC members with access to MCH-FP is far greater than that of BRAC members in the comparison area.

Discussion

Concomitant with the steady increase in child survival apparent since the early 1980s is a marked reduction in the gender and socioeconomic disparities in mortality that have long characterized Bangladesh. In Matlab, the gap in mortality between boys and girls has declined by 99% over the period 1982 to 1996. Even when measured against gender-specific norms, there is a greater than 90% improvement in gender equity in child mortality over the period. Although comparison of absolute levels of child mortality for boys and girls indicates that gender disparities no longer exist in 1996, when assessed against sex-specific standards a small but significant degree of female disadvantage still persists (see Fig. 1).

Socioeconomic disparities in child survival have also decreased dramatically over time. During the period 1982 to 1996, an "inverse gradient" is observed whereby interval improvements in child mortality equality are greatest among the lowest socioeconomic strata and lowest among the highest socioeconomic strata (see Table 1 and Fig. 2). A similar inverse gradient is seen when CMR trends are considered by gender and socioeconomic group: Poor girls have the greatest health gains, followed by girls in the middle-income group, with the smallest gains observed among the wealthiest (see Table 2, Fig. 3).

When considering the validity of these findings, two critical questions arise. First, are these trends in mortality among children aged 1 to 4 years indicative of more pervasive improvements in female survival chances across the life cycle? Second, can these findings be generalized beyond Matlab to the rest of Bangladesh?

Figure 6 Child mortality rate by sex in Matlab intervention area and in Bangladesh, 1981–96

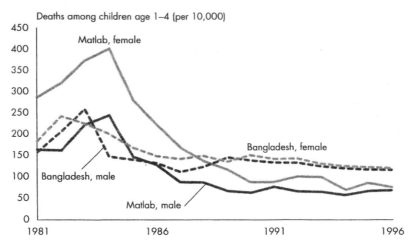

Source: International Centre for Diarrhoeal Disease Research, Bangladesh, Demographic Surveillance System data; Bangladesh Bureau of Statistics.

Based on DSS data from Matlab, the examination of trends in gender differentials in mortality among infants, children aged 5 to 15 years, and adults aged 15 to 44 and over 45 years indicate that the relative gains by females are as great as or even greater than in the 1 to 4 year age group (Bhuiya and Ansary 1998). Indeed, in 1996, the 1 to 4 year age group is the only one in which female mortality continues to exceed male mortality.

The applicability of these findings to the rest of Bangladesh is indicated by the comparison of mortality trends in Matlab to national-level Sample Registration Survey data (BBS 1990). Despite the known inadequacies of national-level data, it appears that the experience of Matlab reflects broader trends in Bangladesh (see Fig. 6). Although data from both Matlab and Bangladesh as a whole indicate a marked decline in child mortality over the period 1981 to 1996, CMRs for girls in Matlab were persistently higher until 1988, when a cross-over occurred to levels below national figures. Indeed, the sharp increase in female mortality due to the shigella outbreak in 1984 makes even more apparent the survival disadvantage of girls compared with boys in this age group (Bennish and Wojtyniak 1991).

What lies behind the encouraging trends described above? One hypothesis relates to preexisting differences in the cause of death structure between socioeconomic groups. Less affected by diseases of poverty such as tuberculosis and measles, the wealthy might be expected to experience a lower rate of improvement in CMR than the poor groups benefiting from public

health programs such as childhood immunization (Bourgeois-Pichat 1981). Alternatively, secular reductions in the severity of poverty may be responsible for the remarkable gain in child survival among the poorest. In either case, the role of social and economic development policies and programs appears critical to understanding gains in equity. As summarized in the conceptual framework of the social basis of health (see chapter 2), a policy-relevant understanding of the determinants of these trends must go beyond the consideration of change in social position and exposure and address the larger social-structural context in which these changes have occurred.

An examination of state development policies reveals an ongoing commitment to improving health care, reducing poverty, and increasing the status of women. Adopted in 1973, Bangladesh's Constitution enshrines women's right to equality and mandates state responsibility to help secure for its citizens the necessities of life (i.e., food, clothing, shelter, education, and medical care). Reflecting these tenets, subsequent national development plans have consistently emphasized a concern for poverty alleviation, employment generation, and women's involvement in the development process (Ahmed and Karim 1998).

In the absence of a formally adopted national policy on health, state development plans have provided the main basis for identifying strategies and priorities for health. Other policies in the areas of education, nutrition, agriculture, rural development, social welfare, and women's affairs have also been instrumental in their commitment to improving the health and well-being of the rural poor and women in particular. Starting in 1973, initial 5 year plans focused on expanding primary health care coverage in underserved rural areas. This focus was given further impetus as Bangladesh embraced the Alma Ata declaration on Primary Health Care in 1978 and, later, UNICEF's Expanded Program on Immunization in 1985. The fourth 5 year plan (1990–1995) had as its priorities the expansion of program efforts in MCH-based family planning, immunization and communicable disease control, human resource development (paramedical training and so forth), and improvement of the physical infrastructure at tertiary and secondary levels.

The degree of success in translating policy commitments to health equity for women and the poor is more difficult to evaluate. Overall, per capita allocations to health and population sectors have increased over time, from U.S. $0.5 in 1986 to U.S. $1.25 (constant price) in 1997, although they constitute only 1.5% of the GNP (Ministry of Health and Family Welfare 1998). With the exception of family planning services, however, as much as 70% of all health-related expenditures are urban based, with a disproportionate amount allocated to secondary and tertiary health systems. Notwithstanding this urban bias, a pro-poor, or progressive, orientation to the distribution of benefits from government expenditures is apparent based on current patterns of utilization. Benefits from public health spending as a proportion of income appear highest among the poorest (2.9%), declining in an almost linear fashion to 0.2% in the upper two income deciles (Begum 1997).

Programmatic successes include the aggressive family planning program, which, proponents claim, has accounted for a rise in the use of modern contraceptive methods among currently married women aged 15 to 45 years, from 5% to 42% in the period 1975 to 1997. Its detractors argue, however, that the fiscal, political, and programmatic emphasis on family planning has inhibited the development of an integrated and effective primary health care system (Ross et al. 1996).

A rise in the national coverage rate for childhood immunizations has also occurred, from 2% in 1981 to over 60% in 1997 (Expanded Program on Immunization [EPI] 1998). Distribution systems for oral polio vaccines and supplemental vitamin A have been equally successful, reaching 80% and 90% of children under 5 years of age, respectively (Mitra et al. 1997; EPI 1998).

Contrary to these positive developments, field studies indicate that the percentage of acute illness treated in the public sector has declined from 20% in 1984 to only 12% in 1995, a trend that is independent of poverty status. Among the hard-core poor (or the lowest two income deciles), 45% seek treatment for acute illness from untrained allopathic doctors, 9% from traditional healers and homeopaths, 18% from drug shops, and only 13% from licensed medical doctors (Begum 1997). Several explanations for the underutilization of public health care services have been offered, the large majority of which are supply-related factors such as inadequate provider–client interaction, doctor absenteeism, the nonavailability of essential drugs, lack of accountability and personnel management, and limited responsiveness to client needs (Begum 1997; Perry et. al. 1998).

Another distinguishing feature of the broader sociostructural context of Bangladesh is the degree of organized collaboration between the state and nongovernmental organizations (NGOs). Currently, 80% of rural subdistricts in Bangladesh have been brought under the umbrella of NGO programs. In addition to intensive activity in the areas of poverty alleviation, female education, and microcredit, over 4000 international, national, and local NGOs work in the areas of health, nutrition, and population, many in partnership with the government. Compared with highly bureaucratized state structures, the greater flexibility and result-oriented management style of NGOs gives them a comparative advantage in terms of program innovation and delivery (Ahmed and Chowdhury 1999).

This chapter examines the impact of two such NGO-facilitated programs with a view to understanding the independent and synergistic impact of intensive health extension (MCH-FP) versus rural development activities (BRAC) on socioeconomic and gender differentials in child survival. In general, it appears that exposure to ICDDR,B's intensive MCH-FP health extension program has conferred a persistent survival advantage to children over the last 15 years (see Table 3). Curiously, however, absolute survival gains, or the rate of improvement in survival over the same 15-year period, are greatest in the comparison area, where only government health services are received (see Table 3).

Improvements in gender and socioeconomic equity are also apparent in both MCH-FP and comparison areas (see Tables 3 and 4). Although absolute levels of child mortality are higher in the comparison area, gains in gender equality are greatest in this population (see Table 3). In both the MCH-FP and comparison area, gains in child mortality are also greatest in the lowest socioeconomic group. It should be noted, however, that this equity-enhancing trend is more pronounced across socioeconomic groups in the MCH-FP area (see Table 4).

Overall, the most marked net health improvements (irrespective of area) are experienced by the poor. It remains difficult to ascertain, however, the extent to which survival gains can be attributed to public health campaigns such as immunization coverage and the promotion of oral rehydration therapy (Chowdhury and Cash 1996) or represent the inevitable outcome of secular changes in poverty, behavior, education of mothers, and environmental exposure, among other factors.

Study findings also indicate a survival advantage associated with participation in BRAC's Rural Development Program. These results must be interpreted cautiously, however, given the possible influence of selection bias on the outcome of interest. According to this argument, although BRAC members and poor nonmembers may be of equivalent socioeconomic status according to BRAC's selection criteria, other nonmeasured attributes or prior endowments may make them distinct such that certain individuals self-select into BRAC's programs.

Although it is possible that among these predisposing factors are ones that confer a survival advantage, to disentangle them from the socioeconomic and psychosocial benefits arising from membership is far from straightforward. A number of studies that investigate the issue of selection bias have been undertaken in the context of the larger BRAC-ICDDR,B Joint Project, the results of which suggest that prior differences between groups only partially account for the beneficial effects of participation (Evans et al. 1998; Mahmud and Huda 1998; Zaman 1998). In short, it appears that participation in socioeconomic development activities has positive health and survival benefits that are real, yet remain poorly understood.

The chapter also provides evidence of the synergy between health and socioeconomic development activities in promoting child survival. Together, a greater survival advantage is attained than with either input alone (Fig. 4). Evidence of synergy also supports the argument for the multiple and complex determinants of health and the importance of a broad-based policy approach that extends beyond the health sector in efforts to improve the health of women and the poor.

An ironic consequence of the apparent benefit of intensive health and socioeconomic interventions is the lessening of socioeconomic inequities in child survival between the poor beneficiaries of these programs and the relatively better off, on the one hand, but the widening of disparities between beneficiary households and the poor who do not benefit, on the other. Clearly, further consideration of the factors that hinder participation of the poor and marginalized are urgently needed in an effort to extend the equity benefits of these programs across the socioeconomic spectrum.

The data used in this study were drawn from the joint project of BRAC and ICDDR,B: Centre for Health and Population Research in Matlab, which has been generously supported by the Ford Foundation, Aga Khan Foundation, International Center for Research on Women, and USAID. The Rockefeller Foundation, through the Global Health Equity Initiative, and SIDA supported the research summarized in this chapter. Special thanks are due to the Demographic Surveillance System of ICDDR,B for the use of their database and to members of the BRAC-ICDDR,B Joint Project team for their valuable contributions at various stages of the research. The authors also gratefully acknowledge the statistical and research input of Mr. Mohammad Mostafa, Ms. Saira Ansary, and Ms. Ami Shah and the valuable conceptual and technical contributions of Dr. Timothy Evans. Finally, we express our gratitude to Dr. Demissie Habte and Mr. F.H. Abed for their unwavering encouragement and support in undertaking the BRAC-ICDDR,B Joint Project.

References

Ahmed S.M., Adams A.M., Chowdhury M., Bhuiya A. 2000. Gender, socioeconomic development and health-seeking behavior in Bangladesh. *Social Science and Medicine* 51:361–371.

Ahmed F., Karim E. 1998. Status of Health and Health Equity in Bangladesh: Policy Perspective. Report prepared for the Global Health Equity Initiative (GHEI) Meeting, December 11–17, Dhaka, Bangladesh.

Ahmed S.M., Chowdhury A.M.R. 1999. *Health scenario of Bangladesh*. In: Ahmed M. (ed), Towards 2000, pp 55–78. Dhaka: Community Development Library.

Anand S. 1993. Inequality Within and Between Nations [mimeograph]. Cambridge, MA: Center for Population and Development Studies, Harvard University.

Anand S., Sen A.K. 1995. *Gender Inequality in Human Development: Theories and Measurement*. Working Paper Series No. 95.05. Cambridge, MA: Harvard Center for Population and Development Studies, Harvard University.

Bangladesh Bureau of Statistics (BBS). 1990. *Patterns, Levels, and Trends in Mortality and Regional Life Tables for Bangladesh: Evidence from Sample Vital Registration System, 1981–88*. Dhaka: Bureau of Statistics, Ministry of Planning.

BBS. 1996. *Bangladesh Health and Demographic Survey: Summary Findings, 1994 and 1995*. Dhaka: Bureau of Statistics, Ministry of Planning.

BBS. 1997. *Progotir Pathey: Achieving the Goals for Children in Bangladesh*. Dhaka: Bangladesh Bureau of Statistics, Ministry of Planning.

Begum S. 1997. *Health and Poverty in the Context of Country Development Strategy: A Case Study on Bangladesh*. Macroeconomics Health and Development Series No. 26. Geneva: World Health Organization.

Bhuiya A., Ansary S. 1998. Status of Health and Health Equity in Bangladesh. Report prepared for the Global Health Equity Initiative (GHEI) Meeting, December 11–17, Dhaka, Bangladesh.

Bhuiya A., Chowdhury M. 1995. *The Impact of Social and Economic Development Programs on Health and Well-Being: A BRAC-ICDDR,B Collaborative Project in Matlab*. Working Paper No. 1, Dhaka: International Centre for Diarrhoeal Disease Research: Bangladesh.

Bhuiya A., Streatfield K. 1991. Mother's education and survival of female children in a rural area of Bangladesh. *Population Studies* 45:253–264.

Bhuiya A., Wojtyniak B., D'Souza S., Nahar L., Shaikh K. 1987. Measles case fatality among the under-fives: a multivariate analysis of risk factors in a rural area of Bangladesh. *Social Science and Medicine* (24)5:439–443.

Bhuiya A., Wojtyniak B., Karim R. 1989. Malnutrition and child mortality: are socioeconomic factors important? *Journal of Biosocial Science* 21(3):357–364.

Bourgeois-Pichat J. 1981. Measuring infant mortality. I. Principles and methods. In: Selected Papers No. 6, National Institute for Population Studies (INED). Paris: INED. (Translated from *Population*, No. 2, 1951), pp. 1–17.

BRAC. 1997. *Annual Report 1996*. Dhaka, Bangladesh: BRAC.

Chen L.C., Huq E., D'Souza S. 1981. Sex bias in the family allocation of food and health care in rural Bangladesh. *Population Development Review* 7(1):55–70.

Chowdhury A.M.R., Alam A. 1997. BRAC's poverty alleviation program: what it is and what it achieved. In: Wood G., Sharif I. (eds), *Who Needs Credit: Poverty and Finance in Bangladesh*. Dhaka: University Press.

Chowdhury A.M.R., Cash R. 1996. *A Simple Solution: Teaching Millions to Treat Diarrhea at Home*. Dhaka: University Press.

Chowdhury M., Bhuiya A., Vaughan P., Adams A., Mahmud S. 1995. Effects of Socioeconomic Development on Health Status and Human Well-Being: Determining Impact and Exploring Pathways of Change. Proposals for phase II of the BRAC-ICDDR,B Matlab joint project 1996–2000 A.D. BRAC-ICDDR Working Paper No. 6. Dhaka, Bangladesh: International Center for Diarrhea Disease Research.

D'Souza S. 1984. Small area-intensive studies for understanding mortality and morbidity processes: two models from Bangladesh—the Matlab project and the Companiganj health project. In: *Databases for Mortality Measurement*. Papers of the Meeting of the United Nations/World Health Organization Working Group on Data Bases for Measurement of Levels, Trend and Differentials in Mortality, October 20–23, Bangkok. New York: United Nations Department of International Economic and Social Affairs, pp. 146–158.

D'Souza S., Chen L.C. 1980. Sex differentials in mortality in rural Bangladesh. *Population and Development Review* 6(2):257–270.

Evans T.G., Adams A.M., Mohammed R., Norris A.H. 1998. Demystifying nonparticipation in micro-credit: a population-based analysis. *World Development* 27(2):419–30.

Expanded Program on Immunization (EPI). 1998. *Findings of the National Coverage Survey. Expanded Program on Immunization*. Dhaka: Directorate General of Health Services, Government of the People's Republic of Bangladesh.

Fauveau V. 1994. *Matlab: Women, Children and Health*. Special Publication No. 35. Dhaka: International Centre for Diarrhoeal Disease Research, Bangladesh (ICDDR,B).

Islam M.S., Becker S. 1981. Interrelationships among certain socioeconomic variables in a rural population of Bangladesh. Working Paper No. 18. Dhaka: International Centre for Diarrhoeal Disease Research, Bangladesh.

Koenig M.A., D'Souza S. 1986. Sex differentials in childhood mortality in rural Bangladesh. *Social Science and Medicine* 22(1):15–22.

Lovell C.H. 1992. *Breaking the Cycle of Poverty: The BRAC Strategy*. West Hartford, CT: Kumarian Press.

Mahmud S., Huda S. 1998. Participation in BRAC's Rural Development Program and the Impact of Group Dynamics on Individual Outcomes. Working Paper No. 24. Dhaka: BRAC-ICDDR,B Joint Research Project, BRAC Research and Evaluation Division.

Ministry of Health and Family Welfare. 1998. *Health and Population Sector Programme, 1998–2003: Programme Implementation Plan Part I*. Dhaka: Ministry of Health and Family Welfare, Government of the People's Republic of Bangladesh.

Mitra S.N., Al-Sabir A., Cross A.R., Jamil K. 1997. *Bangladesh Demographic and Health Survey 1996–1997*. National Institute of Population Research and Training (MIPORT), Mitra and Associates, and Macro International, Dhaka and Calverton, MD.

Perry H., Weierbach R., Hossain I., Islam R. 1998. Childhood immunization coverage in zone 3 of Dhaka City: The challenge of reaching impoverished households in urban Bangladesh. *Bulletin of the World Health Organization* 76(6):565–573.

Razzaque A., Nahar L., Sarder A.M., van Ginneken J.K., Shaikh M.A.K. 1998. *Demographic Surveillance System—Matlab: 1996 Socioeconomic Census*. Vol 29, Scientific Report No. 83. Dhaka: International Centre for Diarrhoeal Disease Research, Bangladesh (ICDDR,B).

Ross J.L., Chowdhury S.N.M., Mirza T. 1996. *Health Gender Sexuality: Bangladesh Country Report*. Special Publication No. 50. Dhaka: International Centre for Diarrhoeal Disease Research, Bangladesh.

Sen A. 1990. More than 100 million women are missing. *New York Review* December 20, pp. 61–66.

Sen A. 1992. *Inequality Reexamined*. Oxford: Clarendon Press.

United Nations Development Programme. 1997. *Human Development Report 1997*. New York: Oxford University Press.

UNDP. 1999. *Human Development Report 1999*. New York: UNDP.

van Ginneken J., Bairagi R., de Francisco A., Sarder A.M., Vaughan P. 1998. *Health and Demographic Surveillance in Matlab: Past, Present and Future*. Special Publication No. 72, Dhaka: International Centre for Diarrhoeal Disease Research, Bangladesh.

Waldron I. 1983. The role of genetic and biological factors in sex differences in mortality. In: Lopez A., Ruzicha L.T. (eds), *Sex Differentials in Mortality: Trends, Determinants and Consequences*, pp. 141–164. Canberra: Department of Demography, Australian National University.

World Health Organization. 1984. *World Health Statistics*. Geneva: WHO, p. 184.

World Health Organization. 1996. *World Health Statistics*. Geneva: WHO, p. B718.

Zaman H. 1998. Who participates and to what extent: an evaluation of BRAC's microcredit programs. DPhil thesis, University of Sussex.

C H A P T E R

1 7

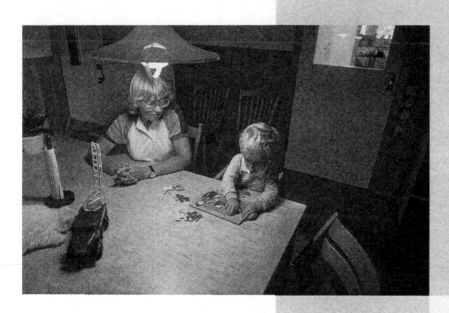

A daycare worker and child in Sweden.
Source: Joe Rodriguez/Black Star Publishing/Picture Quest.

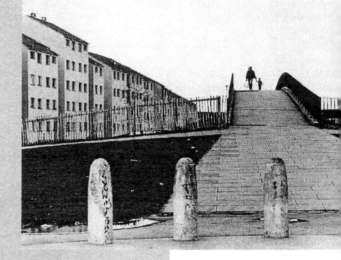

Sweden and Britain: The Impact of Policy Context on Inequities in Health

FINN DIDERICHSEN, MARGARET WHITEHEAD, BO BURSTRÖM,
MONICA ÅBERG, AND PIROSKA ÖSTLIN

Why Is Health Equity Important in North-European Welfare States?

Concern for health equity as a research and policy issue in Europe has grown against a background of unprecedented economic, cultural, and political shifts over the past two decades (Drever and Whitehead 1997; Acheson et al. 1998; Mielck et al. 1994; SOU 1998; National Board of Health and Welfare 1998). Not the least of these shifts has been the break up of the former Union of Soviet Socialist Republics, resulting in the redrawing of the map of Europe, with violent conflicts erupting at many points around the region during the process.

These dramatic developments have been superimposed on an already worsening macroeconomic climate. Over the last 20 years, there has been a growth in mass unemployment in market economies, and Europe has been particularly hard hit (Michie and Wilkinson 1994). The relatively affluent countries in the European Union have experienced a rapidly changing labor market in response to the worsening economic climate. Downsizing of industry, for example, has been associated with collapsing demand for less skilled labor, growth in joblessness, widening income gaps and the reemergence of poverty and social marginalization for the most disadvantaged sections of the population (Nickell and Bell 1995). The cost-containment policies pursued in the face of the European Monetary Union have also had similar effects.

Compounding the effects of these macroeconomic developments, the very extensive social welfare systems built up by these countries in the post-war period are under severe strain. Their continuing challenge is to address the new economic insecurities and risks faced by working-age families because of the rapidly changing labor market, high divorce rates, and single parenthood, while simultaneously sustaining the post-war social insurance programs that now support an expanding elderly population (Diderichsen 1995). A picture is emerging in which a global economy is creating domestic problems that national welfare states are less free to remedy with social policies of their own choice. With a narrower space for policy options, there is a growing need to formulate an effective strategy.

An effective policy strategy will be sensitive to the social context in the country and the varying effects of social position on health. We need to have a better understanding of the pathways leading from social context and policy to social position and on to ill health. This includes being able to assess what impact existing policies in various sectors are having on the health and

Sweden

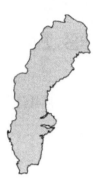

Total population (millions), 1997	8.9
Human development index, 1999	0.923
Human development index rank, 1999	6
Infant mortality rate (per 1,000 live births), 1997	4
Real GDP per capita (PPP$), 1997	19,790
Public spending on health	
as percentage of GDP, 1995	7.1

Source: UNDP 1999. [Human Development Report]

United Kingdom

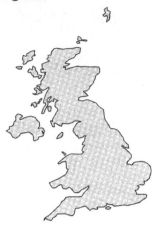

Total population (millions), 1997	58.5
Human development index, 1999	0.918
Human development index rank, 1999	10
Infant mortality rate (per 1,000 live births), 1997	6
Real GDP per capita (PPP$), 1997	20,730
Public spending on health	
as percentage of GDP, 1995	5.9

Source: UNDP 1999.

well-being of different sections of the population and what aspects would lead to improvements in the future.

This chapter has a dual purpose: first, to set out a general approach to exploring the pathways to health inequities and what can be done about them; and second, to illustrate how we have applied this approach in our case study of class, gender, and health in Britain and Sweden. The chapter concludes with a discussion of the implications of this line of enquiry for future research and policy development in Europe.

A Conceptual Framework

In attempting to understand the root causes of health inequities and the most effective ways of tackling them, there are a number of conceptual and practical issues to address. What we mean by "inequities in health" are systematic and important differentials in health between different groups in society that are both potentially avoidable (preventable) and also considered unacceptable (unfair) (Whitehead 1990). In an empirical study of the causes of socioeconomic differences in self-reported health, it is of course not a priori given that all the differences in health we observe are inequitable.

They have, however, been chosen because we judge them to be important and systematic health differences. At least some of these health differences are potentially preventable and widely considered unacceptable in both Britain and Sweden. We therefore refer to them as "inequities" throughout this chapter.

In this analysis, we have used a simplified version of the conceptual framework developed by Diderichsen and Hallqvist (1998) to study and quantify the role of different mechanisms and pathways that generate inequities in health. At a theoretical level, it provides a way of conceptualizing the mechanisms through which the social positions of individuals and the social context of societies influence health. At an empirical level, it gives indications of how some of the various pathways and mechanisms could be measured quantitatively. Finally, for policy purposes, it provides a framework for understanding how policies may influence the mechanisms responsible for inequities in health and for making health impact assessments of policies on population health, including health inequities.

Two important mechanisms with the potential to generate health inequities in individuals should be distinguished (Hallqvist et al. 1998). First, the impact of social position on health may be through *differential exposure*, that is, people in more disadvantaged social positions may have greater exposure to health hazards and risk factors and hence are more likely to fall ill than are other groups with low or no exposure. Second, there may be an impact on health through *differential susceptibility*, that is, people in more disadvantaged positions may be more vulnerable or susceptible when exposed to a given level of health hazard than are their more advantaged counterparts due to the interaction of other adverse conditions associated with their more disadvantaged circumstances.

At the level of society, the impact of social context (including policy context) has three main entry points. First, society influences the social stratification process, for example, the process through which individuals end up in different social positions (defined by gender, occupational class, ethnicity, and so forth). The stratification process influences the amount of social mobility that there is in a society, including the direct and indirect health-related selection into social positions (Kouvusilta et al. 1995). The education system and family policies, for example, may influence what opportunities people have to move up the social scale and, indeed, can influence how wide the gulf is between people in different social positions.

Second, most health policies that have been implemented thus far to combat inequities in health operate at a different entry point: They aim to prevent people in disadvantaged positions from being exposed to poverty, unhealthy housing, dangerous working conditions, nutritional deficiencies, and so on. For example, income distribution, the labor market, and the redistributive policies of taxes and social security benefits will determine the proportion of different groups exposed to poverty. Likewise, a broad range of protective and regulatory policies governing the work environment, housing, traffic, or other health promotion issues will influence exposure levels to many risk factors. Furthermore, these policies will often be designed to have a greater impact on some groups than on others. If one important risk factor is lack of control over living conditions, then the basic societal mechanisms that create and reproduce power will play a fundamental role.

Third, at the aggregate level, several studies have indicated that social context in terms of social deprivation of the local area, or income distribution within a society, may have an impact on mortality and self-reported health. Just as social integration at the individual level appears to buffer the effect of other risk factors (Cassel 1976), it is reasonable to hypothesize that social context in terms of social trust and social cohesion may modify the effect of (i.e., interact with) individual causes of illness. Specific policies may act not only by influencing the risk of being poor or unemployed (second entry point) but also by interacting with the health effects of those risks factors (at a third entry point). For instance, living in a society with strong safety nets, active employment policies, or strong social cohesion may make day to day life less threatening, relieving some of the social stress involved in having very small financial margins or being unemployed.

An Empirical Example: Pathways to Health Inequities in Britain and Sweden

We use this framework to study the pathways to social inequities in health in Britain and Sweden with an integrated class and gender perspective. Social position is measured in terms of social class based on occupation/employment. Nearly all social class schemes used in Europe are based on employment and occupation. Employment opportunities and labor market policies form an important aspect of the social context in a country (at a particular point in time), helping to shape access to material and social resources, life chances, and ultimately to health. Both the context and the impact, however, may be different for men and for women, and thus it is important to look at them separately as well as together, especially when considering policy implications and making comparisons (Macintyre 1997). This should help us understand whether the pathways to social inequities in health are similar or different for men and for women, leading to different implications for policy.

Contextual Differences Between the Countries

The dominant trend in post-war Europe was one of a slow but steady decline in income inequality. Since the late 1970s, however, there has been a reversal of this trend in many countries, and the gap between the richest and poorest households has grown. In a recent review of the evidence on changes in the distribution of income across countries in the Organization for Economic Cooperation and Development, Gottschalk and Smeeding (1998) found that income inequality had increased in 12 of the 17 nations examined. Interestingly, from this case study's data, the largest change in income inequality, in both absolute and percentage terms, occurred in the United Kingdom, while Sweden experienced a slower increase and from a much lower base (see Table 1).

Table 1 Trends in income inequality in Sweden and the United Kingdom, 1975–94

Year	Gini coefficient		Index (1975 = 100)	
	Sweden	United Kingdom	Sweden	United Kingdom
1975	0.228	0.250	100	100
1980	0.201	0.265	88	106
1985	0.216	0.293	95	117
1990	0.226	0.353	99	142
1994	0.230[a]	0.357	114	143

Note: The Gini coefficients were derived using equivalent household income, with an equivalent factor of 0.5 (the square root of household size). The Gini coefficient is a measure of inequality. The higher the value of the Gini, the greater the income inequalities.
a. Data refer to 1995 because 1994 was an atypical year as a result of tax reform.
Source: Gottschalk and Smeeding 1998, Table A-2 and Figure 2.

In the United Kingdom, the rise in income inequality has been accompanied by a large increase in differentials in earnings for those who work, with a widening of the gap between high and low pay. This was due in part to dramatic increases in executive pay awards in the 1980s. At the same time, various laws designed to weaken the trade unions were introduced, which have resulted in a decline in union power. This, combined with high levels of unemployment, has helped keep "low pay" low (Hills 1998).

In Sweden, with centralized labor markets and a continued high degree of unionization (85% to 90% of the Swedish labor force are in a union), the growth in wage dispersion has been much less pronounced than in Britain. Of equal importance has been the reform of the Swedish tax system. This has led to less progressive taxation, with a decreased redistributive effect on household incomes (Gustafsson and Palmer 1997).

Taxation policy in Britain has been relatively neutral. The price indexing of social security levels, however, has meant that those reliant on social security have automatically fallen further behind the rest of the population (Hills 1998). While British spending on social insurance during the post-war period grew slowly, and was still on a low level, Sweden expanded its spending dramatically as the system increasingly included the growing middle classes and a growing number of employed women. Tax spending on social insurance has for many years been more than three times greater in Sweden than Britain, and this has had implications for income distribution (Gottschalk and Smeeding 1998). These features of the British social security system, in combination with the underlying low level of social security benefits, has resulted in another important difference between the United Kingdom and Sweden. In Britain, the rise in income inequality has been accompanied by growth of the proportion of the population in poverty, while in Sweden this does not appear to be the case.

Using data from the Luxembourg Income Study, Smeeding (1997) examined trends in poverty across 15 developed nations. The study used a relative concept of poverty, that is, the percentage of people living with incomes below half of median income. Table 2 presents data on the trends in poverty for different groups in Sweden and the United Kingdom. Overall levels of poverty in Sweden remained fairly stable despite the change in income distribution. There has been a change in the composition of the poor, however, with improvement in the position of children and a more pronounced deterioration among the elderly. Generally, the social security system in Sweden has been effective in protecting the living standard of those at the lower end of the income distribution. This is in marked contrast to the situation for the United Kingdom.

Unemployment has become a serious problem for many established market economies, but Europe has been particularly affected. The unemployment rate in the European Union rose from less than 3% in the beginning of the 1970s to around 11% (over 18 million people) by the mid-1990s (Martin 1998). The Commission of the European Union acknowledged that "unemployment remains the major economic—and social—problem confronting the Union" (European Commission 1995). Table 3 shows the trends in unemployment in the United Kingdom and Sweden, illustrating the growth in unemployment in both countries, but with very different rates.

Table 2 Poverty rates in Sweden and the United Kingdom, selected years, 1979–92

(percentage living on less than half the median income)

Country and year	Elderly (age 65 and older)	Adults (age 18–64)	Children (age 0–17)	Total population
Sweden				
1981	2.7	6.6	4.5	5.4
1992	6.4	8.1	3.0	6.7
United Kingdom				
1979	21.6	6.3	9.0	9.2
1991	23.9	10.7	18.5	14.6

Source: Smeeding 1997, Table A-4.

Most countries in the North are suffering from a dramatic decrease in the demand for unskilled labor, affecting men in particular. The situation, however, has been tackled in different ways in different countries. Some have chosen to reduce labor supply through early retirement, keeping women's employment low, and minimizing immigration. Others have focused on reducing labor prices, lowering wages for unskilled jobs, and removing minimum wage standards, coupled with deregulation and increasing flexibility. Still others have tried to solve the problem by maintaining or increasing public employment or upgrading labor value through training programs and rehabilitation (Esping-Andersen 1995).

Britain in the 1980s went down the route of deregulation and greater labor market flexibility, while keeping wages low. Controlling inflation was given greater priority than keeping unemployment down. This resulted in Britain developing what Prime Minister Tony Blair recently called "the most lightly regulated labor market in Europe"(Department of Trade and Industry 1998). It was, he also pointed out, increasingly "unfair" due to the greatly reduced employment protection and growth in job insecurity. In the late 1990s, there were attempts to redress the imbalance and reintroduce some of the lost protections, with a recently introduced "Fairness at Work" policy (Department of Trade and Industry 1998). In contrast, Sweden throughout the 1980s had active programs attempting to maintain full employment and re-training. Since 1991, when the economic recession struck, the country has been struggling to maintain these policies, but has not been able to prevent a dramatic increase in unemployment, which has reached the same levels as in Britain and the rest of the European Union. Both countries have also encouraged early retirement, leading to a dramatic rise in economic inactivity among older men in both countries and also among women in Sweden.

Over the same period as the collapse in demand for male unskilled labor, there has been a general rise in women's employment throughout Europe, but again, policies and patterns have been quite different in the two countries. Sweden has had a strong gender equality movement since the 1960s, which resulted in concerted attempts to give men and women equal opportunity for paid employment. There has been an emphasis on all adults working, including those caring for young children, with complementary arrangements for extensive public child care provision and family-friendly employment policies, developing into what has become known as the parent-worker model. The explicit national aims of promoting full employment and gender equality has led to job creation in the public sector, particularly in the health and social sectors. This

Table 3 Trends in unemployment rates in Sweden and the United Kingdom, 1975–95

(percent)

Year	Sweden	United Kingdom
1975	1.4	4.1
1980	1.4	6.8
1985	2.5	11.8
1990	1.6	5.9
1995	7.7	8.3

Source: International Labour Organization data.

strategy served several purposes: it created jobs per se, especially for women, and jobs that, because of their service and child care orientation, released women in other sectors from their caring responsibilities so that they could take up jobs. Britain lagged behind in child care provision and other family-friendly employment policies until 1998, when the government started to address some of these deficiencies.

The differences, as they looked in the early 1990s, can be briefly analyzed as follows, including some hypotheses on what impact they may have on inequities in health:

- The high employment opportunities in Sweden, due to expanding public employment and access to child care facilities, have prevented increasing long-term unemployment and poverty rates among less qualified labor. One would thus expect larger class differentials in exposure to poverty and unemployment in Britain than in Sweden, at least among women.
- The high employment rates in Sweden may lead to employment of people who are more susceptible to different job-related exposures, who would otherwise be selected out of a labor market with stronger competition for jobs. This may contribute to larger occupational inequities in health among the employed population in Sweden and a stronger susceptibility to risk factors such as occupational hazards, unemployment, and poverty.
- The labor market in Britain is more deregulated and flexible than the market in Sweden. This has led to larger income inequalities, but may also have increased the incidence of both job creation and unemployment. This may, however, also lead to a higher degree of health-related selection out of the labor market in Britain, especially for less-qualified labor. In the competition for a new job, low education and ill health may act synergistically against employment chances. That may lead to larger social inequities in health among those who are not employed than among the employed in Britain.
- A welfare system that is somewhat more universal (especially in relation to women) and a society with a more egalitarian income distribution, such as Sweden's, may be protective against the effects of being unemployed and poor. We could therefore, expect different health effects of these conditions and thus a different role played in generating inequities in health in countries such as Sweden and Britain with contrasting systems.

The outcomes of these policies in terms of economic growth, employment levels and income distribution are hotly debated. What, however, has been the effects on the health of populations and on the inequities in health between different groups within the population? This question urgently needs to be addressed. We can start by looking at different groups within the two societies. How have men and women in different socioeconomic groups fared under the changing macroeconomic conditions and the differing policy contexts in the two countries? What impact has this had on health equity?

Data Sources and Methods

The empirical study used to illustrate these issues is based on the British General Household Survey (GHS) and the Swedish Survey of Living Conditions (ULF)

BOX 1: DEFINITIONS OF VARIABLES AND DATA ANALYSIS

Health Outcome Measures

General Health Status

Britain: Over the last 12 months, would you say your health has on the whole been good, fairly good, or not good?
Sweden: How do you consider your general health? Is it good, bad, or something in between?

Long-Standing Limiting Illness

Britain: Do you have any long-standing illness, disability, or infirmity? Does this illness or disability limit your activities in any way?
Sweden: Do you have any long-standing illness, effect of injury, disability, or other ailment? Does this illness affect your ability to work (or, if not working, your daily activities)?

Other Measures

Social Position
Social position is measured in Sweden with the existing social classifications used in the ULF–Swedish Socio-economic Classification–SEI (Statistics Sweden 1982: 4) and in the British GHS Socio-Economic Groups (SEG) from the Standard Occupational Classification of the Registrar General. Men and women are coded according to their own job if they have one, otherwise according to their previous job before they left the labor market. If they never had a job, married women are coded according to their husband's job.

Specific Exposures

In Britain poverty is measured using self-reported income, including transfers and benefits, and in Sweden on linked data from tax authorities. They are deflated and adjusted to household size in the same way in the two countries. The OECD and European Union definition of poverty is income below 50% of the median income. Less than 2% of the high-level Swedish employees are poor according to this definition, however, which leaves us with very little power. We have therefore in both countries defined poverty as having below 60% of the median income. Unemployed is defined as those who are without a job and are seeking a job.

Confounding Factors

Age is classified in eight 5 year age groups. Marital status is classified in three groups: single (never married); married or cohabiting; and divorced, separated, or widowed. In Sweden, ethnicity is classified as those born in Sweden and those born in other countries independently of their present citizenship. In Britain the coding divides the population according to self-defined ethnic origin into five categories: white, Afro-Caribbean, South Asian, Chinese, and other.

Data Analysis

Age-standardized prevalences (European Standardized Rates [ESRs]) are calculated by direct age standardization using the European standard population (Armitage and Colton 1998), and 95% confidence intervals are calculated according to the methods of Rothman and Greenland (1998). Other adjustments for confounders and mediating factors are done using logistic regression.

A measure of *explained fraction* (XF) is calculated to estimate the proportion of excess risk explained by mediating risk factors (Hallqvist et al. 1998). If the excess health risk expressed as odds ratio before adjustment is OR′ and after adjustment for potential mediating factors is OR″, then the explained fraction is $[(OR' - 1) - (OR'' - 1)]/(OR' - 1)$.

A measure of interaction between two causes such as social position (A) and poverty (B) is calculated as a measure of susceptibility. If the odds ratio for those exposed to both is OR_{AB} and those exposed to only one of them is OR_A or OR_B, a *synergy index* (SI) can be calculated as $(OR_{AB} - 1)/([OR_A - 1] + (OR_B - 1])$. It thus expresses the odds among those who are exposed to the two risk factors in relation to the added effect of the two exposures (Rothman and Greenland 1998; Lundberg et al. 1996).

during 1992–1995 for both countries. Both studies are annual cross-sectional surveys that employ face to face interviews with respondents in a nationally representative sample of households. Nonresponse rates in Sweden have been slowly increasing from 15% in 1975 to 20% in 1995. In the British GHS, non-response has remained fairly constant at around 18%. This study includes men and women aged 25 to 59 years. The numbers of adults interviewed in this age range are about 12,000 per year in Britain and 4000 per year in Sweden.

The analysis reported here is part of a larger comparative study over the 20 year period from 1975 to 1995, encompassing several aspects of social policy and inequities in health. Two outcome measures are focused on: general health perceived as less than good; and prevalence of self-reported, long-standing limiting illnesses. Social position is measured by social class (based on occupation) and gender. Two specific exposures are studied: relative poverty and unemployment. These two conditions are investigated because they are closely linked to the outcome of welfare and economic policies, and they have been at the forefront of discussions concerning causes of social inequities in health, particularly in Britain. Several other factors contribute

to the social gradients in health in the two countries, but we have here chosen to illustrate the analytical approach with these two. Definitions of variables and data analysis are given in Box 1.

The Relationship Between Social Position and Self-Reported Health

The basic starting point for this analysis is, of course, the inequities in health between different social classes and genders. Figures 1 and 2 show the age-standardized prevalence of limiting long-standing illness and fair/poor health across socioeconomic groups in the two countries.

It can be clearly seen that there is a relationship between health status and indicators of social position. For example, both British and Swedish men from semi-skilled and unskilled occupations are nearly twice as likely to report having a limiting long-standing illness than men from professional and managerial occupations. Similar social differentials are found for women, although the gradient across different socioeconomic groups is less marked than for men, and less marked among British women than among Swedish women.

Figure 1 Age-adjusted prevalence of limiting, long-standing illness among adults age 25–59 by sex and socioeconomic group in Britain and Sweden, 1992–95

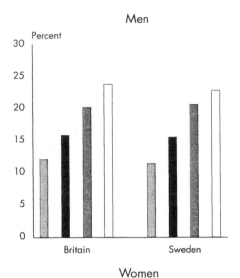

Men

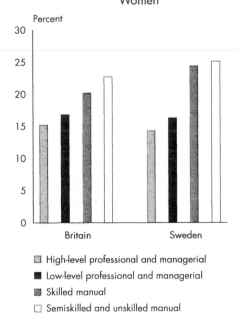

Women

☐ High-level professional and managerial
■ Low-level professional and managerial
▨ Skilled manual
☐ Semiskilled and unskilled manual

Source: British General Household Survey and Swedish Survey of Living Conditions, both for 1992–95; authors' analysis.

Figure 2 Age-adjusted prevalence of fair or poor health among adults age 25–59 by sex and socioeconomic group in Britain and Sweden, 1992–95

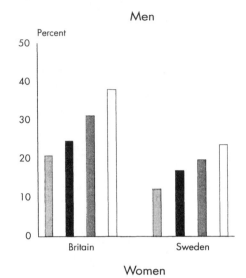

Men

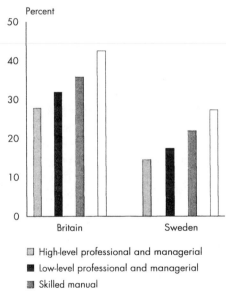

Women

☐ High-level professional and managerial
■ Low-level professional and managerial
▨ Skilled manual
☐ Semiskilled and unskilled manual

Source: British General Household Survey and Swedish Survey of Living Conditions, both for 1992–95; authors' analysis.

Potential Mediating Factors for Social Class Differentials in Health: Poverty and Unemployment

The next step is to examine whether poverty and unemployment are mediating factors in the observed relationship between socioeconomic group and health. Before performing this step, it is important to consider how these factors might operate as a source of bias. Employing a cross-sectional study design, reverse causation may be a source of bias; that is, ill health may lead to poverty and unemployment rather than these factors being a cause of ill health. To minimize this occurrence, all groups not currently working, other than those who were unemployed or housekeeping (not employed outside the home), were excluded from the

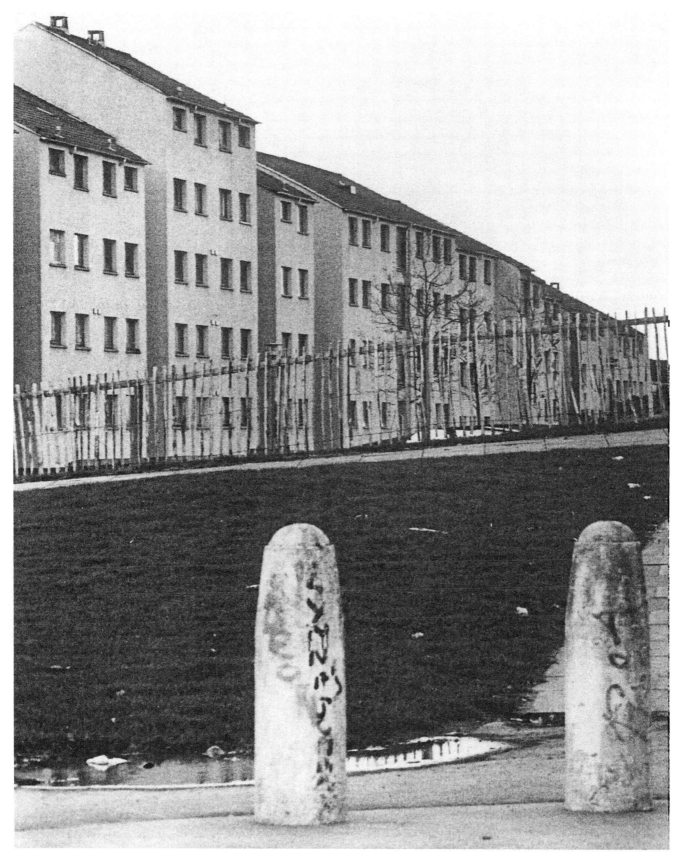

Wester Hailes housing estate, Edinburgh, United Kingdom.
Source: Paul Smith/Panos.

Table 4 Odds ratios for ill health among adults age 25–59 by socioeconomic status in Sweden and Britain, 1992–95

| | Limiting illness | | Fair or poor health | |
Country and socioeconomic status	Women	Men	Women	Men
Sweden				
Poor	1.15 (0.92–1.43)	1.24 (1.00–1.54)	1.05 (0.85–1.30)	1.32 (1.07–1.63)
Unemployed	1.20 (0.95–1.52)	1.34 (1.08–1.67)	1.41 (1.13–1.77)	1.70 (1.39–2.11)
Not employed outside the home	1.60 (1.19–2.17)	n.a.	1.56 (1.16–2.09)	n.a.
Britain				
Poor	1.50 (1.36–1.65)	1.69 (1.52–1.87)	1.50 (1.39–1.61)	1.47 (1.35–1.60)
Unemployed	2.05 (1.74–2.41)	1.84 (1.67–2.14)	1.40 (1.21–1.62)	1.61 (1.45–1.79)
Not employed outside the home	1.68 (1.53–1.85)	n.a.	1.56 (1.44–1.68)	n.a.

n.a. Not applicable.

Note: The odds ratios (with 95 percent confidence intervals in parentheses) are adjusted for age, marital status, ethnicity, and socioeconomic group. "Poor" is defined as having less than 60 percent of median income, with the nonpoor as reference. For "unemployed" (which for women also includes those not employed outside the home), the employed are the reference group. "Not employed outside the home" is synonymous with "housekeeping" in this context.

Source: Based on data from British General Household Survey and Swedish Survey of Living Conditions, both for 1992–95.

analysis. Most of them were permanently sick (defined in Sweden as early-retired with a limiting illness).

Table 4 shows that poverty, unemployment, and (for women) housekeeping are all associated with a higher prevalence of ill health in both countries. The odds ratios show that being poor increases the chances of having limiting long-standing illness and fair/poor health, more so for British men and women. Swedish women who are poor are exceptional, in being no more likely than women who are not poor to report fair/poor health.

The odds ratio for limiting illness among unemployed men and women is somewhat higher in Britain than in Sweden. In both countries, women who are classed as housekeepers report more illness than their employed counterparts. These higher risks of ill health apply to only a small proportion of Swedish women (4% are classified as "housekeeping"), however, while they apply to nearly a one-fourth (21%) of British women.

Can housekeeping be regarded as a risk factor in the same way that unemployment is? Some women may choose to stay at home and keep house, while for others housekeeping may conceal "hidden" unemployment, that is, they would like to have paid work but cannot obtain it due to lack of job opportunities or lack of day care for children. Still others may be in this category because they are unable to work due to permanent sickness, but they are not officially registered as such because they do not qualify for sickness benefits. We cannot entirely exclude the possibility that a selection effect of this nature is playing some role in the high morbidity rates among women who are classed as

"housekeeping," but, apart from excluding those listed officially as "permanently sick," we are unable to reduce this possible source of bias still further.

How Much of the Social Class Differential in Health Is Accounted for by Differences in Poverty and Employment Status?

Table 4 shows that employment status and poverty are strongly associated with self-reported health in both countries. How important are these two mediating factors in explaining the observed differentials in health between the various socioeconomic groups? Does their importance differ for men and for women and in the two countries?

Using regression analysis, we can estimate the extent to which poverty and unemployment contribute to the excess in ill health among lower socioeconomic groups by observing how much the excess risk (expressed as odds ratios) is reduced when adjusting for these factors. As can be seen from Table 5, both of these factors play some role in explaining the health differentials between socioeconomic groups. To quantify how large that contribution is, the *explained fraction* was calculated for each factor as detailed in Box 1.

When this is done, we find that the contribution of each factor is different for men and for women and for each country. Table 5 shows that poverty explains 15% of the excess risk of fair/poor health among women in

Table 5 Odds ratios for fair or poor health among adults age 25–59 by sex and socioeconomic group, and effects of mediating factors, in Sweden and Britain, 1992–95

Socioeconomic group and factor	Women		Men	
	Sweden	Britain	Sweden	Britain
High-level professional and managerial group (reference group)	1.00	1.00	1.00	1.00
Other socioeconomic groups (model 1)[a]	1.95	1.41	2.04	1.56
Controlling for unemployment as well (model 2)	1.93	1.32	1.99	1.50
Explained fraction for unemployment (percent)[b]	2	23	5	10
Controlling for poverty as well (model 3)	1.94	1.27	1.99	1.48
Explained fraction for poverty (percent)[b]	–1	15	0	6

Note: Data exclude employers and the self-employed. The odds ratios are adjusted for age, sex, ethnicity, and marital status.
a. Low-level professional and managerial and manual.
b. The explained fraction shows the percentage reduction in the odds ratios in model 2 compared with model 1, and in model 3 compared with model 2.
Source: Based on data from British General Household Survey and Swedish Survey of Living Conditions, both for 1992–95; authors' analysis.

the lower nonmanual and manual occupations in Britain, but none of the excess risk of ill health among Swedish women from the same socioeconomic groups. Poverty explains only 6% of the excess risk of ill health among British men employed in the lower nonmanual and manual occupations and none of the excess risk for their Swedish counterparts.

Table 5 also shows a marked contrast between British and Swedish women in terms of the role played by joblessness (unemployment plus housekeeping) in accounting for the health differentials between the socioeconomic groups. Joblessness explains 23% of the excess risk of ill health among British women in the lower nonmanual and manual groups, but much less (2%) of the excess risk in their Swedish counterparts. In contrast, there is little difference between British and Swedish men in the role played by unemployment. In both countries, unemployment only explains between 5% and 10% of the excess risk among men from lower nonmanual and manual groups.

Why Do Poverty and Unemployment Play Different Roles in Explaining the Health Differential Between Socioeconomic Groups in Britain and in Sweden?

The interaction between social context and poverty/unemployment

The first possibility already discussed is that the effect of poverty may be weaker in Sweden than in Britain. In other words, being poor in Sweden may be less damaging to health than being poor in Britain. There may be other aspects of living in Swedish society that are more supportive for poor people, such as more affordable and comprehensive public transport and child care, which make the experience of poverty less stressful and damaging. Conversely, there may be aspects of the social and policy context in Britain that add to and reinforce the negative experience of being poor—a synergistic effect between social context and poverty. We cannot adequately explore this possibility empirically with our data because the absolute levels of morbidity are difficult to compare, but there is a hint from the results in Table 4 that this mechanism may be coming into play. It can be seen from the odds ratios in Table 4, for example, that the excess risk of limiting longstanding illness linked to poverty was 15% for women and 24% for men in Sweden, but was higher in Britain: 50% and 69% respectively.

For fair/poor health, there is an excess risk of 50% for British women who are poor, while Swedish women who are poor have no additional risk. In both countries, and for men and women, unemployment seems to be strongly related to self-reported health.

Differential exposure

The second possibility is that the social and policy context in the two countries modifies the level and distribution of poverty and joblessness, influencing the degree to which the population as a whole and different socioeconomic groups within society are exposed to these factors. This can be explored further with our data by examining the patterns of exposure to poverty and joblessness among different groups in the population.

Figure 3 Age-adjusted prevalence of poverty among adults age 25–59 by sex and socioeconomic group in Britain and Sweden, 1992–95

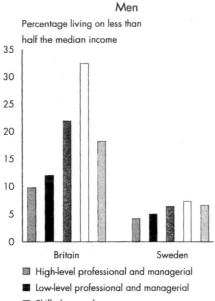

Men

Percentage living on less than half the median income

■ High-level professional and managerial
■ Low-level professional and managerial
▨ Skilled manual
□ Semiskilled and unskilled manual
▨ All men age 25–59

Women

Percentage living on less than half the median income

■ High-level professional and managerial
■ Low-level professional and managerial
▨ Skilled manual
□ Semiskilled and unskilled manual
▨ All women age 25–59

Source: British General Household Survey and Swedish Survey of Living Conditions, both for 1992–95; authors' analysis.

As can be seen from Figure 3, there are major differences in poverty rates between the two countries. For adults of working age as a whole, the poverty rate in Britain is nearly four times greater than in Sweden and slightly higher for British women than for British men. One of the most striking points illustrated in this figure, however, is the steep gradient in the prevalence of poverty among British men and women in different socioeconomic groups. One-third of the men and women in semiskilled and unskilled manual occupations are poor, diminishing to around 10% in the higher nonmanual group. In Sweden, not only is the overall level of poverty much lower, but there is much less of a differential in poverty across the socioeconomic groups.

Figures 4 and 5 show prevalence of unemployment and housekeeping and reveal marked differences in exposure by class, gender, and country. For the population as a whole, the unemployment rates are fairly similar in the two countries and somewhat higher for men than for women. Across occupational classes, however, there is a more than threefold differential among British men in the risk of being unemployed, while there is much less of a gradient among Swedish men (see Fig. 4).

Figure 4 Age-adjusted prevalence of unemployment among men age 25–59 by socioeconomic group in Britain and Sweden, 1992–95

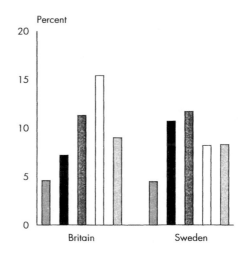

Percent

■ High-level professional and managerial
■ Low-level professional and managerial
▨ Skilled manual
□ Semiskilled and unskilled manual
▨ All men age 25–59

Source: British General Household Survey and Swedish Survey of Living Conditions, both for 1992–95; authors' analysis.

Figure 5 Age-adjusted prevalence of unemployment and nonemployment outside the home among women age 25–59 by socioeconomic group in Britain and Sweden, 1992–95

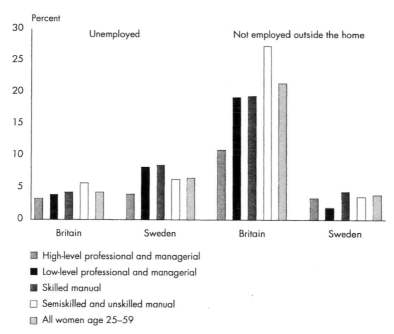

Source: British General Household Survey and Swedish Survey of Living Conditions, both for 1992–95; authors' analysis.

For women the relationships between employment and socioeconomic status are similar but less pronounced. For British women, unemployment rates increase gradually with each occupational group, while in Sweden it is only the highest occupational group that is relatively protected from unemployment (see Fig. 5). The same pattern holds true for Swedish men.

There is, however, a very large differential in prevalence of housekeeping among British women—under 11% of women in the higher nonmanual group are classified as keeping house compared with 27% of women in the semiskilled and unskilled manual group. There is no corresponding gradient in housekeeping among Swedish women, who, as mentioned above, report a very low level of housekeeping. When added together to consider the extent of "joblessness" among women in the two countries, the much higher jobless rate among British women and the marked social gradient in the chances of being in or out of paid employment become apparent. The absence of these social differentials among Swedish women is also highlighted. This illustrates once more the importance of unraveling the

data by class and gender to fully analyze pathways to ill health in different contexts.

These findings also need to be linked back to those in Table 5, which showed that poverty and joblessness accounted for a greater proportion of the social inequities in health among British women than among Swedish women. As such, differential exposure to poverty and unemployment by class seems to be one of the important contributory mechanisms underlying the marked health inequities in Britain but not in Sweden.

Differential susceptibility

The third possibility is that the mechanism of *differential susceptibility* between social groups is operating and, additionally, is more prevalent in one country than another. As discussed earlier, there are theoretical and empirical reasons to believe that the effect of poverty or unemployment may depend on social position, that is, gender and class. Susceptibility to specific exposures may differ between social groups, and policies intended to lessen the effects of those exposures in general may nevertheless have a differential effect on individuals in high and low social positions. For example, in the work environment, people in all occupational groups may be equally exposed to the strain of high demand, but, in addition, people in lower occupational positions may have little control over how they can meet those demands. Under these conditions, the risk factor of "low control" may make them more susceptible to the health-damaging effects of high demand (Hallqvist et al. 1998).

In a similar way, low social position may make individuals more susceptible to the effects of poverty or unemployment on health. We explored the possibility that differential susceptibility was coming into play by analyzing the existence of interactions between social position and the specific exposures, poverty and unemployment, calculating the synergy index with methods described elsewhere (Lundberg et al. 1996). The only indication of differential susceptibility emerging from the synergy index was related to poverty in Britain. The synergy index was 1.71 (CI 1.0–3.1), which means that the risk of poor health among British men and women exposed to both manual occupation and poverty was 71% higher than the added effect of the two factors. For unemployment, the synergy index did not provide evidence of differential susceptibility among men and women in either of the two countries.

Conclusions

We started out with a description of the major differences in income distribution and social policies in Britain and Sweden. We have shown empirically, as have other authors, that in terms of both average levels of adult self-reported health and social inequities in health, the two countries show surprisingly similar patterns. We take this not as an argument that policy and the macroeconomic environment do not matter, but as a challenge to dissect the pathways that lead from the social context (macroeconomics and social policy) to the individual mechanisms linking social position with health. We have adopted a unifying model for studying the health impact of the social and policy context and used it to explore in greater detail two potential mediating factors between social position and health outcomes—poverty and unemployment. Both of these factors may be influenced greatly by public policy and social context in the two countries.

Findings from the empirical analysis indicate, first, that poverty explains more of the social class inequities in health in Britain than in Sweden. Poverty in Britain initially has an impact through the mechanism of dif-

ferential exposure. There is a much higher overall level of poverty and a much steeper gradient across the social classes in Britain than in Sweden. Another mechanism also seems to be coming into play with regard to poverty. The results indicate that there may be greater susceptibility in the British population overall to the health effects of poverty compared with their Swedish counterparts and, within Britain, a greater susceptibility among the lower socioeconomic groups than the higher.

Second, unemployment is an important risk factor for health in both countries, but it explains little of the differences in health between social classes within Sweden. In Britain, however, unemployment explains much more of the health differences between classes, as the social gradient of unemployment and joblessness is much stronger in Britain. Third, the analysis shows that the health effects of unemployment among British men and women is partly mediated through poverty. In Britain, a larger part of the excess risk associated with unemployment was accounted for by poverty than in Sweden. When entering poverty into the model after unemployment, the excess risk associated with unemployment was reduced by one-third for women and nearly one-half for men (results not shown). In Sweden, poverty accounted for none of the health disadvantage associated with unemployment. Fourth, we found some evidence of differential susceptibility across social classes for poverty in Britain.

Several other exposures to health damaging factors may be important to explain the social gradient in health in the two countries. Behaviors such as smoking have been shown to be important for mortality gradients. In this study on self-rated health, smoking explains none of the social gradient and only slightly confounds the effect of unemployment (data not shown). Most likely, however, smoking is an effect of unemployment and should not be treated as a confounder. Other health behaviors are not measured in the surveys we used.

Other possible mediating factors in both countries include differentials across social classes and gender in exposure and/or susceptibility to health hazards in the work environment. These include not only occupational risks linked to the physical work environment but also psychosocial risks linked to lack of control over working conditions and job insecurity. In addition, the multiple roles associated with being both a paid worker and a parent, particularly in Sweden, may be more or less stressful in health terms depending on social position. We are now seeking to develop a better understanding of these factors in order to refine policy development in the future.

Data from the British General Household Survey were made available through the Office for National Statistics and the Economic and Social Research Council Data Archive.

References

Acheson D., Barker D., Chambers J., Graham H., Marmot M., Whitehead M. 1998. *Report of the Independent Inquiry into Inequalities in Health.* London: The Stationery Office.

Armitage P., Colton T. (eds). 1998. *Encyclopedia of Biostatistics.* New York: John Wiley.

Cassel J. 1976. The contribution of the social environment to host resistence. *American Journal of Epidemiology* 104:107–123.

Department of Trade and Industry. 1998. *Fairness at Work.* London: The Stationery Office.

Diderichsen F. 1995. Market reforms in health care and sustainability of the welfare state. *Health Policy* 32:141–153.

Diderichsen F., Hallqvist J. 1998. Social inequalities in health: some methodological considerations for the study of social position and social context. In: Arve-Parès B (ed.). *Inequality in Health—A Swedish Perspective.* Stockholm: Swedish Council for Social Research, pp. 25–39.

Drever F., Whitehead M. (eds) 1997. *Health Inequalities—Decennial Supplement.* Office for National Statistics Series, DS No. 15. London: The Stationery Office.

Esping-Andersen G. (ed). 1995. *Welfare States in Transition.* London: Sage Publications.

European Commission. 1995. *Employment in Europe.* Luxembourg: European Commission.

Gottschalk P., Smeeding T. 1998. Empirical evidence on income inequality in industrialized countries. In: Atkinson A.B., Bourgignon F. (eds), *The Handbook of Income Distribution.* Amsterdam: North-Holland.

Gustafsson B., Palmer E. 1997. Changes in Swedish inequity: a study of equivalent income 1975–91. In: Gottschalk P., Gustafsson B., Palmer E. (eds), *Changing Patterns in the Distribution of Economic Welfare: An International Perspective.* Cambridge: Cambridge University Press.

Hallqvist J., Diderichsen F. et al. 1998. Is the effect of job strain on myocardial infarction risk due to interaction between high psychological demands and low decision latitude? *Social Science and Medicine* 46:1405–1415.

Hills J. 1998. *Income and Wealth: The Latest Evidence.* York: Joseph Rowntree Foundation.

Kouvusilta L., Rimpelä A., Rimpelä M. 1995. Health status: does it predict choice in further education? *Journal of Epidemiology and Community Health;* 49:141–38.

Lundberg M., Fredlund P., Hallqvist J., Diderichsen F. 1996. A SAS program calculating three measures of interaction with confidence intervals. *Epidemiology* 7:655–656.

Macintyre S. 1997. The Black Report and beyond: What are the lessons? *Social Science and Medicine* 44:723–745.

Martin R. 1998. Regional dimensions of Europe's unemployment crisis. In: Lawless P., Martin R., Hardy S. (eds). *Unemployment and Social Exclusion.* Regional Policy and Development Series, 13. London: Regional Studies Association.

Michie J., Wilkinson F. 1994. The growth of unemployment in the 1980s. In: Michie J., Smith J.G. (eds). *Unemployment in Europe.* London: Academic Press, pp. 11–31.

Mielck A., Giraldes M., do Rosario C. (eds). 1994. *Health Inequalities: Discussion in Western European Countries.* New York: Waxmann.

National Board of Health and Welfare. 1998. *Sweden's Public Health Report 1997.* Stockholm: National Board of Health and Welfare.

Nickell S., Bell B. 1995. The collapse in demand for the unskilled and unemployment across the OECD. In: Alyn A. and Mayhew K. (eds). *Oxford Review of Economic Policy: Unemployment* 11:40–62.

Rothman K.J., Greenland S. 1998. *Modern Epidemiology*, 2nd ed. Philadelphia: Lippincott-Raven.

Smeeding T. 1997. *Financial Poverty in Developed Countries: The Evidence From LIS.* Final Report to UNDP. Maxwell School of Citizenship and Public Affairs Working Paper No. 155. New York: Syracuse University.

SOU. 1998. *Hur skall Sverige må bättre?* Delbetänkande av Nationella folkhälsokommittén. [Promoting health in Sweden. Preliminary report of the National Public Health Commission.] Sweden (in Swedish).

Statistics Sweden. 1982. *The Swedish Socio-Economic Classification—SEI.* Report on Statistical Co-ordination. 1882:4. Stockholm: Statistics Sweden.

United Nations Development Programme (UNDP). 1999. *Human Development Report 1999.* New York: UNDP.

Whitehead M. 1990. *The Concepts and Principles of Equity and Health.* Copenhagen: World Health Organization.

BUILDING EFFICIENT, EQUITABLE HEALTH CARE SYSTEMS

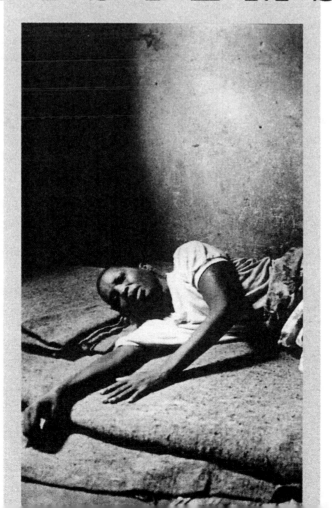

As articulated in the preceding conceptual chapters and demonstrated empirically in the in-depth country analyses, the antecedents of health inequities are often located in the broader social and economic arena. The role of the health care system itself in reducing ill health and suffering, redressing inequities, and preventing future inequities, however, is critical. Furthermore, in the short term, the health sector may be one of the more feasible points of entry for policies to redress health inequities. This section addresses in greater depth the aspects of the health sector that affect health equity, introducing the issue of health care financing and presenting two in-depth country analyses that address health systems reform issues—Mexico and Vietnam.

Global Aspects of Health Systems

Health system reform is a global phenomenon, influenced by market ideology, resource constraints, and prescriptions of international financial institutions such as the World Bank and the International Monetary Fund. Following World War II widespread support for the idea of the welfare state led to national governments taking more responsibility for providing and financing health care. In the last 20 years, however, there has been progressive erosion of support for government involvement in health care, corresponding to the belief that market forces bring greater efficiency to health delivery systems and make them more affordable for cash-strapped governments. The increasing costs of health care in the North, "structural adjustments" of debt-ridden countries in the South, and the implosion of the socialist economies in the late 1980s have unleashed private forces in health care globally. This dwindling of state roles has been accelerated by another pervasive global trend, namely, "decentralization"—often a code word for any number of more specific trends including privatization and commercialization. Health systems reform has come to be characterized by a sort of re-structuring of the public sector organization and procedures (often, decentralization) and reform of the financing strategies (Gilson and Mills 1995).

In studying health systems across countries, common trends that ultimately affect the equity of health outcomes may be observed. For example, many have noted that health care at all levels (primary through tertiary) and public health interventions are more likely to be accessed by the rich than by the poor—the so-called inverse care law (Tudor Hart 1971). In general, the health needs and priorities of the poor differ from those of the rich—and the rich have access to greater preventive, protective, and curative potential than the poor (Chen et al. 1999). Even in Nordic countries, often touted as models for their commitment to equity, it has been noted that the existence of universal coverage does not guarantee equity of access in practice (Guning-Schepers and Stronks 1999).

Health care insurance systems and providers have also moved beyond national borders in search of the global market. In Latin America, reform of health systems encouraging greater private sector participation has led to the market entry of a number of American insurance and managed care giants (Stocker et al. 1999). From an equity perspective, concerns are being voiced about the tendency of the private sector to be selective in providing coverage for healthier and wealthier populations, leaving the underfunded public systems for the chronically ill, elderly, and rural poor. In such situations its not hard to see why "health care for the poor" is often considered synonymous with "poor health care."

With the introduction of private health care services, accelerated tiering of health care systems has occurred within countries along social class and geographical axes. At the same time, transnationalization of health care and its clear stratifying effects according to ability to pay suggests that particular tiers of health systems may have more in common with one another across systems than within nations (Barillas 1999).

The significance of this recent history is that health systems globally have shifted in response to an external set of ideological prescriptions aimed at the state in general with little or no explicit recognition of health system needs such as fairness in distribution. The health care sector, therefore, has played a "follow the leader" role with priorities corresponding to general social sector prescriptions such as cost-cutting and decentralization of services. Gilson and Mills (1995) argue that health sector reform must be adapted to a wider policy context rather than imposed blindly from above. They argue that contextual factors such as pre-existing institutional capacity, socioeconomic inequalities, community attitudes toward risk-sharing, and professional ethics must be considered in shaping health sector reforms.

Standing (1997) emphasizes the variety and diversity of health care reforms. Although health systems are generally focused on financial and institutional reforms, context has tempered the generalized prescriptions. In the Americas the reforms have occurred in the context of strong states and active civil society, focusing on decentralization and reform of social security systems. On the other hand, in sub-Saharan Africa, where reforms are occurring in the context of (and because of) weak state capacity, severe crises in health sector budgets, and limited civil society involvement, the focus of reform is improvement of human resource management and different approaches to financing.

The Chapters in This Section

The conceptual chapter on health care financing introduces financing as one aspect of the health system that affects health equity. The configuration of financing, defined as both the mobilization of financial resources and the allocation of those resources to the population, will affect health outcomes in two important ways—first, by determining, in part, the availability of health care and who has access to it, and second, by dictating the degree of financial protection offered against catastrophic costs of illness. The authors emphasize the point that although financing issues often tend to dominate debates and prescriptions for health systems reform, methods of financing are but one aspect of a broad health system that involves institutions, policies, and human resources.

The case of Mexico, presented in this section, reveals the fact that district/provincial expenditures in health care are inversely related to need, a case in point of the "inverse care law." Mexico is a middle-income country facing a double burden of infectious and chronic disease and engaged in health sector reform and decentralization. Using the marginality index, developed by the Mexican government, the authors employ a policy-relevant mechanism for highlighting disparity and mapping the intersection of marginality, membership in an indigenous group, and rural poverty. As Julio Frenk (1999) points out, middle-income countries like Mexico face a formidable list of obstacles to proper health systems performance—factors experienced by low income countries such as inequity and insufficient resources, *as well as* impediments typically faced by high-income countries such as inefficiency, inadequate quality of care, patient dissatisfaction, and inflation. The authors point to several aspects of current Mexican health sector reforms that hold promise for meeting the differential needs more equitably in marginalized areas, populated by indigenous groups.

The Vietnamese case study presented in this section is written by the Vice Minister of Health and other colleagues in the Ministry of Health. As such, this case study provides a unique look at policy makers' commitment to equity in health in the face of multiple political and economic pressures. The Vietnamese have had a traditional focus on equity and in the early years of the nation created a health infrastructure that "extended throughout the country, including remote rural areas, and provided health care to the entire population" (Hien et al. 1995). Vietnam's overall health performance is remarkably high given its level of economic development. In 1989, the legislature implemented *Doi Moi* (meaning change to the new), dramatically transforming the social, political, and economic context in Vietnam as the country became a transitional economy. *Doi Moi* resulted in the decollectivization of the agricultural system, the privatization of trade and social services (including health), and the opening of markets to promote investment. It also meant financial reforms in keeping with structural adjustment prescription, including cuts in public spending, the reduction of state subsidies, and public revenue generation via fees for public services (Hien et al. 1995). All of these seismic changes were accompanied by the disappearance of the traditional inflows of resources from the Soviet bloc. Faced with these challenges, this section's chapter or Vietnam presents the policy makers' approaches to developing a financing system that will be both equitable and efficient.

In the concluding section of this book, Part V, Whitehead and colleagues put great emphasis on equity as a pillar of health care systems and the consequent need to assess the impact of any reform on the underlying equity objectives.

References

Barillas E. 1999. The global transformation of national health systems. *Development* 42(4):76–77.

Chen L.C., Evans T.G., Cash R.A. 1999. Health as a global public good. In: Kaul I., Grunberg I., Stern M. (eds), *Global Public Goods: International Cooperation in the 21st Century*. UNDP. New York: Oxford University Press.

Frenk J. 1995. Comprehensive policy analysis for health system reform. In: Berman P. (ed), *Health Sector Reform in Developing Countries: Making Health Development Sustainable*. Boston: Harvard School of Public Health, pp. 335–362.

Gilson L., Mills A. 1995. Health sector reforms in sub-Saharan Africa: lessons of the last 10 years. In: Berman P. (ed), *Health Sector Reform in Developing Countries: Making Health Development Sustainable*. Boston: Harvard School of Public Health, pp. 277–316.

Guning-Schepers L., Stronks K. 1999. Inequalities in health: future threats to equity. *Acta Ontologica* 38(1):57–61.

Hien N.T., Ha L.T.T., Rifkin S.B., Wright E.P. 1995. The pursuit of equity: a health sector case study from Vietnam. *Health Policy* 33:191–204.

Standing H. 1997. Gender, vulnerability and equity in health sector reform programmes: a review. *Health Policy and Planning* 12(1):1–18.

Stocker K., Waitzkin H., Iriart C. 1999. The exportation of managed care to Latin America. *New England Journal of Medicine* 340:1131–1136.

Tudor Hart J. 1971. The inverse care law. *Lancet* i:405–412.

CHAPTER
18

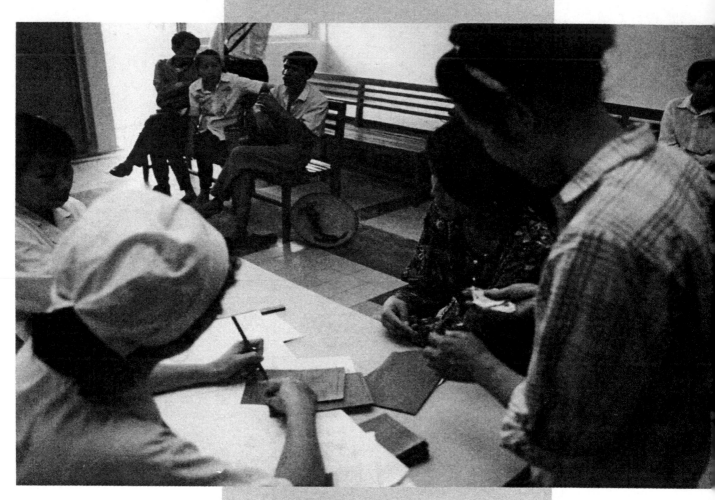

Health clinic, Hanoi, Vietnam, 1995.
Source: Richard Lord/L&I.

Health Care Financing: Assessing Its Relationship to Health Equity

WILLIAM C. HSIAO AND YUANLI LIU

Our ability to learn, work, achieve our full potential, and enjoy our lives depends on our health condition. Thus, adequate health care becomes a fundamental necessity for human well being. From an equity perspective, health care financing is important for two reasons. First, financing determines the availability of health care as well as who has access to it. Second, financing mechanisms dictate the degree of financial protection offered against catastrophic costs of illness. While the probability of a given person being struck with a serious accident or illness is small and uncertain, the medical costs of treating misfortunes are beyond the financial means of most households. As a result, most households would be impoverished should a serious illness strike unless they are insured or have access to subsidized health services. Studies have found that in many low- and middle-income nations with underdeveloped health care financing systems, spending for serious illnesses has thrust many households into poverty.

Health care financing has two definitions, one narrow and one broad. Under the narrow definition, financing pertains only to the mobilization of funds for health care. Under the broad definition, health care financing covers the following three issues: first, the mobilization of funds for health care; second, the allocation of the funds to regions and population groups and for specific types of health care; and third, the mecha-

nisms for paying for health care. In this chapter, we use the broad definition because all three issues are closely interrelated.

This chapter analyzes two issues: equity in health care financing and its relationship to equity in health. At least five methods have been developed to finance health care: general revenue/earmarked taxes, social insurance contributions, private insurance premiums, community financing, and direct out-of-pocket payment. Each method distributes the financial burdens and benefits differently, and each method affects who will have access to health care and financial protection. In short, each method has different equity implications.

We begin the chapter with a description of the five health care financing methods and a table that summarizes each method's equity implications. Next, we examine the relationship between health care financing and health care, health care and health outcomes, and equity in health. This line of inquiry is an effort to link equity in health care financing to the larger issue being addressed in this book—equity in health. Methods of financing affect the availability of health care, its distribution, and who will have access to health care. In turn, health care should affect health outcomes through prevention and treatment of diseases to avoid premature death and disability. In the fourth, fifth, and sixth sections, we review the "state of the art" in terms of how equity in health care financing is being defined and measured. We also summarize some of the empirical findings. Finally, we assess the known and unknown and suggest a research agenda to advance our knowledge about equity in health care financing.

Health Care Financing Methods

High-income and low-income countries alike finance health care using a mixture of five possible sources: taxes, social insurance contributions, private insurance premiums, community financing, and direct out-of-pocket payment (e.g., user fees and patients' direct payment to private providers). Most health care financing schemes are designed to serve two purposes: to ensure equal access to health care and to protect patients from catastrophic losses due to illness (financial protection), thus preventing poverty. We briefly describe the main features of these financing methods (Liu et al 1998).

General tax revenues have long been used in every nation to finance a major portion of health care. Low-income nations often rely on general taxes to finance health care more than high-income nations because technical and administrative complexities make social and private insurance infeasible. Low-income nations also, however, have less of a tax base and less capability to collect taxes. A recent International Monetary Fund study (InterAmerican Development Bank 1996) reports the average national income collected as tax revenue is 18% for low-income countries as opposed to 48% for high-income nations. Low tax ratios often translate into insufficient public finance for health care. Some governments may "earmark" a particular tax for health purposes. An advantage of this source of financing is that it is possible to assign a tax to fund certain priority programs. Abel-Smith et al. (1991) observed that it might be practical to earmark for health the taxes on certain goods and activities that may have adverse health implications (e.g., alcohol or tobacco use). The problem with such taxes, however, is that they are often difficult to administer, may be politically unpopular, and are regressive.

Social insurance has two characteristics that distinguish it from private insurance. First, social insurance is compulsory. Everyone in the eligible group must enroll and pay a specified premium contribution in exchange for a set of benefits. Second, social insurance premiums and benefits are described in social compacts established through legislation. Premiums or benefits can be altered only through a formal political process.

Private insurance is a private contract offered by an insurer to exchange a set of benefits for a payment of a specified premium. Private insurance is marketed by either nonprofit or for-profit insurance companies, and consumers voluntarily choose to purchase an insurance package that best matches their preferences. Private insurance is offered on individual and group bases. Under individual insurance, the premium is based on that individual's risk characteristics. The major concern in private insurance is buyers' adverse selection, that is, unhealthy people are more likely to purchase than are healthy ones. Under group insurance, the premium is calculated on a group basis. Often the members are divided into two groups: single persons and families. For each category, the risk is pooled across age, gender, and health status. Thus, there is significant income transfer under group insurance compared with individual insurance from low-risk groups to high-risk groups (e.g., from younger workers to older workers).

Direct out-of-pocket payment is made by patients to private providers at the time a service is rendered. Although such payments have always been used by private providers to obtain revenue, in the past public sector providers rarely charged patients a significant fee. This changed in the mid-1980s, however, when the World Bank adopted a policy of pushing the low-income nations to charge significant user fees for public health services. In this chapter, the term *user fees* refers only to the fees the patients have to pay to public hospitals, clinics, and health posts, not to private sector providers. The proponents of user fees believe that the fees can increase revenue to improve the quality of public health services and expand coverage (Litvack and Bodart 1993). The major objection raised to user fees has been on equity grounds, in particular that the poor would not be able to afford to pay for, and thus would decrease their use of, "necessary services" (Reddy and Vandemoortele 1996).

Community financing is a term loosely applied to many different activities, but the best schemes are based on three principles: community cooperation, self-reliance, and prepayment. The members of a community pay a contribution (in cash or in kind) to a community-organized entity in advance for a package of basic benefits. In exchange for the advance payment, the community entity organizes and provides preventive care, primary health care, and drugs when members need them. Unlike insurance financing, provision and financing of primary health care are integrated under community financing. The fund may also serve as financial protection by covering some inpatient services. Community financing is organized and managed by the community, although the government may have to encourage it, subsidize it, and provide technical assistance to establish it. Among the most successful examples of community financing are Indonesia's *Dana*

Sehat (Suwandono 1995), the Health Card System in Thailand (Creese 1991), and the Cooperative Medical System in China (Hsiao 1984; Liu et al. 1995). In Box 1, we describe *Dana Sehat* in greater detail to illustrate the function and operation of community financing.

Equity in Health, Health Care, and Health Care Financing

Health care financing is a means to an end. While we are concerned about the equity of financing and expenditures, we are equally concerned about how effective a given financing method is in improving equity of health outcomes and general human well-being. There are multiple pathways by which health care financing affects the availability, distribution, and efficiency of health care. This is illustrated in Figure 1.

The financing scheme and design chosen are a major determinant of how much money will be available for health care. In allocating the funds for specific services, financing influences what services are made available. In its allocative determination as to which region,

community, or population group should receive the funds, the financing scheme affects who will have access to the services and the equity of health care. The financing agency must also decide how to pay health practitioners, clinics, and hospitals and drugs. The payment method gives financial incentives to providers, encouraging them to alter their health practices and work patterns in response. In sum, the financing scheme determines how much money will be mobilized, how the funds will be used and managed, how efficiently the services will be delivered, and what type of services will be available and to whom.

In health care, money has to be transformed into services. How effectively funds can be transformed into efficacious services depends, in part, on how the health delivery system is organized. For example, the government can deliver health care by funding, organizing, and directly managing immunization programs, health posts, and hospitals, an organizational structure that creates public monopolies. Such operations are influenced by politics, and their management tends to rely on inefficient bureaucratic rules. Alternatively, the delivery of health care can be organized and operated by private for-profit or nonprofit organizations. Each

---

BOX 1: COMMUNITY FINANCING: INDONESIA'S *DANA SEHAT*

Since the 1970s, Indonesia has promoted community-based health funds called *Dana Sehat*. Financing relies primarily on prepayments from members, often supplemented by government subsidies and funds from community agriculture cooperatives. These monies ensure members access to a basic benefit package of health care services.

Dana Sehat schemes are premised on the broader Indonesian policy of promoting community action to ensure social equity, quality, and prevention measures. Through a government initiative that systematically emphasizes community involvement, authorities have been able to double the population covered by *Dana Sehat* from 6 million in 1988 to 12 million in 1994, representing 13% of Indonesian villages.

The central feature of *Dana Sehat* is community involvement, supervised and monitored by local authorities. A *Dana Sehat* is run by the community itself, through such institutions as the "family welfare movement," the village cooperative, and religious organizations.

The government plays an enabling role in the establishment of *Dana Sehat*. Usually, government officials initiate the process of organizing meetings between health providers, local authorities, religious sectors, and key persons in the

community, including communitywide meetings. The next step generally is a community self-survey. Government officials help to train surveyors as well as assist with analysis and presentation of the results to the community.

A second round of community meetings is then facilitated by government authorities. The goals are to select a communitywide health package and commit, as a community, to its implementation. A government technical assistance team presents a precalculated menu of health care benefit designs and their financing requirements. Community members then choose the services to be covered by the fund, balancing their needs against their ability and willingness to finance the package. Poor rural communities often choose a package of basic outpatient and curative care, combined with free preventive services. The community also chooses teams to be responsible for managing and overseeing implementation of the *Dana Sehat*.

Many communities can complete these preliminaries and initiate the *Dana Sehat* in a period of about 6 months. Thereafter, the local government continues to supervise, monitor, and guide fund management. Usually at the close of the fund's first year, a community self-assessment is conducted to evaluate and improve the fund.

Figure 1 Relationship between health care financing and equity in health in a broad context

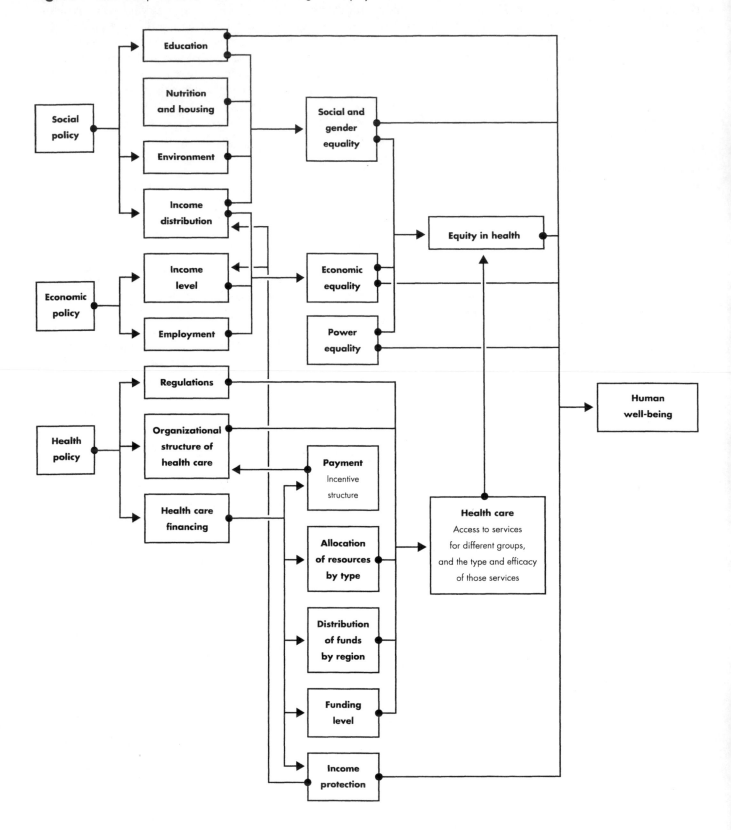

alternative has significant implications as to how efficiently the funds are transformed into services.

While these logical relationships are clear, it is difficult to empirically study the impact of different combinations of these components of financing on equity in health. The reason is simple. The observational unit for such a study is likely to be a country. Collecting uniform data from many nations would require the cooperation of many countries and would be expensive and time consuming. No one has attempted it yet. Nonetheless, many partial studies have been done to examine the impacts of separate components of the various financing schemes.

Our knowledge about the pathways by which health care financing influences health is only partial. For instance, it has been shown that the health status of the population depends partly on the ability of those who "need" it to obtain health care. Because health care financing determines availability, distribution, type, and accessibility of health care for the population, it is clear that financing will have an effect on equity of health. We do not, however, know all the pathways, the interactions between the various factors, or the relative impacts of the pathways. We can express this set of complex relationships and their plausible sequence in the following functional expressions, which indicate how variables on the left are determined by the variables on the right and how they are sequenced (boldface indicates the direct components of *financing* that play a role in determining outcomes):

1. Well-being = G (health, **income protection**, education, gender equality, social equality, income, environmental conditions, and so forth)
2. Equity in Health = G (**access to health care**, education, nutrition, housing, social equality, income, environmental condition, and so forth)
3. Availability and Distribution of Health Care = G (**method of financing, resource allocation, payment method**, organization, national income level, income distribution, and so forth)
4. Income Protection = G (**method of financing, coverage of risks**, and so forth)

This set of expressions shows how human well-being may be affected by health care financing. We do not, however, know the strength of these causal relationships because the results vary by cultural, institutional, and managerial conditions. Studies have consistently found that various components in health care financing schemes have a measurable impact on the availability of health care and people's access to health care. In general, research has focused on the relationships in equations 3 and 4, neglecting the relative effectiveness of health care in producing health and well-being. The relationships between the nonhealth care factors influencing equity in health and well being are much more complex and involve theories from many disciplines. Unfortunately, our current knowledge is limited in this regard.

Figure 1 illustrates some of these complex relationships and their plausible sequences in greater detail. The desired "end" is human well-being (on the far right in Fig. 1) with health and nonhealth care policies contributing to that state of well-being. In the broader context (depicted at the top left of Fig. 1), well-being is determined by social and economic policies that influence such factors as education, income, environmental conditions, health equity, income protection, nutrition, housing, social and gender equality, and so on. At the same time, health policy (represented in the lower half of Fig. 1) influences the availability and distribution of health care and arrangements for financial protection, which in turn govern equity in the health care system. Health care then contributes to the wider outcomes of equity in health and human well-being. It should be noted that in Figure 1, health care financing appears early in the chain of events depicted and is only one of many factors that affect equity in health.

Definition and Measurement

Health care financing schemes are often designed to couple the source of funding with the party eligible to receive benefits. The redistributive effects are built into both the source of funding and the benefit side. As a result, equity in financing needs to be evaluated on a comprehensive basis. Several authors have suggested that equity should be assessed on the basis of its net benefit (Zschock 1989; Hoare and Mills 1986). Among the rich body of empirical analysis on equity in health care financing, however, most have been partial analyses. These analyses only assessed equity by source of financing and ignored the benefit side. Consequently, their findings could be erroneous. We found only a few studies of small population groups that assessed the monetary value of the direct health care benefit received net of the amount paid. These studies had, however, overlooked the value of another benefit, that of protection against high medical costs. In this section, we summarize the literature on equity in mobilization of financial resources, which represents only one dimension of health care financing. The equity issues for the benefit side are analyzed later.

Equity in Mobilizing Financial Resources

Definition

Studies of equity in health care financing have largely followed the principles and methods developed in the field of public finance. Financing is defined in a narrow sense and pertains to mobilizing financial resources only (hereafter, we will refer to it as *resource mobilization*). Under this narrow definition, equity is analyzed by examining the question of who paid the taxes or premiums and whether the pattern is "equitable."

Public finance literature distinguishes between two competing principles: the benefit principle, requiring payments to be related to benefits received; and the ability to pay principle, requiring that payments be related to ability to pay. A comparison of policy statements and empirical studies on equity in the finance of health care reveals that the benefit principle commands little support in health care systems. It is not regarded as an equity principle (Wagstaff and van Doorslaer 1993). Instead, there seems to be a broad measure of support for the idea that health care ought to be financed according to ability to pay (Hurst 1985, 1991; Gottschalk et al. 1989; Wagstaff and van Doorslaer 1993). To give this ethical premise empirical content, a definition of "ability to pay," therefore, is required. Russell (1996) has questioned the validity of the published research that assumed that willingness to pay for medical care is synonymous with ability to pay. Russell argues that households may pay for care when a member suffers from acute pain or life-threatening conditions, but sacrifice other basic needs such as food and education and face serious consequences later. Many households may also go into debt to pay for care.

According to the principle of ability to pay, equity should be measured in two ways: vertical equity, requiring households with greater (lesser) ability to pay to contribute a greater (lesser) portion of their income for health care, and horizontal equity, requiring households of the same ability to pay to make the same contribution. In vertical equity, a system is considered to be progressive when higher income households pay a greater portion of their income for health care, whereas a regressive system is one in which payments fall as a proportion of income when income rises. A proportional system is one in which payments account for the same proportion of income for people of all income groups. To be defined as equitable, how progressive should a system be? Typically, empirical studies have avoided making such explicit value judgments and focused simply on quantifying the degree of progressivity (Hurst 1985; Christiansen 1993; Nolan and Turbat 1993; Baker and van der Gaag 1993; Wagstaff and van Doorslaer 1993).

Measurement

In the published literature, measuring equity in resource mobilization is synonymous with measuring how progressive a system is. Empirical work on progressivity in resource mobilization has been based on either a proportional method—comparing the share of total health care expenditure paid by a group with its share of national income—or an index approach, as described below. After describing these more standard approaches, we go on to argue that in addition to measuring the equity of resource mobilization, the equity of benefits must also be assessed.

The proportional method. Under the proportional method, the population is divided into income groups. The proportion of total health spending paid by an income group is compared with the proportion of national income received by that income group. For example, Gottschalk et al. (1989) compared the health care financing systems of the Netherlands, the United Kingdom, and the United States. They concluded that the U.S. system was regressive because the share of total health expenditure paid by the lower income groups exceeded their portion of the national income, while the share borne by the top income groups was less than their share of the national income (see Fig. 2).

Index of progressivity. A more comprehensive approach to measuring progressivity is to employ indices (Wagstaff et al. 1989), particularly in relation to vertical equity (Kakwani 1977; Suits 1977; Lambert 1989). Recent work attempts to measure and compare both the vertical and horizontal effects (Aaronson et al. 1994; Wagstaff and van Doorslaer, 1993, 1997). As an illustration of the essence of these indices, we briefly describe Kakwani's index, which has been extensively used in studies conducted for high-income nations (Wagstaff and van Doorslaer 1993).

Kakwani's index of progressivity. Kakwani's index measures the extent to which the tax burden borne by each income group departs from proportionality. This index is best explained by illustration (see Figure 3). The Lorenz curve labeled "income share" plots the cumulative proportions of the population (ranked according to pre-tax income) against the cumulative proportions of income. The second curve, labeled "payment concentration," plots the cumulative proportions of the population (ranked according to pre-tax income against the cumulative proportions of payment for health care). If health care payments are levied in pro-

Figure 2 Distribution of the health care financing burden across income deciles in the United States, 1988

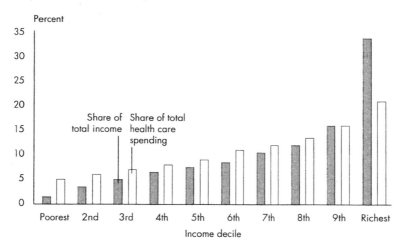

Source: Gottschalk, Wolfe, and Haveman 1989.

portion to income, the payment concentration curve and the pre-tax income share curve coincide. If the financing system is progressive (i.e., the payment rate rises faster than income), the payment concentration curve lies outside the income share curve. If the health care payment rate is regressive (i.e., the payment rate decreases with income), the payment concentration curve lies inside the income share curve. The degree of pro-

Figure 3 Kakwani's index of equity in health care spending

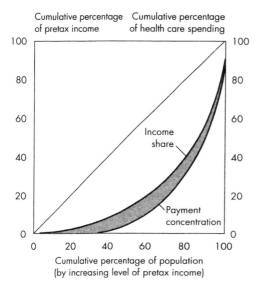

Note: The area of the shaded region is the level of Kakwani's index.
Source: Adapted from Wagstaff and van Doorslaer 1993.

gressivity is measured by the size of the area between the payment concentration and income share curves. The value of Kakwani's index of progressivity ranges from −2.0 (most regressive) to 0.0 (payment is proportionate to income) to 1.0 (most progressive). Figure 3 depicts a progressive health care finance system.

Results for high-income nations

Using Kakwani's index of progressivity, Wagstaff and van Doorslaer (1993) found that general taxes for health care are typically a progressive means of raising revenue under standard incidence assumptions. Social insurance, in contrast, is proportional, unless the amount that a worker has to contribute is capped, at which point it tends to be slightly regressive. Private insurance is more regressive because social insurance contributions are assessed proportional to wages, whereas private insurance is not. Premiums for individual private insurance are adjusted for risk. Because the financially worse off tend to be sicker, these premiums tend to be negatively related to income. Private group insurance also tends to be regressive because employees pay the same amount of premium regardless of their income. Out-of-pocket payments tend to be substantially more regressive than other methods of financing.

Although there has been no systematic study on how progressive community financing systems are, they can arguably be rendered more progressive than user fees and individual private insurance because the prepayment is typically uniform within the same communities without being adjusted for risk (Liu et al. 1995; Bennett et al. 1997). Wagstaff and van Doorslaer (1993) found that tax-financed health care systems, such as those operating in Ireland and the United Kingdom, tend to be mildly progressive; social insurance systems, such as those operating in France and Spain, are mildly regressive; and the predominantly private insurance systems, such as the U.S. and Swiss systems, tend to be regressive (see Fig. 4). These empirical results have clear implications for some of the health care reforms undertaken in many countries. A greater reliance on out-of-pocket payments, recently instituted in France and other countries in the Organization for Economic Cooperation and Development (OECD), is likely to make health care financing more regressive (Wagstaff and van Doorslaer 1993).

Results for developing nations

Typically, governments of developing nations have a scarcity of general revenues because they have a very small tax base, compounded by a limited capacity to collect taxes. Yet, these governments face many meritorious demands for public financing such as education, agricultural development, and roads. Thus, many governments devote only a modest portion of their total budget to health care, ranging from 5% to 15%. Many poor nations rely on donors to finance a significant portion of their total health expenditures.

The government's spending is financed through direct or indirect taxes, inflation (printing money), or budgetary deficits supported by domestic and foreign borrowing. Each revenue source has a different equity impact in terms of who bears the burden. Most nations also organize and manage public clinics and hospitals to deliver the services funded by the government. User fees have played a minor role in generating resources for health care in most low-income countries.

Providing affordable health care to all citizens has been the main justification for heavily subsidized public health services. Theoretically, if the public health services are financed by progressive taxes and the services are used mostly by the poor and low-income households, then the public health services serve a major redistributive function and can help to correct some of the inequities in a nation. In practice, however, it has been difficult to achieve the equity objective by publicly financed and delivered health care. Experiences of developing countries indicate two major problems. First, tax evasion is highly correlated with the progressivity of the tax rate. Ahmad and Stern (1991) cited a personal income tax evasion rate of over 60% in Pakistan, whose tax system is purportedly progressive. Second, progressive redistribution has seldom taken place under government financing. Most governments of developing nations allocated the largest

Figure 4 Kakwani's index of equity in health care spending in selected high-income countries

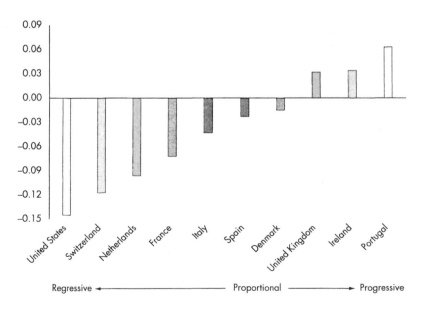

Note: The data refer to various years between 1980 and 1987.
Source: Wagstaff and van Doorslaer 1993.

share of their health budget to subsidize tertiary and hospital services. These publicly funded health services tend to be located in the nation's capital and large cities, where the higher income households who demand these services live (Grosh 1995; Demery et al. 1995). Such an urban bias in demand for tertiary health care results in the majority of public health sector funding benefiting the wealthy.

Because developing nations have limited capacity to tax or to establish social or private insurance, they must search for other sources of funding to support public health services. In the mid-1980s, the World Bank (1987) advocated user fees for public health services, and as a result many developing countries implemented user fees in the following years (Nolan and Turbat 1993). Studies have been conducted for sub-Saharan African nations to evaluate the equity and efficiency implications of their user fee implementation. Studies consistently found that user fees reduce the utilization of health services by the poor more than by the rich (Waddington and Enyimayew 1990; McPake et al. 1993a,b). These findings are supported by econometric investigations that have found the demand for health care by the poor and low-income households, compared with that of higher income groups, to be much more sensitive to the level of fees they are required to pay (Gertler et al. 1986). A study in Burkina Faso found that while the overall demand for health care was not very sensitive to the fees charged, the demand for services for infants and children was highly sensitive (Sauerborn et al. 1996).

On a positive note, Diop et al. (1995) found that user fees could improve equity if the revenue generated from the fees was retained and used by the facilities to improve the quality of services. This study discovered that the availability of drugs seemed to be the key factor that encouraged low-income households to use public health services. Litvak and Bodart (1993) found that the probability of the poorest quintile seeking care at public facilities increased after user fees were increased. Abel-Smith and Rawal (1992) observed that "if services are so bad that poor must resort to the private sector, user fees may be less inequitable than free care."

In implementing user fees, some countries have taken equity into consideration by exempting the poor and low-income households. Malawi included low-income exemptions in phases—first in central hospitals, then in district hospitals, and finally in health centers (Shaw and Griffin 1995). In Tanzania, a study found 90% of hospitals and 20% of dispensaries exempted the disabled; approximately 30% of the facilities also exempted children under 5 years of age and the chronically ill. Most health facilities also accepted deferred payment or alternative forms of payment—payment in kind with crops or temporary employment without pay (Hussein and Mujinja 1997).

McPake et al. (1993b) reviewed a group of five African nations initiating user fees as part of the Bamako Initiative and found all of the countries had some exemption mechanism. The criteria were usually very stringent with exception only for those with physical or mental disability. Deferred payment was frequently allowed in most of the countries reviewed. Unfortunately, some studies found that exemption schemes were not widespread. A survey of official cost-recovery policies in African countries suggested that exemptions were remarkably uncommon (Nolan and Turbat 1993). Even the existing exemption schemes were subject to distortion and abuse by those who have the power to grant an exemption. There is evidence indicating that relatives and friends of the administrators of the exemption program benefited more than the needy and the poor. This has been documented in countries such as Lesotho (Shaw and Griffin 1995), Ghana (Waddington and Enyimayew 1990), and Bangladesh.

The major barriers in implementing equitable user fees are defining who is poor, working out an acceptable formula for providing subsidies, and effectively administering exemptions. Empirical evidence seems to suggest that means testing at the point of service is likely to be less fair than a formal, prospective means test such as that used in Vietnam and Thailand (Barnum and Kutzin 1993). In these countries, subsidized "health cards" are given out to the poor, whose entitlement to the cards (a form of voucher for purchasing health care services) is determined jointly by the governments and local representatives (e.g., the Village People's Committee).

Overall, the evidence indicates that user fee schemes are, for the most part, regressive. Creese (1997) conducted a review of the impact of user fees and concluded that they had widened the gap in access to health care by different socioeconomic groups. From an efficiency perspective, studies found the administrative costs for collecting and processing the fee revenue to be substantial (Jimenez 1987).

Equity in Health Care Benefits

Definition

Culyer and Wagstaff (1993) highlighted the linkage between equity in health care financing and equity in health care benefits, noting that "an ethical interest in the equity in health care financing is motivated first and foremost by an ethical concern about the distribution of health care." How do we define and measure equity in health care? Unlike equity in terms of who pays for health care, equity takes on different meanings in terms of who benefits from health care spending depending on the underlying ethical theories. For example, equity defined in terms of "need" would be different from equity defined by income class, potential to benefit from health care, or gender. In addition, we must address the fundamental question of how health care should be defined. Further development of the definition and measurement of equity in health care benefits is clearly needed.

For developing nations, many studies have used a simple definition for equity in health care: equal *use* of health care. Studies have been conducted to assess the equity of health care benefits by comparing the immunization rates and the numbers of visits and hospital days by income classes, region, and gender. This definition and measurement method only gives a limited picture because we cannot compare immunization with hospital stays. This limitation, for example, led van Vliet and van de Ven (1985) to argue that we should define equity in health care based on expenditures for each income group.

Measurement

Equity in the mobilization of financial resources emphasizes vertical equity (people with unequal ability to pay should be required to pay differently). In contrast, studies measuring equity on the benefit side tend to focus on horizontal equity where people with equal "need" should receive equal health care benefits. van Vliet and van de Ven (1985) proposed a method to standardize health expenditures for each income group. They assumed that each income group has the same morbidity rate (in reality, however, low-income groups usually have higher morbidity rates). Then the standardized expenditures can be interpreted as the expenditures each income group would receive if it had the age distribution and the morbidity of the population as a whole. From the standardized expenditure shares for the various income groups, one can plot a standardized expenditure concentration curve (g_{exp}^+) (see Fig. 5). Under an egalitarian benefit system, the standardized expenditure shares will be equal to each group's share. In this case, the expenditure concentration curve (g_{exp}^+) will coincide with the diagonal line. The extent of inequality in health care benefits (HI_{wvp}) is measured as the area between the expenditure concentration curve (g_{exp}^+) and the diagonal. When the index (HI_{wvp}) is greater than zero, it means that the health expenditure is distributed regressively while a

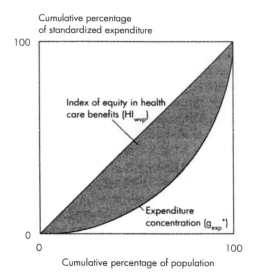

Figure 5 Standardized health expenditure concentration curve

Source: Van Vliet and van de Ven 1985.

negative value indicates a progressive distribution. Figure 5 depicts a regressive distribution.

Results for high-income nations

Employing this index of the extent of inequality in health care benefits (HI_{wvp}), Wagstaff and van Doorslaer (1993) estimated the extent of inequities in health care benefits for some OECD countries. Figure 6 lists indices of equity in funding (Kakwani) and in benefits (HI_{wvp}) for eight countries. When the two indices are compared, we cannot detect any direct relationship between the two. Judging by the signs of Kakwani (negative values mean more regressive) and HI_{wvp} indices (negative values mean more progressive), only half of the countries examined exhibited a consistent pattern in equity in funding and equity in benefits. While the United States and Spain appear to have both funding and benefits that favor the rich, Ireland has a system in which both tend to favor the poor. In Spain, however, there appears to be inequity in health care benefits favoring the rich even when there is a relatively equitable, tax-financed universal and comprehensive insurance coverage. In the other countries depicted in Figure 6 (Denmark, Italy, Switzerland, the Netherlands, and the United Kingdom), inequities in funding and benefits take different directions. Thus, we argue that simply judging the equity of a health financing system based on the Kakwani index (equity in resource mobilization) may be misleading; a measure of the equity in distribution of the benefits of health financing is also necessary.

Figure 6 Comparing equity in health care finance and benefits

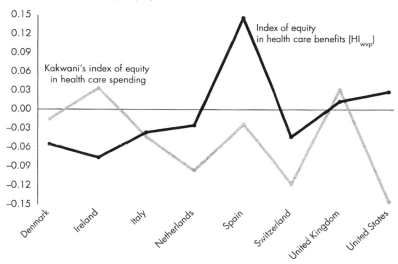

Note: For the index of equity in benefits, a negative value indicates a more progressive outcome; for Kakwani's index of equity in spending, a negative value indicates a more regressive outcome.

Source: Wagstaff and van Doorslaer 1993.

Results for developing countries

Many developing countries use tax revenues (a financing source that tends to be progressive) to fund public health care, where services are free. This is intended to ensure equal access for the poor and low-income households. Some incidence analyses, however, indicate that the public expenditures tend to benefit the rich disproportionately in most nations (see Table 1).

These findings suggest that progressive funding (or resource mobilization) alone is not an adequate indicator of the overall equity in a health care financing system. Progressivity in funding does not necessarily mean that health care benefits are distributed equitably (in other words, according to need).

Equity in Financial Protection

Another major purpose of health care financing is financial protection. The aim is to protect households from financial ruin arising from serious illnesses that may drive the family into poverty. This financial protection benefit, however, is often overlooked by studies on equity in health care.

The *World Development Report 1993* (World Bank 1993) provides a good illustration of the incomplete understanding of the roles of health care financing. It recommended that public funds should be allocated to various health services only on the basis of cost effectiveness in producing health outcomes. This recom-

Table 1 Share of public health spending benefit received by poorest and richest quintiles in selected countries, various years, 1979–95

(percent)

Country	Year	Poorest quintile	Richest quintile
Sri Lanka	1979	30	9
Jamaica	1989	30	9
Malaysia	1989	29	11
Brazil	1985	17	42
Egypt	1995	16	24
Kenya	1993	14	24
Vietnam	1992	12	29
Indonesia	1989	12	29
Ghana	1992	11	34

Source: Alailima and Mohideen 1983; Demery and others 1995; Grosh 1995.

mendation ignored the need for financial protection and the role of public financing schemes in securing such protection (Kutzin 1995; Hammer and Berman 1996). If a nation had followed this policy recommendation, its people would be exposed to financial catastrophe arising from uncertain high-cost medical care. For example, studies in poor rural Chinese counties found that the primary cause of poverty was households' expenditures for serious illness. Thus, health care financing has strong implications for poverty alleviation. Ironically, World Bank's study entitled *Voices of the Poor* identifies catastrophic health care expenditures as a leading cause of impoverishment (Narayan et al. 1999).

Measurement

Development of a measure to assess extent of financial protection embedded in health care financing systems is an essential tool for assessing equity in health care finance. Mark McClellan and Jonathan Skinner (1997) have developed a measurement that relies on the economic theory of risk aversion and the imperfect insurance market. Their method of measurement is quite theoretical and may be useful for the United States, but it is unlikely to be useful for other nations. For many high-income countries, equity in financial protection is not a significant issue because all high-income nations (other than the United States) have provided financial protection to their citizens through National Health Services (e.g., United Kingdom) or universal health insurance. For those developing nations that provide financial protection, it is often done through means other than insurance, such as the provision of "free" public hospital services to those who need it.

Issues for developing nations

For developing nations, the magnitude of impoverishment arising from health care expenditure has not been systematically or widely studied. Studies of some African nations (Sierra Leone, Tanzania, Kenya, Nigeria, Burundi, and Guinea) found that when households had no cash to pay for health care, they borrowed and/or sold food stocks, belongings, and livestock (McPake et al. 1993b; Mwabu et al. 1995).

As mentioned earlier, a recent study on China's poor rural areas, covering 150 million people, indicated that high medical expenses had become the primary cause of poverty (Liu et al. 1995). Those with modest incomes must spend one-third of a person's weekly average income to pay for village doctors and prescriptions and nearly double that for a visit to a township health center. A poor farmer would have to spend 1.2 years of his disposable income to pay for an episode of

hospitalization at a county hospital. The authors found that 18% of the households that used any health services in 1993 had incurred health expenditures that exceeded their total household income. Of the 11,000 rural households interviewed, 25% of the households that used any health care had borrowed or become indebted to pay for health expenses in that year. Another 6% sold or mortgaged properties to pay for health care. In the China study, 47% of the medically indebted households reported having suffered from hunger. These findings led the authors to conclude that health expenditure can have a substantial impact on household income and indebtedness. The interaction between health and income could start a vicious cycle of illness, poverty, and further illness.

Risk pooling under social or private group insurance has another equity impact that is often overlooked. Risk pooling merges the health risk for a group of people who have different levels of health care need and different incomes. Meanwhile, the benefits are provided on the basis of need within that group. Thus, the less healthy people and the low-income households have the potential of benefiting more from risk pooling. In other words, the expenditure side of insurance could be progressive.

Given the equity benefits embedded in risk pooling, how extensively has this been used among the developing nations? A World Bank survey of 37 developing countries found that 15 countries had formal social insurance systems in place. Although four countries had some kind of employer-provided health care program, 18 countries had no such health care programs in place. Coverage ranged from less than 10% of the population in most countries to about 15% in Burundi and Senegal and 25% in Kenya (Nolan and Turbat 1993). The proportion of the population insured is small because social or private insurance can only be used effectively as a financing mechanism for workers in the formal sector. Thus, overall coverage will be low since developing nations have only a small portion of their population employed in the formal sector (Hsiao 1998).

For the rural residents in low-income nations, community financing has been successfully established in several nations, pooling health risks and providing primary care. Members can pay the premium at optimal or high cash flow periods such as just after a harvest season. When a community has any form of cooperative, the members of the cooperative can be organized and covered by a community financing plan; premiums are then deducted from crop sales. This method is used in countries like India, Indonesia, and China (Suwandono 1999; Liu et al. 1995). Collecting a contribution when cash incomes are highest can help ensure that the members have ongoing access to health care and thus limit the effects of fluctuations in seasonal income on people's ability to pay for health care. This prepayment scheme is gaining increasing attention as a way to finance and organize health services in rural areas (Korte et al. 1992).

Although community financing has been practiced for decades, it has not spread widely among developing countries. The problem seems to be a lack of knowledge and governments' unwillingness to relinquish some power to the community level. Establishing and operating prepaid schemes requires knowledge, information, and technical know-how, such as benefit design, bookkeeping, and payment techniques. The success of schemes in Indonesia (e.g., *Dana Sehat*) is, to a large extent, attributed to extensive efforts on the part of the government to develop the human resources and to organize local stakeholders in designing and managing schemes suitable to the local conditions (Suwandono 1999). Furthermore, rural residents have shown their reluctance to prepay unless they trust that the organization will use the funds for their benefit.

As we have explained above, the five methods of health care financing have different distributional effects. Each method may place the financial burden and the benefits on different population groups. The comparative advantages and disadvantages of each method of health care financing, as gleaned from our literature review and from an equity perspective, are summarized in Table 2.

Research Agenda

Based on our literature review, we conclude that there are gaps in knowledge of equity in health care financing and its relationship to equity in health. The areas about which we have substantial knowledge are defining and measuring equity in resource mobilization and equity outcomes among high-income nations; measuring equity of health care benefits by expenditures according to income classes and the results for many high-income and developing nations; allocating resources according to the population's health needs, and tar-

Table 2 Equity outcomes of different methods of financing

Financing method	Mobilization of funds	Access to health care	Financial protection
General revenue			
High-income countries	Tends to be progressive	Other than the United States, all nations provide equal access	Equal under universal insurance or national health service (except in the United States)
Developing countries	Highly varied. Income tax is progressive; value added tax is regressive unless food is exempted	Depends on resource allocation; tends to be regressive	Progressive when public hospitals provide free services
Social insurance	Proportional; slightly regressive when the taxable wage base is capped		
High-income countries		Progressive	Equal under universal coverage
Developing countries		Covers only high- and middle-income classes; overall, it is regressive	Protects only insured workers in the formal sector
Private insurance			
Individual insurance	Very regressive	Insured have equal access	For insured only
Group insurance	Regressive	Insured have equal access. Within group, tends to be progressive	For insured only
Direct out-of-pocket and user fees	Very regressive unless the poor are exempted	Regressive	No protection
Community financing	Regressive unless significantly subsidized by general revenue	Equal access for members. Regressive when there is cost sharing	Progressive for members

geting public resources to vulnerable groups to enhance equity.

The areas in which we have insufficient knowledge include measuring equity in resource mobilization for developing nations, taking into account their data limitations; defining health care benefits based on "need" criteria and measuring the equity of the benefits for high-income and developing nations; defining and measuring access to health care and equity in access to health care; defining and measuring quality of health care; and measuring the benefits of financial protection and its equity in distribution.

Several major unresolved issues regarding equity in health care financing are especially noteworthy. First, how should equity be defined when we are assessing health care benefits and financial protection? The current literature primarily uses the income gradient to define and measure equity of health benefits. This criterion seems appropriate for measuring who bears the financial burden, but inappropriate for equity in health care benefits and financial protection. A health "need" criterion seems more appropriate, but measuring need is a formidable challenge. Second, there is a trade-off between equity in health care benefits and financial protection; this issue has not been clarified and analyzed systematically. Finally, there is a fundamental conflict between equity and efficiency among the alternative methods of health care financing. There has been little work done to analyze and quantify the trade-offs.

We believe it is more cost effective for future research to focus first on those critical gaps in our knowledge that have high value for policy makers. Currently, we have no practical standard method to measure the equity in resource mobilization among developing nations. Second, we have no commonly accepted definition and measurement method for the benefit side of health care financing. As a result, we cannot examine and compare equity in health care financing, especially for developing nations. The lack of quantitative measurements and benchmarks impairs our ability to set goals and monitor progress.

As for high-income nations, we have solid knowledge about equity in resource mobilization. We are quite ignorant, however, about the equity of benefits. The next logical step is to expand research to examine the equity of health care financing in *net benefit* terms. Of course, the benefit side should include the financial protection benefit of financing methods.

Understanding the relationship between equity in health care financing and equity in health will require further research. As we acknowledged earlier, we lack adequate theories to hypothesize the relationships between the various determinants of well-being, especially since many factors overlap and interact with each other.

It is also possible that many important variables have been omitted in this framework. Nonetheless, this research is exceedingly important for policy making because adequate evidence-based information is required to design financing policies that are effective in improving equity in health. As we have emphasized, health care financing is just one of many determinants of well-being. It is a mechanism, however, often seized upon by policy makers and others as a panacea for health system ills. At the very least, equity concerns demand that analyses of health care finance assess the full impact of health care financing; it is not sufficient to assess equity based solely on the progressivity of resource mobilization. The net benefits (payment minus benefit), the allocation of health care resources according to need, and financial protection must be made integral parts of health care financing equity assessments.

References

Aaronson J.R., Johnson P., Lambert P.J. 1994. Redistributive effect and inequal tax treatment. *Economic Journal* 104:262–270.

Abel-Smith B., Rawal P. 1992. Employer's willingness to pay: the case for compulsory health insurance in Tanzania. *Health Policy and Planning* 9(4):409–418.

Abel-Smith B., et al. 1995. *Choices in Health Policy: An Agenda for the European Union*. Brookfield, VT: Dartmouth Publishing Co.

Ahmad E., Stern N. 1991. *The Theory and Practice of Tax Reform in Developing Countries*, pp xvii, 344. Cambridge: Cambridge University Press.

Alailama P., Mohideen F. 1984. Health sector expenditure flows in Sri Lanka. *World Health Statistical Quarterly* 37(4):403–420.

Baker J.L., van der Gaag J. 1993. Equity in the finance and delivery of health care: evidence from five developing countries. In: van Doorslaer E., Wagstaff A., Rutten F. (eds), *Equity in the Finance and Delivery of Health Care*. London: Oxford University Press, pp. 356–394.

Barnum H., Kutzin J. 1993. *Public Hospitals in Developing Countries: Resource Use, Cost, Financing*. Baltimore: Johns Hopkins University Press.

Bennett S., Quick J.D., Velasquez G. 1997. Public–Private Roles in the Pharmaceutical Sector: Implications for Equitable Access and Rational Drug Use. *Health Economics and Drugs*. DAP Series No. 5. WHO/DAP/97.12. Geneva: World Health Organization, Action Program on Essential Drugs.

Christiansen T. 1993. Equity in the finance and delivery of health care in Denmark. In: van Doorslaer E., Wagstaff A., Rutten F. (eds), *Equity in the Finance and Delivery of Health Care: An International Perspective*. New York: Oxford University Press, pp. 101–115.

Creese A. 1991. User charges for health care: a review of recent experience. *Health Policy and Planning* 6(4):309–319.

Creese A. 1997. User fees [editorial]. *British Medical Journal* 315(7102):202–203.

Culyer A.J. 1989. Cost containment in Europe. *Health Care Financing Review Suppl* 21–22.

Demery L., Chao S., Bernier R., Mehera K. 1995. The incidence of social spending in Ghana, 1989–92. Draft of unpublished report, Ghana Extended Poverty Study, the World Bank, Washington, DC.

Diop F., Yazbeck A., Bitran R. 1995. The impact of alternative cost recovery schemes on access and equity in Niger. *Health Policy and Planning* 10(3):223–240.

Garner P. 1989. The Bamako Initiative: financing health in Africa by selling drugs. *British Medical Journal*. 299:277–278.

Gertler P., van der Gaag J. 1990. *The Willingness to Pay for Medical Care*. Baltimore: John Hopkins University Press.

Gottschalk P., Wolfe B., Haveman R. 1989. Health care financing in the U.S., U.K. and Netherlands: distributional consequences. In: Chiancone A., Messere K. (eds), *Changes in Revenue Structures*. Detroit: Wayne State University Press, pp. 351–373.

Grosh M. 1995. Toward quantifying the trade-off: administrative costs and incidence of targeted programs in Latin America. In: van de Walle D., Nead K. (eds), *Public Spending and the Poor. Theory and Evidence*. Baltimore: The Johns Hopkins University Press for the World Bank, pp. 450–458.

Hammer J.S., Berman P. 1995. Ends and means in public health policy in developing countries. *Health Policy* 32(3):29–45.

Hoare G., Mills A. 1986. Paying for the Health Sector: A Review and Annotated Bibliography of the Literature on Developing Countries. Evaluation and Planning Center (EPC) for Health Care, Publication No. 12, London School of Hygiene and Tropical Medicine. London: EPC.

Hsiao W.C. 1984. Transformation of Health Care in China. *New England Journal of Medicine* 1984;310:932–936.

Hsiao W.C. 2000. Economic transition and health transformation. In: Pham Manh Hung, Minas I.H., Liu Y., Goran Dahgren G., and Hsiao W. (eds) *Efficient equity-oriented strategies for health: International perspectives—focus on Vietnam*. Chapter 21. Melbourne: The Center for International Mental Health, pp. 353–367.

Hurst J.W. 1985. *Financing Health Services in the United States*. London: King Edward's Hospital Fund.

Hurst J.W. 1991. Reforming health care in seven European nations. *Health Affairs* 10(3):7–21.

Hussein A.K., Mujinja P.G. 1997. Impact of our user charges on government health facilities in Tanzania. *East African Medical Journal* 74(12):751–757.

InterAmerican Development Bank. 1996. *Economic and Social Progress in Latin America*: 1996 Report. Baltimore: John Hopkins University Press.

Jimenez E. 1987. *Pricing Policy in the Social Sectors: Cost Recovery for Education and Health in Developing Countries*, pp vi, 170. Baltimore: Johns Hopkins University Press for the World Bank.

Kakwani N.C. 1977. Measurement of tax progressivity: an international comparison. *Economic Journal* 87:71–80.

Korte R., Richter H., Merkle F., Gorgen H. 1992. Financing health services in sub-Saharan Africa: options for decision makers during adjustment. *Social Science and Medicine* 34(1):1–9.

Kutzin J. 1995. The Consequences of Health Financing Change: A Framework for Analysis. Unpublished draft report. Geneva: WHO.

Lambert P.J. 1989. *The Distribution and Redistribution of Income: A Mathematical Analysis*. Cambridge, MA: Basil Blackwell.

Litvack J.I., Bodart C. 1993. User fees plus quality equals improved access to health care: results of a field experiment in Cameroon. *Social Science and Medicine* 37(3):369–383.

Liu Y.L., Hsiao W.C., Li Q., Liu X.Z., Ren M.H. 1995. Transformation of China's rural health care financing. *Social Science Medicine* 41(8):1085–1093.

McClellan M., Skinner J. 1997. The Incidence of Medicare. National Bureau of Economic Research Working Paper 6013. Cambridge, MA: National Bureau of Economic Research.

McPake B., Hanson K., Mills A. 1993a. *Community Financing of Health Care in Africa: An Evaluation of the Bamako Initiative*. London: Health Economics and Financing Program, London School of Hygiene and Tropical Medicine.

McPake B., Hanson K., Mills A. 1993b. *Implementing the Bamako Initiative in Africa: A Review and Five Case Studies*. London: Health Policy Unit, Department of Public Health and Policy, London School of Hygiene and Tropical Medicine.

Mwabu G., Mwanzia J., Liambila W. 1995. User charges in government health facilities in Kenya: effect on attendance and revenue. *Health Policy and Planning* 10(2):164–170.

Narayan D., Chambers R., Shah M., Petesch P. 1999. *Global Synthesis: Consultations with the Poor*. Prepared for the Global Synthesis Workshop, September 22–23, 1999. Poverty Group, PREM, World Bank. Washington, DC: World Bank.

Nolan B., Turbat V. 1993. Cost Recovery in Public Health Services in Sub-Saharan Africa. Mimeograph. Washington, DC: Economic Development Institute, Human Resources Division, World Bank.

Reddy S., Vandemoortele J. 1996. *User Financing of Basic Social Sciences: A Review of Theoretical Arguments and Empirical Evidence*. New York: Office of Evaluation, Policy and Planning, UNICEF.

Russell S. 1996. Ability to pay for health care: concepts and evidence. *Health Policy and Planning* 11(3):219–237.

Sauerborn R., Adams A., Hien M. 1996. Household strategies to cope with the economic costs of illness. *Social Science and Medicine* 43(3):291–301.

Shaw R.P., Griffin C.C. 1995. *Financing Health Care in Sub-Saharan Africa Through User Fees and Insurance*. A Directions in Development Book. Washington, DC: World Bank.

Suits D. 1977. Measurement of tax progressivity. *American Economic Review* 67:747–752.

Suwandono A. 1995. The Indonesian Experiences on Rural Health Financing. Presented at the International Seminar on Financing and Organization of Health Care for the Poor Rural Population in China, October 8–10, Fragrant Hill Hotel, Beijing Medical University.

Suwandono A. 1999. Indonesia's Dana Sehat. Presented at the International Conference on Health Equity, April 5–8, Hainan, Vietnam.

van Vliet R., van de Ven W.P.P.M. 1985. Equity in health care, an international comparison. *European Economic Review* 28:637.

Waddington C., Enyimayew K.A. 1990. A price to pay, part 2: the impact of user charges in the Volta region of Ghana. *International Journal of Health Planning and Management* 5:287–312.

Wagstaff A., van Doorslaer E. 1993. Equity in the finance of health care: methods and findings. In: Wagstaff A., van Doorslaer E., Rutten F. (eds), *Equity in the Finance and Delivery of Health Care: An International Perspective*. New York: Oxford University Press, pp. 20–49.

Wagstaff A., van Doorslaer E. 1997. Progressivity, horizontal equity and reranking in health care finance: a decomposition analysis for the Netherlands. *Journal of Health Economics* 16(5):499–516.

Wagstaff A., van Doorslaer E., Paci P. 1989. Equity in the finance and delivery of health care: some tentative cross-country comparisons. *Oxford Review of Economic Policy* 5:89–112.

World Bank. 1987. *Financing Health Services in Developing Countries: An Agenda for Reform*. Washington, DC: World Bank.

World Bank. 1993. *World Development Report 1993: Investing in Health*. New York: Oxford University Press.

Zschock D.K. 1989. Health sector disparities in Peru. *Bulletin of the Pan American Health Organization* 23(3):323–336.

CHAPTER 19

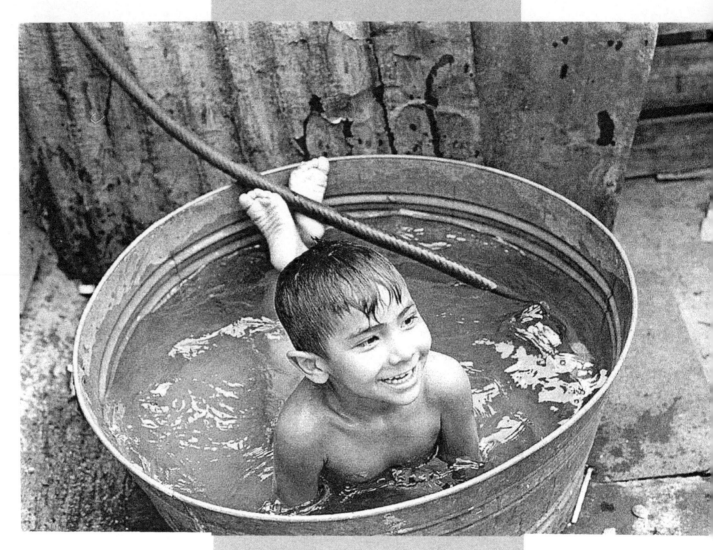

A Mexican boy playing in a galvanized steel tub.
Source: Jésus Quintanar, La Jornada.

Mexico: Marginality, Need, and Resource Allocation at the County Level

RAFAEL LOZANO, BEATRIZ ZURITA, FRANCISCO FRANCO,
TERESITA RAMÍREZ, PATRICIA HERNÁNDEZ, AND JOSÉ LUIS TORRES

Mexico is a country of contrasts and contradictions—urban concentration coexists with rural dispersion, and democratic change confronts old political practices and structures. The growth in formal employment has not kept up with the increasing size of the labor force, resulting in an expansion of the informal labor market. An emerging economy, Mexico currently ranks twelfth in size and tenth in exports worldwide. Annual per capita income is low, however—$3670 (US$ 1997)—ranking forty-third in the world. Mexico is among the 12 countries in which 80% of the world's poor are concentrated (González 1998).

In the 1990s, Mexico opened its economy and accepted more foreign investment, embarked on government deregulation, placed greater constraints on public expenditure, and imposed measures to reduce inflation from 30% in 1990 to 7% in 1994. These measures have stimulated macroeconomic growth, with the gross national product (GNP) increasing from 5% in 1994 to 6% in 1997 (Comisión Económica para América Latina y el Caribe [CEPAL] 1997a). These macroeconomic changes have also, however, had a negative impact on the well-being of many Mexicans (CEPAL 1997b). A polarization in household income developed between 1984 and 1994 as the proportion of total income held by the lowest quintile diminished from 5% to 4%, while the proportion of total income held by the highest quintile increased from 50% to 55% (Instituto Nacional de Estadística Geographía e Informatica [INEGI] 1990, 1995). This skew in the distribution of economic growth has only accentuated unfavorable social conditions among the most deprived groups. The result is an economic growth that is partial and precarious in the face of an increasing concentration of poverty (Consejo Nacional de Población [CONAPO] 1993).

It is within this complex context that, since 1996, Mexican health care reform has been taking place. Among the most important aims of reform policies is to increase equity and efficiency in the health care system through wider coverage (1996) and to decentralize (1997). The effects of the health reform will be visible in the near future and will need to be assessed in order to evaluate the policy initiatives.

The purpose of this chapter is to present the empirical evidence on health inequalities and inequity in health in Mexico at the county level (called a "municipality" in Mexico) as a baseline to be used for further assessment of the reform. Inequalities between counties in life expectancy, infant mortality, and probability of death between birth and age 5 years and between

277

Mexico

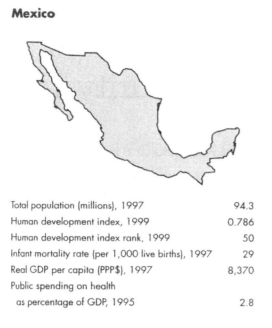

Total population (millions), 1997	94.3
Human development index, 1999	0.786
Human development index rank, 1999	50
Infant mortality rate (per 1,000 live births), 1997	29
Real GDP per capita (PPP$), 1997	8,370
Public spending on health as percentage of GDP, 1995	2.8

Source: UNDP 1999. [Human Development Report]

ages 45 and 60 years are examined. This analysis is extended using the "years of life lost" (YLL) measure to determine the relationship between level of county marginality and causes of premature mortality (group I, communicable disease; group II, noncommunicable disease; or group III, injuries; as defined by Murray and López 1997). Once differences in need are determined, we analyze how equitably health care resources are distributed. Finally, the chapter concludes with policy recommendations and comments on the adequacy of current health reform policies.

The Context: Health Status and Health Care Inequalities in Mexico

At the beginning of the twentieth century, Mexicans had a life expectancy of only 30 years (Cabrera 1966). By 1990 life expectancy had reached nearly 72 years. Likewise, at the start of the twentieth century, 40% of children did not reach the age of 5 years; today, this figure has been reduced to 4%. Despite these vast im-

Figure 1 Counties by level of marginality in Mexico, 1990–96

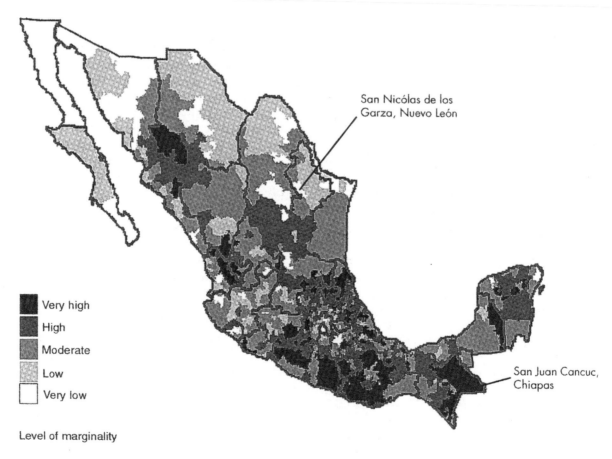

Level of marginality

Source: Authors' calculations

Figure 2 Premature mortality from all causes, by county, in Mexico, 1990–96

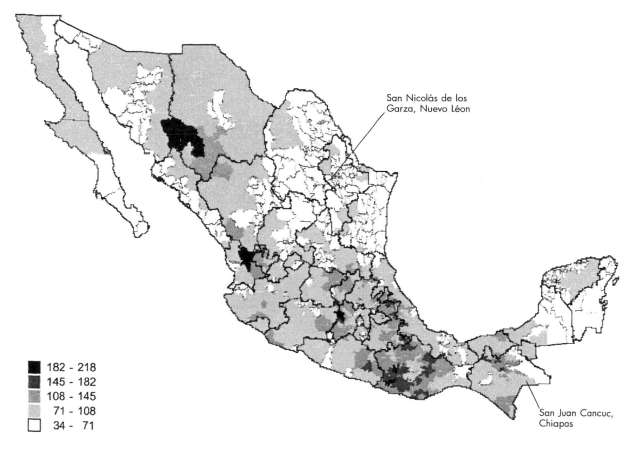

San Nicolás de los
Garza, Nuevo Léon

San Juan Cancuc,
Chiapas

- ■ 182 - 218
- ▨ 145 - 182
- ▨ 108 - 145
- ▨ 71 - 108
- ☐ 34 - 71

Years of potential life lost per 1,000 people
Source: Authors' calculations

provements, the Mexican health care system still faces many challenges, including gaps in coverage, equity, and efficiency. Mexicans living in extreme poverty—8 million people in 1994—do not have regular access to health services. This figure could increase to 30 million (one-third of the total population) if existing economic and organizational barriers in the health system are taken into account. It is estimated that approximately 5% of households in the lowest income group spend more than half of their available income (household income after food expenses) to pay for medical services (Frenk et al. 1994).

As expected, Mexicans living in extreme poverty suffer from a burden of largely preventable, communicable diseases. An aging population and the proliferation of unhealthy lifestyles, however, place additional burdens of noncommunicable diseases and injuries on the system and exacerbate health inequalities. Thus, Mexicans living in poverty face a triple burden of commu-

nicable and noncommunicable disease as well as injuries. In 1995, 26% of the 91 million Mexicans lived in rural settlements (localities with less than 2500 inhabitants) under marginal conditions—deprivation or structural poverty. Between 1990 and 1996, about 16 million Mexicans (18% of the population) lived in counties with a "high" or "very high" level of marginality, areas that are concentrated in the southeast and central areas of the country. More than half of the population from the states of Oaxaca, Chiapas, and Guerrero lived in these high marginality counties. In contrast, the northern areas of the country had a greater proportion of counties with lower levels of marginality. The states of Baja California, Mexico City, and most of Nuevo León are composed of low marginality counties (see Fig. 1).

The link between county-level marginality and membership in an indigenous group is quite strong in Mexico. Of the 10 million indigenous people in the country, most live in deprived and rural areas. Roughly 58% of their households lack running water, 88% do not have sewage, and 35% lack electricity (Instituto Nacional Indigenista [INI] 1999). Overall, there are 56 ethnic groups, with more than half of these groups concentrated in four states of the country (INI 1999). Almost half of the indigenous people are illiterate, and it is estimated that counties with over 70% indigenous populations contain approximately 80% of the population below the poverty line (Psacharopoulos and Patrinos 1994). Overall, the indigenous population is more likely to live in areas or conditions that expose them to greater risk of ill health.

There is a gradient in mortality across the counties, measured as YLL due to premature mortality. The northern portion of the country and the Gulf of Mexico, areas with high industrial development, have the lowest number of YLL, while the most deprived areas have rates of YLL seven times as large (Fig. 2). The priorities, infrastructure, and policies of the health system, however, have not adequately reflected this differential need.

Since its creation, the Mexican health system has been segmented. In general, middle- and high-income groups use medical services in the private sector. Workers in companies that are part of the formal economy have access to mandatory public health insurance for their families through the social security system. In Mexico, however, lack of employment in the formal sector is a major barrier to access to health care (Frenk et al. 1998). The poor, who are not covered by the so-cial security system, mainly use the Ministry of Health Services and other public services, which tend to be less efficient and of lower quality than private services.

Empirical Analysis

For our analysis, an ecological study was conducted in 2429 municipalities (or counties)—the smallest geopolitical units in Mexico. Inhabitants per county range from 270 to 1.5 million people. The range in county population sizes posed a challenge in achieving an adequate population size for studying mortality in all counties. To increase the population size in the smallest counties, similar neighboring counties in the same state were aggregated to form microregions with a minimum size of 20,000 people (Black et al. 1996), and larger counties were divided so as to obtain a maximum population size of 250,000 people. To build life-tables and a mortality profile with an adequate sample of deaths, 6 years of data were aggregated. A resulting total of 713 counties/microregions was used for this analysis.

In the analysis, health policies and macroeconomic variables were not explored, with the exception of those concerning the degree of social deprivation. Microdata from the Population Census (INEGI 1992), the midterm population count (INEGI 1997), and the National Population Register of Births (RENAPO) (INEGI 1990–1996a) were used to create socioeconomic and health indicators for each county/microregion, de-

---

BOX 1: CONCEPTS AND VARIABLES EMPLOYED IN THE ANALYSIS

Concepts

- **Equity in public health systems.** An important aim is to reverse the negative association between need and access to health care, that is, the "inverse care law" described by Tudor Hart (1971). This has been documented in Mexico, where the poor were twice as likely to suffer total activity limitations than the nonpoor, yet were only half as likely to use health services (Lozano et al. 1993).
- **Equity in health care.** Another key aim is access to services according to health needs rather than ability to pay (Frenk 1993). This search for equity should respect the dignity of the individual and should provide access to an essential package of health care interventions that are based on health needs according to the available resources in the country (Frenk 1998).
- **Core conditions for equity.** Increases in the opportunities for the poor and in the potential capability and function-ality of individuals for health and education (Sen 1992) are needed. For emerging economies such as Mexico, economic growth should be achieved by strengthening equity in health and welfare (Hernández-Peña et al. 1991).

Socioeconomic Variables

- **The marginality index (MI)** is a deprivation index constructed from the following six variables:

- The proportion of the population per county that is illiterate
- The proportion with incomplete elementary education
- The proportion earning less than twice the minimum wage
- The proportion living in towns with less than 2500 inhabitants
- The proportion of households lacking running water, electricity, sewage facilities, and a proper floor

- The proportion of households living in overcrowded conditions

The MI is constructed and used by the Mexican government through a principal components analysis. This index has both a standardized z-score version (ranging from −3 to +3) and an ordinal version with five marginality levels ranging from very low to very high marginality (CONAPO 1993). Both versions were used in the analysis. For the county-level gross domestic product (GDP) statistics, we used the National University of Mexico estimates (Sánchez 1998)

- The **ethnicity indicator** is based on census data regarding the proportion of the population speaking a native language. The census does not contain further elements to identify the indigenous population of this country as a distinctive group in society (Bronfman 1994), although it is recognized that language is insufficient to embrace the whole ethnic dimension.

Health Service Availability, Use and Expenditure

- **Availability and use** of health resources in the public sector by county were estimated using data on the number of physicians, nurses, outpatient rooms, and beds, combined with the number of hospital deliveries and outpatients visits.
- **State health expenditure** in public services for 1995 (Zurita 1998) was imputed to counties based on an index of health care personnel (medical doctors, 30%) and facilities for public institutions (beds, 50%; consultation areas, 20%).

Adjustments to Health Variables

- **Number of births.** Numbers were estimated by three different sources and compared. One source was based on estimates of the population born in 1 year in each county, obtained from the CONAPO projections (CONAPO 1995). The second source was the vital statistics for each municipality. The third source was the age-specific fertility rate in each region. The estimation of the county fertility rate for 1990 was based on the census information about the number of live births by female age using the United Nations (1990) Mortpak software and smoothed using the Arriaga method (1994).
- **Infant mortality rate** (IMR). The indirect Brass method was utilized to correct for underregistration of IMR at the county level using 1990 census data to project IMR for the years 1991–1986 (INEGI 1990–1996b).
- **Mortality rates by cause, age, and sex for 98 diseases** (Organización Panamericana de la Salud 1978). To correct for underregistration of mortality for other age groups, mortality was compared with the rates in the West Model of Mortpak (United Nations 1990). Mortality rates for adults over 20 years were smoothed with the logit moving average method (Arriaga 1994). For those over age 60 years, whose mortality was below the expected, the value of the corresponding West Model tables was used.
- **Years of life lost (YLL).** Years of life lost is a measure of premature mortality adjusted by age through the direct method (Murray and López 1996) using the mortality rate data described above.

---

scribed in Box 1. Years of life lost (YLL) is the primary indicator of health inequality used in this study. Statistical techniques used in the analysis are explained in Box 2.

Some of the limitations of the county level analysis should be noted in advance of a description of the results. As described earlier, the analysis is based on aggregated county data. Each county is composed of a variety of households and settlements with varying levels of size and rural/urban composition, a factor that could bias the marginality index and the estimate of the proportion of indigenous peoples in the population. An additional source of bias is introduced by the aggregation of counties to achieve a minimum population size for

---

BOX 2: CONSTRUCTION OF INEQUALITY MEASURES AND STATISTICAL ANALYSIS

Inequality Measures

The inequalities in health by county were estimated by the slope index of inequality (SII), the relative index of inequality (RII), and the concentration curves (Wagstaff et al. 1991). The SII measures the change in the absolute value of the health outcome by level of marginality—the increase in the health outcome per unit change in the marginality index. The RII is a measure of the relative inequality that is calculated by dividing the SII by the average rate of a spe-

cific health indicator for the whole country. The RII measures the relative change in health per unit change in the marginality index. The SII and RII are positive in sign when positive health outcomes (e.g. life expectancy) are disproportionately concentrated among the poor but negative in sign when negative health outcomes (e.g. IMR) are disproportionately concentrated among the poor.

The SII and RII were estimated using a weighted least squares model. These indexes were used to assess inequalities in life expectancy, infant mortality, and the probability of dying in certain age groups (see Table 1) as well as inequalities in YLL by cause of death (see Table 2). A concentration index and concentration curves were calculated according to the methods of Wagstaff et al. (1991).

Estimating the Health Gini and Relative Causes
Multiple regression models were fitted in the following form:

$$\theta = \text{Log (AA)} + \text{Log (IND)} + \text{Log (PHE)} + \text{MI} + \epsilon$$

where θ is cause specific YLL rate or the probability of dying under age five raised to the power of -1.5 to improve normality; AA is the average age of the population in the county; IND is the proportion of indigenous people; PHE is the per capita public health care expenditure; MI is the marginality index in its continuous form; and ϵ is an estimation of random error. Inequality is expressed in terms of the Gini index of the burden of health problem (θ). After fitting this model we calculated the residual Gini by holding each variable (PHE, IND, and AA) constant in turn to assess its impact upon inequality (the Gini) in the burden of disease indicator. In this way, we calculated the reduction in the observed Gini index that could be achieved by eliminating disparities in living conditions or health care resources among counties (brief narrative overview of results included in this chapter).

demographic data. In Mexico, there is a strong relationship between rural counties and impoverishment such that the marginality index is also a measure of how rural the county is—the more rural the county, the more impoverished. The marginality index is not, however, able to properly account for small pockets of the poor in large urban areas or for the poor who are scattered widely in a wealthy county. In fact, it is possible that in a highly populated county the absolute number of poor is higher than in a small county, yet this will not be adequately indicated by the marginality index. Nevertheless, we use the marginality index for two main reasons. First, even with its limitations, the marginality index is still the best available indicator of poverty in Mexico, and second, it is used by policy makers in the development of national policies.

Results

Inequalities in Health by Level of Marginality

The increase in the average life expectancy in Mexico over the past 50 years has been accompanied by a reduction in the variation in life expectancy among the 32 Mexican states, with the difference between the states with the highest and lowest life expectancies dropping from 18 years in 1950 to 6 years in 1994 (Lozano 1997). Use of a smaller unit of analysis (the county), however, highlights substantial disparities in life expectancy that are masked when larger units like the Mexican state are compared. Around 1993, the absolute difference in life expectancy at birth between counties was 14 years, similar to the gap among the Mexican states in 1980.

As a first look at the disparities between extremes in Mexico, Figure 3 compares an extremely well-off county with one of the worst-off counties. San Juan Cancuc, one of the counties with the lowest life expectancy at birth (62 years), is located in the state of Chiapas. It is a small area with very high marginality, 100% indigenous people, 67% illiteracy, 4.2 years of average education, scarce health care resources, and a high IMR of 45 per 1000 live births. It is worth noting that the life expectancy in this county (62 years) is similar to the national life expectancy in 1970. In contrast, the county with the highest life expectancy, Nicolás Gaiza (71 years), is part of the metropolitan area of Monterrey, the capital city of the northern state of Nuevo León, and shows a very low marginality level, 0.1% indigenous people, 8.2 years average education, and good availability of health care resources. The gap in life expectancies between these two counties is 9 years, a range not seen at the state level since the 1980s. Of note, diarrheal diseases predominate, with extremely high rates in the high marginality county, San Juan Cancuc, while cardiovascular diseases predominate in the low marginality county, Nicolás Garza. Interestingly, cardivascular diseases and other noncommunicable diseases (such as cirrhosis and genitourinary diseases) have rates just as high in San Juan Cancuc as in Nicolás Garza.

The following results use the relative and slope indices of inequality between high and low marginality counties to assess the distribution of four health indicators (life expectancy at birth, IMR, and probability of death between birth and 5 years of age and between 45 and 60 years of age). This type of analysis allows us to estimate the additional health "lost" (e.g., years

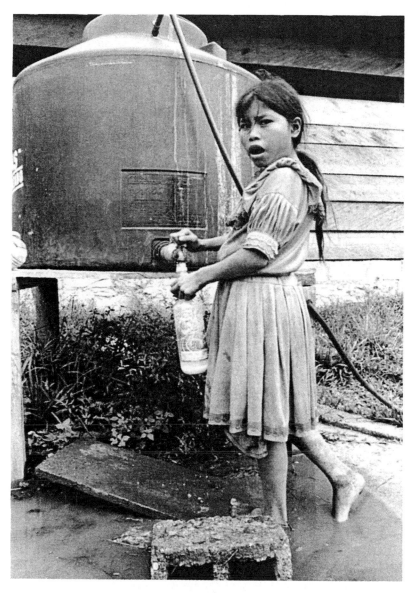

A Mexican girl fetching water.
Source: Francisco Olvera/La Jornada.

Figure 3 Sociodemographic and health conditions in two counties in Mexico, 1990–96

Indicator	San Juan Cancuc (Chiapas)	Nicolás Garza (Nuevo León)
Sociodemographic indicators		
Marginality	Very high	Very low
Population, 1995	27,750	436,603
Indigenous population as percentage of total	100	0.1
Illiteracy rate (percent)	67	2
Average education (years)	4.2	8.2
Households with access to running water (percent)	4	95
Households with access to sewerage (percent)	45	92
Life expectancy (years), 1990–96	62	71
Economic indicators		
GNP per capita (U.S. dollars), 1990	3	43.6
Health expenditures per capita (U.S. dollars), 1995	3	79

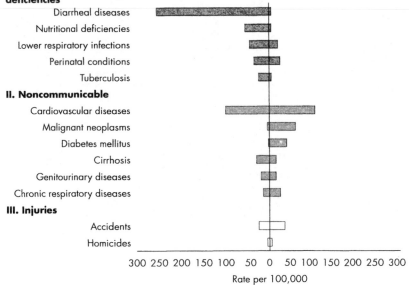

Health conditions

San Juan Cancuc   Nicolás Garza

I. Communicable, maternal, perinatal, and nutritional deficiencies
Diarrheal diseases
Nutritional deficiencies
Lower respiratory infections
Perinatal conditions
Tuberculosis
II. Noncommunicable
Cardiovascular diseases
Malignant neoplasms
Diabetes mellitus
Cirrhosis
Genitourinary diseases
Chronic respiratory diseases
III. Injuries
Accidents
Homicides

300 250 200 150 100 50 0 50 100 150 200 250 300
Rate per 100,000

Source: Authors' calculations.

of life expectancy) for each incremental increase in the level of county marginality (the results are summarized in Table 1).

On an aggregate level, life expectancy at birth for both sexes differs by an average of 3 years between the least marginalized counties (life expectancy of 68 years) and the most marginalized counties (life expectancy of 65 years). This translates into an average reduction of 1.25 years in life expectancy for each unit increase in marginality measured by the slope index of inequality (SII) or approximately a 2% decrease in life expectancy per unit increase in marginality measured by the relative index of inequality (RII) (see Table 1).

Infant mortality rates analyzed by Mexican county reveal even higher inequalities in both absolute and relative terms than were evident in the comparison of life

Table 1 Slope and relative indices of inequality for selected mortality indicators in Mexico, 1990–96

Mortality indicator	Sex	Mean indicator level Very low marginality counties	Mean indicator level Very high marginality counties	Slope index of inequality[a]	Relative index of inequality[b]
Life expectancy at birth (years)	Both	68	65	−1.25 (−1.35, −1.15)	−1.87 (−2.02, −1.72)
	Male	66	62	−1.23 (−1.34, −1.11)	−1.91 (−2.09, −1.72)
	Female	71	67	−1.14 (−1.23, −1.05)	−1.65 (−1.78, −1.52)
Infant mortality rate (per 1,000 live births)	Both	22	39	5.72 (5.23, 6.20)	19.57 (17.89, 21.25)
	Male	24	44	6.37 (5.80, 6.94)	19.51 (17.77, 21.24)
	Female	19	34	5.09 (4.67, 5.51)	19.80 (18.17, 21.44)
Probability of dying between ages 0 and 5 (per 1,000)	Both	24	49	7.98 (7.28, 8.70)	23.98 (21.84, 26.11)
	Male	27	54	8.68 (7.88, 9.47)	23.42 (21.27, 25.56)
	Female	21	43	7.32 (6.69, 7.95)	24.83 (22.69, 26.97)
Probability of dying between ages 45 and 60 (per 1,000)	Both	145	183	10.78 (9.57, 12.00)	6.82 (6.05, 7.59)
	Male	174	215	11.75 (10.06, 13.44)	6.29 (5.39, 7.20)
	Female	120	149	8.37 (7.42, 9.33)	6.45 (5.71, 7.18)

Note: The numbers in parentheses refer to the confidence interval.
a. Predicted absolute change in mortality indicator per unit decline in marginality index (95 percent confidence interval).
b. Predicted percentage change in mortality indicator per unit decline in marginality index (95 percent confidence interval).
Source: Authors' calculations.

expectancy at birth. The IMRs ranged from 22 in low maginality counties to 39 in high marginality counties. Thus, there is a 20% increase in IMRs with each increase in the level of marginality (as measured by the RII). The risk of dying before 1 year of age is nearly twice as high in very high marginality counties as compared to the least deprived counties. It is important to note, however, that even the best-off Mexican counties have on average an infant mortality rate (22 deaths per 1000 live births) that is higher than that observed in most developed countries.

The probability of dying within the first 5 years of life reveals the highest RII by county marginality of all health indicators measured (see Table 1). The RIIs indicate that each unit increase in marginality yields about a 24% increase in the probability of a child death. Data on child deaths among girls reveal a slightly higher level of inequality than that of boys in relative terms. As expected, boys have on average a higher risk of dying within the first 5 years of life than girls, irrespective of the marginality level.

Mortality during middle age is measured as the probability of dying between ages 45 and 60 years. Even in this age group inequalities in both absolute and relative terms are observed according to the marginality level of the counties. Each increment in county marginality is associated with an increase of approximately 7% in the risk of death for both sexes as measured by the RII or approximately 11 more deaths per thousand per year as measured by the SII (see Table 1).

Disease-Specific Burden by County Grouping

To assess the nature of the disease burden in relation to level of marginality, YLL are described according to communicable disease (group I), noncommunicable disease (group II) or injuries (group III; see Figs. 4 and 5). Of the total YLL, group I causes of death account for 30% of the disease burden in low marginality counties, 48% in very high marginality counties, and 58% in counties with a large proportion of indigenous people. Years of life lost in the poor counties can be attributed to four easily avoidable causes of death—diarrheal diseases (13%), pneumonia (9%), nutritional deficiencies (8%), and tuberculosis (2%). These four causes of death represent 40% of YLL in counties with large concentrations of indigenous people compared with 32% in very high marginality counties and only 11% in counties with very low marginality (see Fig. 4). The YLL for group I diseases is twice as great in very high marginality counties and slightly higher for females than in lower marginality counties.

Perinatal mortality includes causes of death that to a great extent reflect problems in access to prenatal care and delivery facilities. For this reason, we would expect that in very high marginality counties perinatal mortality would be higher than in very low marginality counties. We did not, however, find significant differences in rates between the two extremes of marginality. This finding may be influenced by the substantial underregistration of deaths in very high marginality counties, which despite our mortality correction, could not be fully taken into account.

Figures 4 and 5 reveal that as a proportion of total YLL, noncommunicable diseases and injuries are *relatively* more important causes in *low* marginality countries. In these well-off counties, four noncommunicable diseases and injuries (cancers, ischemic heart disease, motor vehicle accidents, and diabetes mellitus) account for one-third of the burden of disease and only 12% of YLL in the marginalized counties.

Among group III diseases (injuries), motor vehicle accidents accounted for three times as large a percentage of the burden of disease in the better-off counties as in the more marginal counties (6% vs. 2%). The percentage of YLL due to homicide and falls is higher in the worst-off counties than in the best-off counties (8% vs. 6%).

The analysis comparing health outcomes between high and low marginality counties was extended to examine premature mortality by sex and cause of death using the slope index of inequality (SII) and relative in-

Figure 4 Premature mortality by disease group and level of county marginality in Mexico, 1990–96

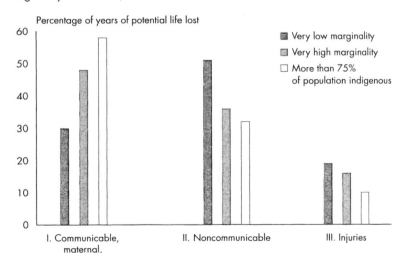

Source: Authors' calculations.

Figure 5 Premature mortality by cause and level of county marginality in Mexico, 1990–96

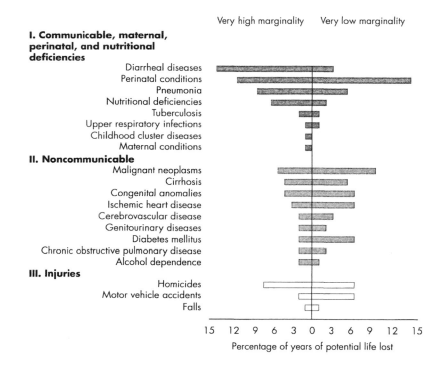

Source: Authors' calculations.

dex of inequality (RII) (see Table 2). First, we considered all causes of premature mortality combined and found that an increase of over 13 YLL per 1000 is observed per unit increase in the marginality index in both sexes. Although females show a greater inequality in relative terms than males (a RII of 19% and 15%, respectively) their YLL are on average between 30% and 40% lower than those of males.

Mortality due to group I diseases—communicable, maternal, perinatal, and nutritional disorders—is highest in the poorest areas and shows the highest inequality between counties by level of marginality. Mortality is approximately 10 YLL per year greater with each level of increasing marginality, equivalent to a 35% increase in risk of death from communicable disease for males and females combined.

The YLL for group II diseases (noncommunicable) is also 15% higher in very high marginality counties: 41 versus 36 per 1000 inhabitants (see Table 2). As for group III conditions (injuries), the marginalized counties also have YLL rates 18% greater. Most striking, however, is the gender disparity in the risk of group

III diseases. Males in very high marginality counties are at much higher risk than males in very low marginality counties, while there are no risk differences for women. As indicated by the SII and RII (see Table 2), the most deprived counties have higher YLL in all three groups of diseases—communicable diseases, as well as noncommunicable disease and injury rates.

Figures 6 and 7 depict concentration curves for specific causes of death, showing the cumulative percentage of YLL for each cumulative percentage of the population (by increasing level of county marginality). Causes of death that are responsible for more premature mortality in worst-off counties are grouped as "higher in the most marginalized counties," while those causes of death responsible for more premature mortality in better-off counties are grouped as "higher in the least marginalized counties." The main inequalities in the distribution of the burden of disease are in avoidable deaths concentrated among the poor, namely, due to childhood-cluster diseases, diarrheal diseases, maternal conditions, malnutrition, tuberculosis, alcohol dependence, and pneumonia. Figure 6 illustrates the

Table 2 Slope and relative indices of inequality by disease group and sex in Mexico, 1990–96

Cause of death by disease group	Sex	Age-adjusted years of potential life lost (per 1,000)		Slope index of inequality[a]	Relative index of inequality[b]
		Very low marginality counties	Very high marginality counties		
All causes	Both	71	114	13.24 (12.05, 14.43)	16.54 (15.06, 18.03)
	Male	87	134	14.57 (13.10, 16.03)	14.89 (13.39, 16.39)
	Female	71	67	11.60 (10.63, 12.57)	18.55 (16.99, 20.10)
I. Communicable, maternal, perinatal, and nutritional deficiencies	Both	21	54	9.97 (9.21, 10.73)	35.62 (32.89, 38.35)
	Male	25	58	9.95 (9.10, 10.79)	31.20 (28.54, 33.85)
	Female	18	50	9.92 (9.23, 10.62)	41.08 (38.21, 43.96)
II. Noncommunicable	Both	36	41	1.49 (1.06, 1.91)	4.03 (2.88, 5.18)
	Male	40	45	1.33 (0.76, 1.90)	3.28 (1.87, 4.69)
	Female	32	37	1.58 (1.26, 1.90)	4.73 (3.77, 5.68)
III. Injuries	Both	13	18	1.78 (1.40, 2.16)	11.86 (9.26, 14.35)
	Male	22	31	3.28 (2.62, 3.96)	12.94 (10.30, 15.57)
	Female	5	5	0.096 (−0.03, 0.22)	1.95 (−0.58, 4.48)

Note: The numbers in parentheses refer to the confidence interval.
a. Predicted absolute change in mortality indicator per unit increase in marginality index (95 percent confidence interval).
b. Predicted percentage change in age-adjusted years of potential life lost (per 1,000) per unit change in marginality index (95 percent confidence interval).
Source: Authors' calculations.

skew in the distribution of causes of death that increase in prevalence with increasing county marginality. Years of life lost due to diarrheal disease are the most unequally distributed by county marginality, while YLL due to stomach cancer appear to be the most equally distributed across counties. For each increase in the level of marginality, there are 4 YLL due to diarrhea and approximately 2 YLL each for malnutrition and pneumonia.

There are also inequalities in the other direction, that is, diseases that are concentrated among wealthier people, including the human immunodeficiency virus (HIV), breast cancer, lung cancer, and diabetes mellitus. In general, HIV, most cancers, and diabetes show a relative inequality, concentrating among the nonpoor. The absolute differences in YLL are, however, very small, at most a half a year per unit increase in the level of marginality (see Fig. 7).

Figure 6 Concentration curves for selected causes of death with higher YLLs in the most deprived counties in Mexico, 1990–96

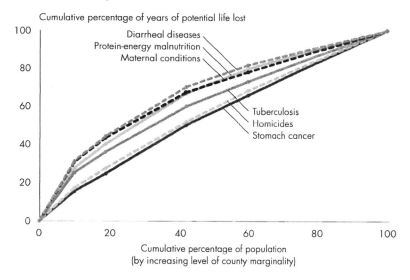

Source: Authors' calculations.

In summary, the epidemiological transition in Mexico is polarized and leads to a triple burden of the three major groups of ill health—communicable diseases, noncommunicable diseases, and injuries—for those in marginalized areas. This burden is concentrated among the poor, with high mortality in young children, significant mortality in young adult males from injuries, and an increasing number of older adults with coexisting noncommunicable and chronic diseases. Given the inequality in health needs, how does the health system respond?

Figure 7 Concentration curves for selected causes of death with higher YLLs in the least deprived counties in Mexico, 1990–96

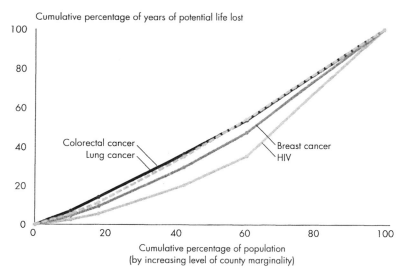

Source: Authors' calculations.

Distribution of Health Resources

In Mexico, improvements in the quality of life and medical care have reduced the rate of selected causes of death and delayed the age of death. Mexico's health gains have made it clear that so-called avoidable deaths can be reduced through the alleviation of deprivation and the access to high quality medical care. Hence, the distribution of health care resources plays a vital role as a health determinant.

The allocation of health resources is, however, inversely related to marginality and to county GNP per capita in Mexican counties (see Fig. 8). Physicians concentrate in areas with little deprivation and higher per capita wealth (16 per 10,000 inhabitants) and are relatively scarce (4 per 10,000) in very high marginality counties (see Fig. 9). The more deprived or poorest counties also have fewer public hospital beds (1 bed per 10,000 in marginalized counties compared with 12 beds per 10,000 inhabitants in better off counties). The

Figure 8 Distribution of health resources among counties by GNP per capita in Mexico, 1990–96

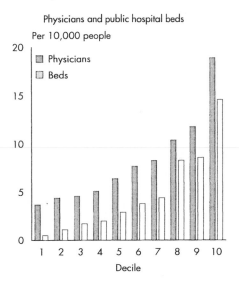

Figure 9 Distribution of health resources among counties by level of marginality in Mexico, 1990–96

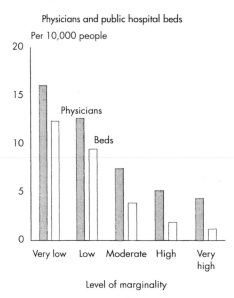

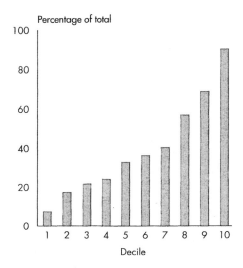

Note: Counties were divided into deciles by GNP per capita from lowest (1) to highest (10).
Source: Zurita et al. 1999.

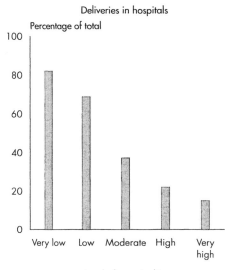

Source: Zurita et al. 1999.

proportion of hospital deliveries is also very low in the marginalized counties (15% compared with 82% in better-off counties). Hence, health resources appear to increase in proportion to the per capita GNP in Mexican counties.

Further analysis by Hernández-Peña et al. (1998) revealed three additional striking dimensions of the inverse care laws:

- The availability of health care resources is higher when the proportion of indigenous people is very low.
- Public expenditure per user is 12 times higher for the insured than for the uninsured.
- The Mexican states with the highest child and adult mortality rates have lower public health expenditures per capita (US$35 to US$44 in 1995) when compared with those states with lower mortality rates (US$74 to US$198).

As in the case of health status, public health expenditures per capita by county also show an even greater variation than is apparent using the state as a unit of analysis. Very low marginality counties have average health expenditures per capita that are almost five times greater (US$96) compared with the very high marginality counties (US$21).

Reduce Marginality or Increase Health Expenditure?

Specific health problems seem to have a differential response to improvements in living conditions or health care expenditures according to the regression models designed (see Box 2; full results not displayed in this chapter). In these models, health inequality is measured using a Gini index. Group I diseases (communicable, maternal, nutritional, and perinatal disorders) are more sensitive to the living conditions as measured by the marginality index. A model of the inequality in YLL for group I diseases shows that if marginality between counties was equally distributed it would reduce the observed inequality by 31%, whereas an equal distribution of health care expenditures would reduce the observed inequality by 17%. Another model for the inequality in YLL from injuries (group III) showed that 20% of the inequality in YLL could be attributed to county marginality and another 8% to inequities in health care expenditures. On the other hand, for group II, or noncommunicable disorders, the observed inequality in YLL could be reduced by 15% each through an equal redistribution of health care expenditures and equalizing marginality across counties.

Inequalities in the probability of dying among those under 5 years of age are also sensitive to socioeconomic or health expenditure improvements. The observed in-

equality for this indicator decreases by nearly 9% when counties are assumed to have a similar proportion of indigenous people. Marginality explains 26% of the inequality observed in the probability of dying before the age of 5 years, whereas unequal public health expenditure explains an additional 7%.

Regression models of health inequality between counties indicate that the most important reduction in years of life lost might be obtained through an improvement in conditions of deprivation or structural poverty as measured by the marginality index. Improvements in education, income level, and housing conditions in the marginalized counties might enable indigenous people to cope with and avoid the impact of inequalities on the quality of life. Correcting current health expenditure inequalities could also reduce the burden of disease.

Discussion

The analysis of health inequalities at the county level reveals differentials in health and in health care access which are not nearly as apparent at the state level. Furthermore, county-level analysis is particularly useful for it is precisely at this geographic level that policies could be implemented in order to reach the more deprived population. Implementation may well be enhanced by the current democratic changes in Mexico, which include a progressive decentralization process that will enable counties to adapt their assigned budgets to their needs and priorities. This change will allow the social development and health programs to be adjusted at the local level and will potentially focus expenditures and programs on the most deprived populations. Since poor and indigenous populations suffer from a dramatic health disadvantage, they should be treated as priority groups by policy makers. Social policies and the health reform have already implemented strategies oriented toward alleviating structural poverty in deprived groups. An assessment of their actual equity impact is, however, still needed.

Specific Proposals Aimed at Reducing Health Inequality

Structural proposals

This study shows an association between poor county-level living conditions and high mortality in Mexico. The most important factors related to changing mortality caused by communicable diseases are associated with "structural factors," highlighting the need to promote socioeconomic equity (Townsend et al. 1992). During the last several years, economic growth in Mexico has been 1.5% lower than the population growth rate. The effects of the fall in oil prices and the recurrent national and international economic crises have eroded purchasing power. To redress health inequities, it could be argued that purchasing power ought to be ameliorated through distributive policies. There is a need to increase complementary wages and earnings and to implement programs that promote employment opportunities and technical assistance, productive credits, microindustries, regional markets, and trade networks. This challenge requires a comprehensive social and economic policy that modifies the current distribution of wealth and health.

Analysis of resource distribution in the present study shows that deprived counties, and those with the lowest GNP, do not obtain the same amount of general social development resources as wealthier ones. At the same time, the public social budget has been affected by public financial shortages. The adoption of a policy of redistribution of resources would increase social development and health and provide a safety net for those living in more marginal conditions. Such a policy should focus particularly on those counties identified in this study as having greater health needs—as measured by their burden of communicable and noncommunicable diseases and injuries. For the most part, these counties are in rural areas located in the south and center of the country. A further exercise should be the prioritization of activities according to the components of the marginality index. In other words, which of the many aspects of marginalization—from access to clean water to education—should be addressed first?

The avoidable causes of death are often associated with the scarcity of adequate environmental conditions that should be provided through social investment policies. Housing policies, for example, have largely benefited urban settlements. Hence, 15% of households still lack water supply to the home, and 25% lack access to sewage systems, representing a gap that should be narrowed (Garduño and González 1998). Water sanitation is a key goal to be jointly implemented by health services and county governments.

Health sector proposals

As is the case with social services in general, analysis of health resource distribution shows that deprived counties, and those with the lowest GNP, do not obtain the same level of resources as do wealthier ones.

BOX 3: PRINCIPAL STRATEGIES AND PROGRAMS OF HEALTH REFORM IN MEXICO

1. **Program to increase coverage:** The Programa de Ampliación de cobertura (PAC) is one of the main strategies of the current health reform. The program provides a basic health care package (13 interventions) in 660 counties in 19 Mexican states. The estimated population without access to health care facilities was 10 million in 1995, but by 1999 it was reduced to 1.7 million. This strategy seeks to use all the available health care infrastructure in public institutions. Additional mobile units provide care to communities that are more than 1 hour away from a health facility. This program is financed by state governments and the World Bank (SSA 1999).

2. **Program for Education, Health and Nutrition:** The Programa de Educación, Salud y Alimentación (Progresa) seeks to reduce poverty for 31 states. It was launched in 1997 and is a targeted intervention for 2.3 million families (13 million individuals) in very high marginality counties. The three components are nutrition and food (for children under 5 years and pregnant women); health (follow-up care for children under 5 years and pregnant and breastfeeding women and other health care through a basic package in public health care institutions); and education for which an increasing monetary incentive is given for children who stay in school beyond the third and up to the ninth grade (the incentive is larger for girls) (SSA 1999; Sedesol 1999–2000).

3. **Program of Support to Indigenous Zones:** The Programa de Apoyo a Zonas Indígenas (PAZI) has operated since 1997 in 300 largely indigenous counties (localities where more than 70% of the population speaks an indigenous language). The program provides medical care through mobile brigades and health centers (SSA 1999).

4. **Child Health Program:** The Programa de Salud del Niño includes preventive and curative activities directed to children under 5 years of age. A recent evaluation of the program found the following successes: 50% reduction in mortality from diarrhea, 80% increase in the use of the oral rehydration therapy, immunization coverage of at least 90% of the population, eradication of poliomyelitis by the year 2000, elimination of neonatal tetanus in 1995, and a halving of the marginality index (Comisión Nacional de Acción a favor de la Infancia 1998).

5. **Better distribution of health expenditures:** Passed in 1998, the reformed Law of Fiscal Coordination outlines a formula to distribute the additional budget of the Health Ministry more equitably (Gobierno Federal 1997).

This discrepancy could be modified through new policies of resource allocation stemming from the decentralization program (see Box 3 for the highlights of the current Mexican reforms). It is important that policy makers work to eliminate the existing barriers to health services and to ensure access to the health system for the most deprived counties, particularly those with high mortality rates due to avoidable causes.

Much of the inequity in health and social services has its roots in ethnic differences and cultural barriers. Hence, activities aimed at promoting respect for the indigenous people and their human rights might enhance their health status as well. It is also important to continue coping with illiteracy. The PROGRESA program, developed to promote education and provide proper nutrition to the most deprived, is a worthwhile effort that should be continued on a permanent basis. It could also be argued that geographic barriers are an important obstacle to good health in rural areas. It is necessary to ensure that roads are in good condition and that public transportation services are available and affordable; to this end, strategic methods of financing necessary investments should be sought. A proper communication network would enable even those populations living in distant settlements to have access to health services.

Special focus should be placed on avoidable causes of death. To eliminate diarrheal diseases, for instance, the health system should promote access to clean water, improved sanitation methods, and proper sewage disposal while simultaneously reinforcing the Child Health Program. Education and health promotion activities should strive to reach the mothers of children under 5 years of age. Because the causes of disease and death are varied, essential packages of medical care should include preventive and follow-up procedures for chronic diseases and injuries, as well as activities for communicable diseases. In highly deprived areas, we would expect a greater impact from such human development programs.

Causes of death in deprived counties are often related to malnutrition. Previous nourishment surveys in rural areas have shown a higher malnutrition rate among the deprived, as well as among indigenous people, when compared with other rural groups (58% vs. 43%) (Instituto Nacional de la Nutrición Salvador Zubirán 1997). Thus, primary health care programs could be oriented towards providing, among other items, nutritional supplements and also close follow-up of disease controls in cases involving tuberculosis, acute respiratory diseases, oral rehydration, and antiparasitic treatment.

The Mexican Health Reform has proposed an increase in coverage and has focused health activities on the vulnerable and deprived populations (see Box 3). It is worth noting that a new health program for the indigenous population (PAZI) was recently developed and designed to include health promotion, preventive measures, and curative activities. This program needs more resources in order to ensure continued coverage and the quality of its activities. In the social security system, a special kind of insurance program has been put into effect to increase coverage for informal workers (Health Insurance for the Family or Seguro de Salud para la Familia). The Ministry of Health (SSa) is attempting to extend coverage of a basic health care package to most of the 8 million Mexicans who lacked access to permanent health services in 1994.

Quality of care is also one of the items addressed by the current health reforms. In terms of equity promotion, the provision of health services is being targeted. Special efforts should now be made to ensure that primary health care achieves the expected benefits. Because of the mixed epidemiological profile, it is imperative to promote comprehensive preventive and curative health services in the rural areas. Also, local health systems need to be linked to a state and national referral network that would ensure access to available and cost-effective complex treatments. Efficiency studies to promote equity are scarce and should also be promoted.

Monitoring and research

Some policies have been implemented to cope with prevailing inequalities. Studies are needed, however, to assess whether coverage has incorporated the most deprived and what impact there has been on the health profiles of the target population. Studies about policies and programs dealing with health inequalities need to assess the inclusion of all groups in greatest need and provide for adequate follow-up of their efficacy and long-term impact. In this sense, policies should be studied for their capacity both to promote health improvements *and* to overcome inequalities.

Alternative low-cost care models with a focus on prevention need to be designed. One of the tools used to increase coverage includes the promotion of an essential package of health care; however, the relevance of its components should be analyzed in accordance with the specific health needs of the population it serves, ensuring coverage for the most deprived groups. Thus, assessment of its adequacy in meeting the local needs and of the specific benefits obtained by county is a key factor in the policy's effectiveness.

People have a potential role in the promotion of their own health and the prevention of illness and early death. Hence, their participation in policies and programs should be encouraged. Participatory programs aimed at reducing health inequalities should also identify local adjustments and specific challenges to participation of the population. In this chapter, health needs were studied mainly through an analysis of mortality, including its causes and the age of death. The study of inequalities in health, however, especially with regard to changes in morbidity and the quality of life (including disability), is a research task that lies ahead.

The real mechanisms through which inequalities are generated and maintained were not fully addressed in this chapter. Interactions between measured variables should be studied in order to identify more detailed interventions. Monitoring of government initiatives would yield valuable data on the effectiveness of various interventions. For example, careful monitoring is needed of the initiative aimed at reallocating public resources among the health services for the uninsured populations at the state level through 16 indicators on health and institutional performance (Gobierno Federal 1997). The application of more sensitive and inequality-specific indicators for health should be incorporated and discussed. Indicators such as SII and RII could be applied to guide operational adjustment of programs.

Health inequalities in Mexico are a complex problem, mediated by ethnicity, geography, and politics. The results of this study point out the usefulness of county-level analysis to highlight gaps in health status that are masked at the state level. Furthermore, the analysis provides some insight into the effects of marginality on health and the disease-specific dimensions of inequities in health. Finally, the analysis of policies and health reforms points to positive steps taken by the Mexican government to protect the marginalized, but notes the need to monitor and evaluate the effectiveness of these reforms.

We thank Gabriel Camacho, Oscar Méndez, Javier Dorantes, Ana Gamble, and Manuel Recio for their statistical and programming assistance; Efrén Motta and Tania Castellanos, who provided secretarial support; and especially Ma. Teresa de Mucha and Finn Diderichsen, for their assistance in the development of this chapter.

References

Arriaga E. 1994. *Population Analysis with Microcomputers: Presentation of Techniques, Vol I.* Washington, DC: Bureau of the Census.

Black R.J., Sharp L., Urquhart J.D. 1996. Analyzing the spatial distribution of disease using a method of constructing geographical areas of an approximately equal population size. In: Alexander F.E., Boyle P. (eds), *Methods for Investigating Localized Clustering of Disease*, pp. 28–39. Lyon, France: International Agency for Research on Cancer Scientific Publications.

Bronfman M. 1994. *La salud de los pueblos indígenas: una conquista impostergable.* Cuadernos de Salud, No.1. México City, México, DF: SSA.

Cabrera G. 1966. *Indicadores demográficos de México a principios de siglo.* México City, México, DF: El Colegio de México.

Comisión Económica para América Latina y el Caribe (CEPAL). 1997a. *Estudio Económico de América Latina y el Caribe, 1996–1997.* Santiago de Chile: Comisión Económica para América Latina y el Caribe.

CEPAL. 1997b. *La Brecha de la Equidad.* Santiago de Chile: Comisión Económica para América Latina y el Caribe.

Comisión Nacional de Acción en favor de la Infancia. 1998. *Programa Nacional de Acción a favor de la Infancia: Evaluación 1997.* México City, México, DF: Comisión National de Acción a favor de la Infancia.

Consejo Nacional de Población (CONAPO). 1993. *Indicadores socioeconómicos e índice de marginación municipal, 1990: primer informe técnico del proyecto: desigualdad regional y marginación municipal en México.* México City, México, DF: Consejo Nacional de Población.

CONAPO. 1995. *Proyecciones de población de la República Mexicana, 1990–2010.* México City, México, DF: Consejo Nacional de Población y Vivienda.

Frenk J. 1993. *La salud de la población: hacia una nueva salud pública,* pp 15–73. México City, México, DF: Fondo de Cultura Económica.

Frenk J. 1998. 20 Años de salud en México. *Nexos Enero,* 21(241): 85–91.

Frenk J., González-Block M.A., Lozano R. 1998. Seis tesis equivocadas sobre las políticas de salud en el combate a la pobreza. *Revista Este País* Marzo 84:28–36.

Frenk J., Lozano R., González-Block M.A. 1994. *Economía y salud: propuestas para el avance del sistema de salud en México. Informe final.* México City, México, DF: Fundación Mexicana para la Salud.

Garduño S.R., González G. 1998. *Los indicadores de bienestar en México 1940–1995.* México City, México, DF: Instituto de Investigación Económica y Social Lucas Alamán AC.

Gobierno Federal. 1997. *Iniciativa de decreto por el que se adiciona y reforma la ley de coordinación fiscal.* México City, México, DF: Presidencia de la República.

González R.A. 1998. Es la economía número 12 del mundo, pero 43 en nivel de ingreso: Banco Mundial. *La Jornada* July 11.

Hernández-Peña P., Zapata O., Leyva R., Lozano R. 1991. Equidad y salud: necesidades de investigación para la formulación de una política social. *Salud Pública de Mexico* 33:9–17.

Instituto Nacional de Estadística Geografía e Informática (INEGI). 1990. *Encuesta nacional de ingresos y gastos de los hogares: ENIGH—1984.* México City, México, DF: Instituto Nacional de Estadística Geografía e Informática.

INEGI. 1992. *IX censo nacional de población y vivienda.* México City, México, DF: Instituto Nacional de Geografía Estadística e Informática.

INEGI. 1995. *Encuesta nacional de ingresos y gastos de los hogares: ENIGH 1994.* México City, México, DF: Instituto Nacional de Geografía Estadística e Informática.

INEGI. 1990–1996a. *Nacimientos registrados en la República Mexicana.* México City, México, DF: Instituto Nacional de Geografía Estadística e Informática.

INEGI. 1990–1996b. *Defunciones Registradas en la República Mexicana.* México City, México, DF: Instituto Nacional de Geografía Estadística e Informática.

INEGI. 1997. *Conteo de población y vivienda, 1995. Resultados definitivos.* México City, México, DF: Instituto Nacional de Geografía Estadística e Informática.

Instituto Nacional Indigenista. 1999. *Información básica sobre los pueblos indígenas de México.* Instituto Nacional Indigenista. Página Electrónica de la SEDESOL. www.sedesol.gob.mx. (11/1/00)

Instituto Nacional de la Nutrición Salvador Zubirán (INNZS). 1997. *Encuesta nacional de alimentación en el medio rural 1996.* México City, México, DF: Instituto Nacional de la Nutrición Salvador Zubirán.

Lozano R. 1997. El peso de la enfermedad en México: avances y desafíos. In: Frenk J. (ed), *Observatorio de la salud: necesidades, servicios, políticas.* México City, México, DF: Fundación Mexicana para la Salud.

Lozano R., Infante C., Schlaepfer L., Frenk J. 1993. *Desigualdad pobreza y salud en México.* México City, México, DF: Consejo Consultivo del Programa Nacional de Solidaridad. El Nacional.

Murray C.J.L., López A. 1996. *The Global Burden of Disease: A Comprehensive Assessment of Mortality and Disability from Diseases, Injuries and Risk Factors in 1990 to 2020, vol 1.* Boston: Harvard University Press.

Murray C.J.L., López A. 1997. Global mortality, disability and the contribution of risk factors: global burden of disease study. *Lancet* 349:1436–1442.

Organización Panamericana de la Salud. 1978. *Clasificación internacional de enfermedades.* Revisión 1975. Washington, DC: Organización Panamericana de la Salud.

Psacharopoulos G., Patrinos H. 1994. *Indigenous People and Poverty in Latin America: An Empirical Analysis.* Washington, DC: World Bank.

Sánchez A.A. 1998. Marginación e ingreso en los municipios de México, 1970–1990. México City, México, DF: Tesis de maestria, Facultad de Ciencias Políticas y Sociales, Universidad Nacional Autónoma de México.

Secretariat de Salud (SSA). 1999. *Principales líneas de trabajo de la Secretaría de Salud 1999.* México City, México, DF: Síntesis Ejecutiva.

Sedesol. Programa de Desarrollo Social y Combate a la Pobreza. 1999–2000. Secretaría de Desarrollo Social. www.sedesol.gob.mx. (11/1/00)

Sen A. 1992. *Inequality Reexamined.* Cambridge, MA: Harvard University Press.

Townsend P., Whitehead M., Davidson N. (eds). 1992. *Inequalities in Health: The Black Report and the Health Divide*, 2nd ed. London: Penguin Books.

Tudor Hart J. 1971. The inverse care law. *Lancet* 1:405–412.

United Nations Development Programme. (UNDP). 1999. *Human Development Report 1999.* New York: UNDP.

United Nations. 1990. *The United Nations Software Package for Mortality Measurement.* Version 3.0/CP. New York: United Nations.

Wagstaff A., Paci P., Doorslaer E.V. 1991. On the measurement of inequalities in health. *Social Science and Medicine* 33(5):545–557.

Zurita B., Colin R., Villoro R., Gamble A., Cruz C. 1995. Situación actual de las necesidades y la oferta de servicios de salud: 227 municipios de extrema pobreza. (mimeo). Dirección General de Estudios en Economía. México City: PASSPA-Secretaría de Salud/Banco Mundial.

Zurita B., Hernández P., Ramírez T., Gamble A., Méndez O., Recio M., Cruz C. 1998. Cuentas nacionales de salud 1995. En: *Iniciativas de Revorma del Sector Salud en Latinoamerica y el Caribe.* Cuaderno 11. México City: Organización Panamericana de la Salud y Oficina Regional de desarrollo Sostenible, Oficina para América Latina y el Caribe.

CHAPTER 20

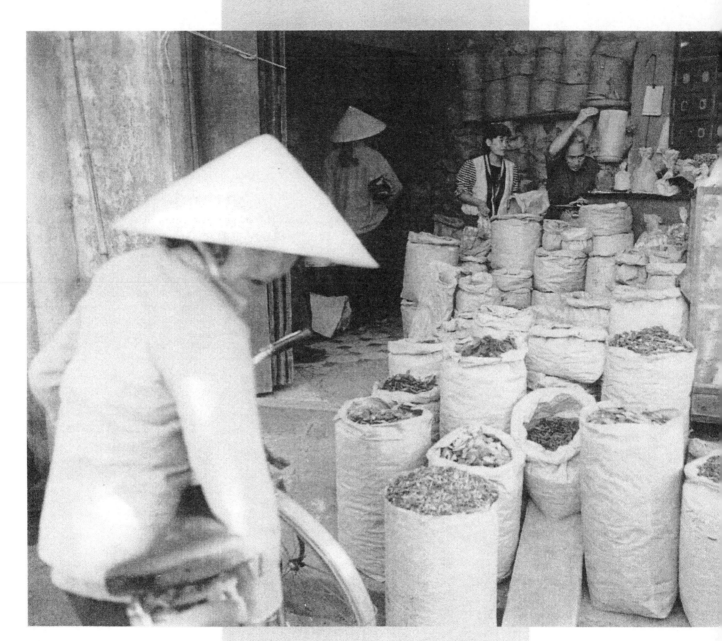

Customers at a traditional medicine shop, Hanoi, Vietnam, 1995.
Source: Lois Raimondo/Associated Press.

Vietnam: Efficient, Equity-Oriented Financial Strategies for Health

PHAM MANH HUNG, TRUONG VIET DZUNG, GÖRAN DAHLGREN, AND TRAN TUAN

Vietnam is unique in terms of health development, with a life expectancy 11 years above what could be expected considering its present level of economic resources. Like other countries, however, social inequities in health exist in Vietnam and are reflected in the substantial differences in mortality and morbidity between economically privileged and poor areas. Vietnam is also experiencing a double disease burden: While many of the communicable diseases still constitute a major threat to people's health, the incidence of noncommunicable diseases is also increasing. Emerging health problems include injuries and tobacco-related diseases. Furthermore, the consequences of 35 war-torn years are still being experienced by the many who suffer from the effects of toxic chemicals and mental diseases related to the war.

Changes in the health panorama influence the need for health services and thus the development of the health care sector. Far more important, however, particularly in a Vietnamese context, are the social and economic changes related to the *Doi Moi* reform process, that is, the transformation from a planned to a socialist market economy.

Within this context, the Vietnamese Government has declared its commitment to developing an efficient, equity-oriented health care system. To achieve this, many challenges must be overcome. The purpose of this chapter is to describe some of the key challenges and to present some of the policy options for the future. The chapter begins by describing the profound transition taking place in the Vietnamese health system. It then outlines five major policy issues related to this transition and the options available to deal with them in the Vietnamese context. Special attention is paid to the need for additional public funding, possibilities for expanding subsidized rural health insurance schemes, and the risks associated with high user fees. A conceptual framework is also presented for the allocation of resources according to the varying needs of different provinces and districts. The final section considers some tentative long-term strategies for the future.

A Health System in Transition

Despite many economic constraints, during the era of Vietnam's subsidized and centrally planned economy, considerable equity in health care was achieved. At that time, Vietnam was often referred to as a good example for many other countries, particularly due to its development of a basic rural health care network. The shift from the subsidized management mechanism to a

Vietnam

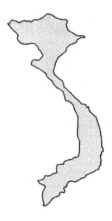

Total population (millions), 1997	76.4
Human development index, 1999	0.664
Human development index rank, 1999	110
Infant mortality rate (per 1,000 live births), 1997	32
Real GDP per capita (PPP$), 1997	1,630
Public spending on health	
as percentage of GDP, 1995	—

— Not available.
Source: UNDP 1999. [Human Development Report]

socialist-oriented market and, in particular, the introduction of fairly high user fees, however, resulted in the growth of social health insurance schemes and private for-profit providers. As a result, inequities in terms of access to hospital care are increasing. The *Doi Moi* process, initiated in 1986, has had an impact on the health sector, including public health services, private providers, traditional healers, and even self-medication. Each of these changes is described below.

Public Health Services

Before 1986, the agricultural cooperatives provided basic health services at the village and commune levels. Village health workers were paid in rice or work points by the cooperative. The cooperative was also in charge of the community health center, where high priority was given to primary prevention. The referral system to higher level care, which was financed by the government, was very strict and the choice of providers limited. The main problem was often the shortage of drugs. This grassroots health service network was often cited by the World Health Organization (WHO) and other agencies as a model for other countries.

The introduction of *Doi Moi* reforms had many positive effects in terms of increased economic growth and reduced absolute poverty, but also negative effects such as increased economic inequities and reduced access to basic health care. Outpatient visits at public health facilities were reduced, for example, by 50% between 1986 and 1990, but have been increasing steadily since 1993 and by 1998 were at a level of 1.5 visits per capita per year (Dzung 1999).

The role of the agricultural cooperatives was drastically reduced when individual farmers began selling their products directly on the emerging market. This lessened—sometimes eliminated—sources of revenue to finance commune health centers and village health workers, and a large segment of the basic health care system collapsed. Since then, the Vietnamese Government has reinforced the health service network at the village and commune levels. It has employed health staff at commune health stations, and village health workers in poor communities are paid from government funds. The network of commune health stations has also been expanded, as illustrated in Figure 1.

The utilization of many public health facilities has, however, changed over time. The better-off groups are utilizing public hospitals and poly-clinics more than less privileged groups despite the fact that the need for professional care is greatest among the poor. The share of total utilization of public hospitals for the poorest 20% of the population has, for example, declined between 1993 and 1998. At the same time, the richest 20% increased their share of total hospital utilization from 36% in 1993 to 45% of all public hospital users in 1998 (LSMS 1998). This pro-rich bias within the public health care system has been reinforced by increasing differences in income combined with the introduction of fairly high direct user fees and a compulsory health insurance scheme primarily available to economically better-off groups.

Community and district health centers, however, are utilized almost equally by all income groups, except for a lower utilization rate among the richest. Strengthening this level of care is thus likely—within the present health care structure—to benefit the poor at least as much as the better-off groups such as civil servants and skilled workers in big industries.

Private For-Profit Providers

Diversification, or the opening up of health care to private for-profit providers, is an important part of the *Doi Moi* reform process in the health sector. The average rate of consultations with private providers in 1998 was 1.8 per capita per year, which is somewhat higher than average annual consultations with public providers. There was, however, a relatively significant

Figure 1 Commune health stations in Vietnam, 1986–98

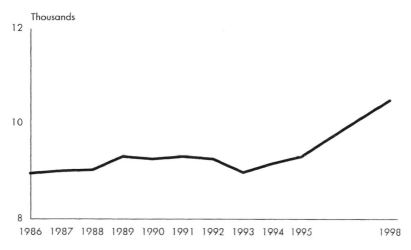

Source: Ministry of Health, *Health Statistics Yearbook,* various years.

decline in the utilization of private health services between 1993 and 1998, in particular among the poorest 20% of the population (from 16% of all contacts to only 9%) (LSMS 1998). The pro-rich bias is thus increased with regard to private for-profit providers as well.

Traditional Healers

Traditional healers have played an important role in providing health services in Vietnam, but currently the average rate of consultation is only 0.3 contacts per capita per year (LSMS 1998). Efforts are being made by the government, however, to reinforce the practice of traditional medicine and to improve the integration between traditional and modern medicine.

Self-Medication

Reduced financial access to public as well as private health care facilities has, in combination with the increased supply of drugs available over the counter without prescriptions, increased the rate of self-medication. The average number of drug vendor contacts per capita was 7.3 visits in 1998 (LSMS 1998). Drug vendors are by far the most common health care contact. The quality of services provided in terms of professional advice, however, is often very low, as the people selling drugs often lack medical or pharmaceutical training. Furthermore, the drug vendors operate in a commercial environment with strong financial incentives to sell as many pharmaceutical products as possible. They tend to sell whatever drugs they can con-

vince people they need, even if it is not in the patient's best interest. The poorest 20% of the population has increased their self-medication, sometimes by buying incomplete courses of medicines such as antibiotics. This is, of course, a very dangerous trend as it reflects an increase in irrational use of drugs and a reduction in professional, medical consultations for those most in need for these health services.

Against this background of increasing inequities in the utilization of public health facilities and very high levels of self-care among poor people, a number of policy issues are of critical importance, as discussed below.

Defining the Role of the State and the Market Within the Health Sector

Defining the role of the state and the market within the health care sector is of particular importance during a transitional period from a planned to a socialist market economy. Four major alternative options can be identified, illustrated graphically in Figure 2.

Alternative 1 is the *Market Approach*, where health services are looked on as a commodity to be sold in a regulated health care market. Key elements of the market approach are high levels of private financing via direct user fees and private health insurance schemes as well as a large private for-profit health care sector. The role of the government is to provide the services that private for-profit providers do not find profitable and thus are not interested in or able to provide (e.g.,

Figure 2 Ministry of Health's conceptual model illustrating four alternative approaches to health sector reform in Vietnam

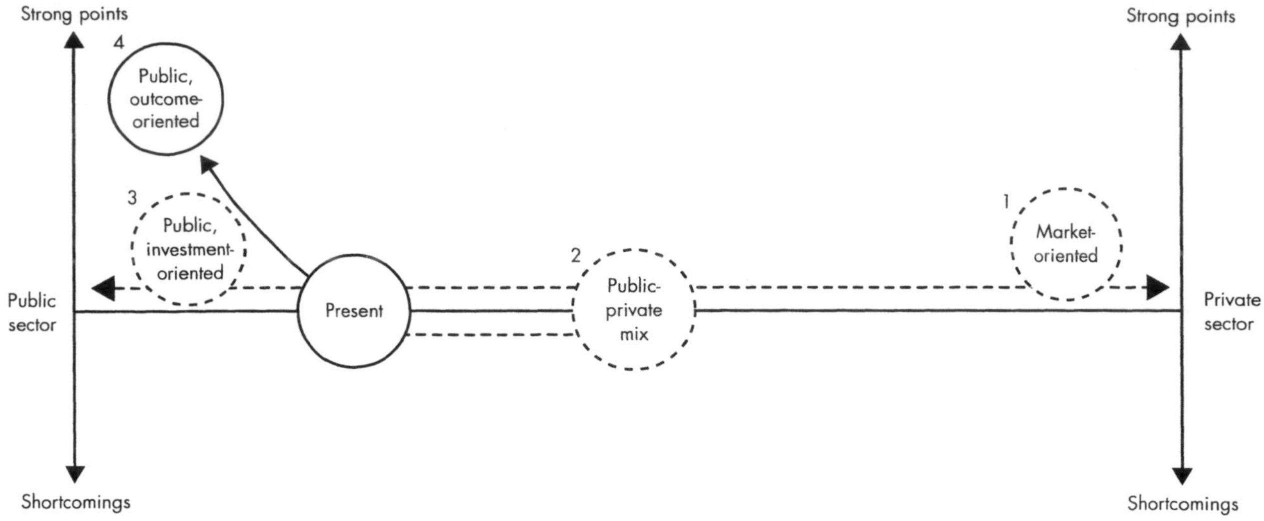

community-based primary prevention programs and curative care for people unable to pay user fees above full-cost recovery levels). As stated in the WHO's *World Health Report* in 1999, international experience clearly indicates that "not only do market oriented approaches lead to intolerable inequity with respect to a fundamental human right, but growing bodies of theory and evidence indicate markets in health to be inefficient as well" (World Health Organization 1999).

Alternative 2 is the *Public–Private Mix Approach*, based on the assumptions that efficiency can be increased in public systems by introducing market elements and that equity can be improved in market models by strengthening the role of the government. An ideal balance between public and private could then be achieved, optimizing the positive and minimizing the negative effects of the two approaches. The experiences of many European countries indicate that any efficiency gained with the introduction of market elements into public systems was often negated by increasing costs (Saltman and Figueras 1997). Equally evident are the difficulties in strengthening the role of the government in commercial health markets. Consequently, the vision of the perfect public–private mix remains elusive.

Alternative 3 is the *Public Approach*, where health services—like education—are looked on as an investment in human development. Key elements of this approach as applied in Vietnam before *Doi Moi* were community responsibility and tax-financed public health care providers. The role of the government would be to guide and control the entire health care system. The public approach for the provision of health

care is found in most fully developed market economies as well as in many low-income countries. Experiences gained are usually quite positive in terms of sustainability, efficiency, and equity. Constraints are scarce public resources and focus on inputs rather than outputs. Private providers, and general practitioners in particular, are often seen as a complement to the public health care system.

Alternative 4 is the *Public Outcome-Oriented Approach*, with the main role taken by the government/public sector, a further development of the public approach presented above. Here, health services are still considered an investment in human development, but the focus is increasingly on outcomes of care. The allocation of public resources is closely related to expected results, and the providers are encouraged to find the best way to achieve these results with given resources. Within this outcome-oriented approach, efforts are also made to assess progress toward stated targets as well as people's satisfaction with the health services provided. Thus, when equity objectives are selected, the outcomes of the system need to be assessed in terms of the progress made towards those objectives. Private for-profit health care providers are seen as a complement to the public health care sector. The role of the government is to control the whole health care sector according to stated objectives and targets.

Alternative 4 is the option chosen by Vietnam. The overall objectives for the health sector have been clearly stated by the government and the party: "The humanitarian nature and socialist orientation of health activities demand equity in the provision of health care. Circumstances where a poor and sick patient is denied medical treatment because of her lack of money should be put to an end" (Vietnam Ministry of Health 1996). Because present trends are not in line with these objectives, the further development of alternative 4 is of critical importance so that efficient, equity-oriented systems for mobilizing and allocating financial resources for health services can be analyzed and developed.

Financial Resources for Health Services

Figure 3 illustrates the main sources of finance for the public health care system in Vietnam at present (Vietnam Ministry of Health 1998). It is often assumed that the most important issue is the amount of resources available for health care services, that is, the size of the "financial pie." More important, however, is the issue of how much is financed by taxes, compulsory health insurance, and user fees, respectively. The reason is that the burden of payment—who is to pay and how much—differs depending on the source of funds and so does the scope for different groups to utilize the available resources. The various financing options for Vietnam are considered in turn below.

Taxes

In a progressive tax system, contributions are made according to ability to pay, and the funds allocated for public health care services can be utilized according to need. This is an ideal method for financing an efficient, equity-oriented health care system, as healthy people contribute to the care of the sick, better-off groups contribute to the care of the poor, and working-age peo-

ple contribute to the care of children and elderly people.

The present public funding of the Vietnamese health care sector is still far below what could be considered adequate. The annual (public) health spending is around US$5 per capita, which is only one-half of the US$12 recommended by the *World Development Report* in 1993 for low-income countries for financing an essential package of health services. To achieve this level of spending, Vietnam would need to spend an additional US$500 million annually on health, most of which must be financed via increased revenues from taxes.

Social health insurance

Compulsory social health insurance. There are many similarities between compulsory social health insurance and tax financing, as both are compulsory prepayment schemes controlled by the government. There are, however, great differences with regards to who pays and who utilizes the funds raised. Contrary to a tax-financed system, there is a direct link between paying (in the form of insurance premiums) and receiving services (only by those insured). This is a problem in low-income countries where social health insurance schemes only cover a small proportion of the total population (in Vietnam, 12.4% of the population in 1997). People with insurance are likely to use more than their share of available resources than are noninsured people. Social health insurance schemes covering only a very limited proportion of the total population are thus very likely to be a major reason why better-off groups actually utilize hospital services—as illustrated above—far more often than noninsured. There is thus an urgent need to expand health insurance coverage to the greatest possible proportion of the population in general and among the poor in particular. Experiences clearly indicate that this is very difficult to achieve by expanding the present compulsory health insurance and by offering voluntary insurance schemes. The way forward seems to be subsidized health insurance cards.

Free health cards for the poor. A step toward expanding health insurance coverage among poor people was taken recently when the government decided to provide—beginning in April 1999—4 million (an estimated 25% of) poor people with free, tax-financed health insurance cards. Although the implementation of this scheme has been somewhat delayed due to financial and other constraints, it is still envisaged that the provision of free health insurance cards will be expanded.

Figure 3 Public health budget funding sources in Vietnam, 1998

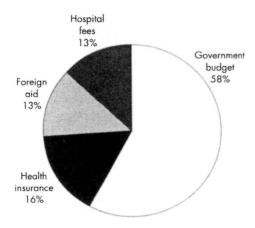

Source: Ministry of Health 1998.

Community-based health insurance schemes. It is also envisaged that community-based health insurance schemes could constitute an important element in an equity-oriented and sustainable financial strategy for public health services. The idea to be further developed and tested is that government funding, and perhaps also foreign aid, could match community contributions to a "health fund" from which social health insurance cards for the whole community could be financed. The proportion to be financed by the community could then be adjusted according to the socioeconomic classification of the commune/district. If foreign aid funds are utilized, it is important that the government initially make a commitment securing a gradual shift from foreign aid to regular government funds. The foreign aid component could be used to increase coverage temporarily while additional government funds for public health services are secured for the long term.

The advantage of this scheme, compared with direct tax financing alone, is that it can mobilize additional funds for health via an organized community-based prepayment scheme. A disadvantage is that community-based insurance schemes are more complicated to implement than is direct government funding of preventive and curative health services. Compared with direct user fee programs, subsidized health insurance schemes are preferred on both equity and financial grounds, as the whole community is covered and thus more money is raised when the whole population, not only the sick, contributes. Furthermore, all experiences indicate that prepayment schemes are far more appropriate and effective for health care financing than sudden unexpected payments via direct user fees when people fall ill.

Private for-profit health insurance schemes

Commercial private health insurance schemes are not a viable option for health care financing in poor countries such as Vietnam, as they have risk-related premiums, that is, the most privileged groups pay the lowest premiums and the poor pay the highest. It is generally only the most privileged who can afford to pay the premiums charged for this type of insurance plan.

Direct user fees

In 1997 in Vietnam, individual households' direct payments for health care (user fees and drugs) constituted 80% of total spending on health, while 19% was paid via taxes and 1% by foreign aid (LSMS 1998). Increasing the user fees for services such as hospital care would add to an already substantial burden of direct payments for people who are sick. Direct user fees without well-functioning exemption schemes in fact constitutes the most regressive form of all types of health care financing. Furthermore, high user-fees are very likely to

- Reduce economic access to essential health services, in particular among the poor
- Allocate resources according to purchasing power rather than need
- Increase inequities in health, as the poor are those most in need of health services and high fees would either deter their use or make them poorer

One argument in favor of user fees is that they increase financial resources for health care and thus increase the possibilities to provide care for the poor. Even when higher user fees increase revenues, however, most of the funds are used for covering the cost of providing care for those able to pay, while at the same time public subsidies to these groups are greater due to higher utilization rates. Increasing user fees at the same time reduces the number of patients able to pay. This is because the higher user fees lead to reduced demand and also increase the number of patients for whom the fees should be waived. On both counts, revenues are reduced.

Yet, increased user fees are often perceived as the only short-term option available for maintaining hospital services during periods of increasing financial constraints. This has been the case in Vietnam where, for people without social health insurance, average total out-of-pocket expenditure for a visit to a public hospital *increased* by 36% in real terms between 1993 and 1998. Over the same period, however, those with social health insurance experienced a *reduction* of 40% in average out-of-pocket expenditure for a hospital visit (LSMS 1998).

It should also be noted that drug prices were reduced between 1993 and 1998, indicating that the increase caused by user fees alone was far above the 36% increase (in real terms) for fees and drugs stated above for noninsured patients (LSMS 1998). The decline in drug prices has, in fact, reduced the share of total household expenditures on health care in all groups but the most affluent. This trend has been accompanied by a growth in irrational and unnecessary prescribing to poor people by private drug vendors. There is thus a somewhat unusual dual picture with regard to direct out-of-pocket expenses for health care: very substantial increases in average hospital fees per visit with a concomitant reduced share of total household consumption for health because of lower prices on drugs.

Shifting from financing health care services through taxation to relying on user fees will mean that the sick, the poor, and the elderly will pay more while the healthy, the rich, and the working-age population will pay less. Waiving fees for the very poor may reduce, but will not eliminate, these negative effects. Equally important to consider fully are the effects of user fees on the utilization of care. Health care users fall into four groups: The first group consists of people who can afford to pay high hospital fees without any major problems. The second group includes very poor people who are offered free care because of their inability to pay. The third group consists of poor people who are forced to take out expensive loans, sell off capital goods such as land or cattle, or take their children out of school in order to pay the hospital bill. A recent survey in four Vietnamese provinces showed that between 43% and 63% of all inpatients in 30 district hospitals had to make these types of sacrifice (Vietnam Ministry of Health 1997). This clearly indicates that high hospital fees are very likely to increase the risk of becoming poor. In China, where user fees in public hospitals are at a much higher level than in Vietnam, high medical expenses have become a major reason for rural people becoming poor. The role of health care fees in exacerbating poverty is rarely recognized within the health sector. Those who pay are simply described as able to pay, regardless of the social consequences of these payments.

The fourth category consists of people who are too poor to pay but not poor enough to receive free care, estimated to be 28 million people in Vietnam out of a total population of 76 million people (Phuong 1999). The size of this group is of course determined by the level of user fees applied. It is sometimes argued that raising user fees increases the possibilities to provide care for those who cannot afford to pay the fee as the better-off subsidize the care of others. The evidence for this assumption must, however, be carefully analyzed on a case by case basis before being accepted. The reason is that usually only a small proportion—if any—of revenues generated from user fees helps provide free care for the poor. Furthermore, the group not able to pay is increasing as user fees are increased, and this will serve to reduce direct payments and increase the need for additional public funds to secure the same level of medical services.

Allocation of Resources Between Provinces/Districts

Several different approaches exist for the allocation of public funds (taxes) between different provinces and districts, including appropriations based on need, population size, and demand:

Need: For the purposes of this discussion, need is determined by the size of the population to be served and the disease burden experienced by different groups of the population.

Population size: When only population size is considered, equal resources are designated per capita.

Demand: Allocations may be made according to demand, expressed by the purchasing power on the commercial health care market.

Figure 4 illustrates the potential outcomes of allocating a given budget between a poor and a rich district with the same number of inhabitants. Prospects for resource allocation for health between districts/provinces in Vietnam differ depending on the perspective chosen. For a long time government funds have been allocated on a per capita basis, with certain adjustments made for differences in assessed need for health services. This provided an equity-oriented approach to resource allocation when almost all resources for health were coming from government funds. More recently, however, this equity effect not only has been reduced but has been replaced by a highly unequal distribution of available funds for the following reasons: Provincial budgets fund an increasing proportion of health care, in particular, curative care. Rich provinces have more funds to allocate than poor provinces from their own local tax revenues. Economically better-off provinces are also favored because the provincial health expenditure allocations are partially based on the number of hospital beds.

Moreover, revenues from compulsory health insurance schemes are much higher in better-off provinces than in poor provinces because of their larger pool of civil servants and skilled workers in large industries. In short, differences in the resource bases for compulsory health insurance create major differences in revenue in different parts of the country.

Revenues from user fees are also higher in better-off regions than in poor regions, partly because of higher utilization rates among the more privileged groups and partly because fewer patients are given "free care." Private for-profit providers add resources to already privileged areas of the country by serving primarily the better-off groups in urban areas.

Thus, the gap between privileged and less privileged areas in terms of per capita resources for health is increasing rapidly, and the Vietnamese system, as a whole, is moving toward resource allocation according to purchasing power. Consequently, there is an urgent need to further develop and adopt a country-specific needs-based index for resource allocation between provinces and districts that takes into account the total resources available, not only government funds but also revenues generated by social health insurance

Figure 4 Three criteria for allocating public health funds between two areas with the same population size—and the outcomes

By need

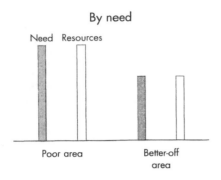

By population

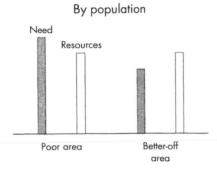

By demand (purchasing power)

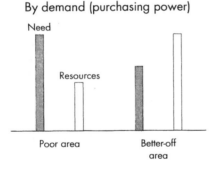

Outcomes

By need: The poor area, with greater need, would receive greater resources than the rich area. But in both areas resources would meet needs.

By population size: Since both areas have the same population, they would receive the same amount of resources. But since need is greater in the poor area, the resources would fall short of need in that area—while exceeding it in the rich area.

By demand: The poor area, where poverty limits effective demand, would receive far too little to meet the need—while the rich area, where demand outstrips need, would receive far too much.

schemes and user fees. Government funds must be reallocated from rich to poor areas if the gap in per capita resources for health is to be reduced, as a major share of the revenues from neither health insurance nor user fees can be reallocated from rich to poor provinces. Increasing public funding would allow a reallocation of government funds to poor areas without any major reductions of existing services in more privileged parts of the country.

Allocating Resources Between Different Types of Services

Public resources for health are very limited and it is of particular importance to recognize "that if services are to be provided for all then not all services can be provided" (World Health Organization 1999). Given that public resources for health are limited, cost-effective services that will improve the health of disadvantaged groups and narrow inequities in health should be provided first.

An efficient, equity-oriented strategy for health must thus give very high priority to primary prevention and health services at village, commune, and district levels. An Asian Development Bank (1999) report on health sector reform in Asia recently acknowledged that almost all essential health services can be carried out within primary health care programs. Despite this, countries in the Asian region typically spend an average of less than 10% of their health care resources on primary care (Dzung 1999). The Asian Development Bank (1999) recommends that "governments should consider allocating fewer resources to expensive hospital based curative care and shift revenues towards public health activities."

This also applies to the Vietnamese health sector, where a high proportion of government funds for health is spent on curative hospital care rather than on primary health care with its focus on prevention. Furthermore, it must be noted that additional revenue from user fees and social health insurance is used almost exclusively for curative care.

In Vietnam, the Ministry of Health has given high priority to already established national health programs to combat communicable diseases as well as emerging non-communicable diseases. Two recent examples of the latter type of intervention are a comprehensive tobacco control policy/program recently approved by the Prime Minister and an expansion of injury prevention/safe community programs. Village, commune, and district health services have also been strengthened, but much remains to be done. A special problem in Vietnam is that available facilities—at the commune level in particular—are underutilized. This underscores the need for improved management and incentive systems directly related to outcome-oriented progress indicators (e.g., as regards primary prevention at village and commune levels).

Diversification of Health Services

The private for-profit health care sector has grown rapidly in Vietnam since the government began promoting a policy of diversification. By 1998, about 50% of all hospital consultations were with a private provider (LSMS 1998). The number of private for-profit hospitals is still limited, but there is privatization occurring "from within" at some public hospitals. Private for-profit providers thus constitute an important source of health care, particularly outpatient care.

It is often assumed that ownership status, whether the provider is public or private, does not matter "provided that health practices and health facilities meet certain quality standards and that they are subject to similar levels of managerial flexibility" (WHO 1999). Empirical evidence for this assumption, however, is difficult to find, as the possibilities to guide and regulate the private for-profit health care sector are far less than within the public health care sector. In defining these differences and possibilities, as well as the limitations for strengthening the regulatory role of the government within the private for-profit health care sector, it is necessary to focus on the following dimensions:

Quality control: Quality control is particularly important for small, low-cost, private, for-profit hospitals and individual private providers. The ability to control the quality of private providers is fairly good when they are recognized and licensed. In Vietnam, however, 4600 of 36,000 private for-profit providers are currently working without a license (Dzung 1999). The capacity to supervise the services provided must be increased.

Type of services: Private for-profit providers are unlikely to engage in activities such as community-based health promotion and disease prevention programs. The possibilities for the government to influence the type of services provided by private providers are limited if they are not financed by public funds. Certain agreements can be made, however, for the limited provision of emergency care at high-budget, private, for-profit hospitals regardless of the patient's ability to pay.

Price of care: Private for-profit providers normally charge higher fees than subsidized public health care providers in order to fully recover costs and achieve profitability. The possibilities to regulate the price of care provided on commercial terms are very limited or nonexistent when reduced fees are a real threat to profitability. Fee levels for private for-profit health care services are thus normally determined by the market and not by the government.

Location of care: Most private for-profit providers are found in urban areas and very few, if any, in very poor rural districts. The possibilities for the government to influence the location of private for-profit providers are almost nonexistent. Instead, the regulatory role of the government is to prevent an expanding urban-based private for-profit health sector from undermining the possibilities of recruiting public doctors to poor rural communes.

Provision of drugs: The negative consequences of a partly unregulated market for pharmaceutical products include an irrational and dangerous use of drugs. Today, Vietnam is among the countries with the highest prevalence of antibiotic resistance. Furthermore, the cost of drugs both for public and private purchasers is unnecessarily high. Stricter government control of the drug market has been given high priority, and a new comprehensive drug law will soon be adopted.

Health information: Private for-profit providers do not usually report on a regular basis with regard to number of consultations, type of treatments, and so forth. The possibilities to include them in the routine health information systems as applied by public health care providers are often very limited, sometimes even nonexistent. This implies that an expanding private for-profit health sector reduces the possibilities to develop a good national health information system.

The very limited possibilities to influence—even with a strong regulatory role of the government—the type, price, and locality of services provided by private for-profit providers must be taken into consideration in order to develope an efficient, equity-oriented health care system.

The Way Forward

The alternative policies presented in this chapter need to be further analyzed before they can be used to inform decision making. The tentative long-term strategies to be further explored in Vietnam are as follows:

- Increase public funding for health care services from US$5 per capita to US$8. This amount would ensure that essential preventive and curative health services are provided according to need and at the same time promote a more equitable distribution of the financial burden for these services. Furthermore, additional public funds are necessary to prevent low- and middle-income households from being exposed to economic ruin as a result of health expenditures.

- Expand social health insurance schemes to rural areas by increasing the availability of subsidized health insurance cards and developing community-based health insurance schemes.
- Reduce high hospital fees as public prepayment schemes for health care financing are developed.
- Allocate public funds between provinces/districts according to need and with due consideration of total resources available, taking into account revenue from provincial funds, social health insurance, and user fees.
- Increase the share of total funds used for preventive programs and primary health care, in particular at village and commune levels.
- Strengthen the regulatory role of the government in order to ensure, as far as possible, that the diversification of health care services contributes to, rather than undermines, opportunities to develop an efficient, equity-oriented health care system.

Provided that these policy options are gradually implemented, the long-term vision could include

- Rural public health care services financed mainly by taxes and community contributions via community-based health insurance schemes and foreign aid.
- Urban public health care services financed largely by taxes, but at a somewhat lower level than rural health services, from revenue from compulsory and voluntary health insurance schemes, and with some additional revenue from hospital fees and foreign aid.
- Private for-profit providers fully financed on commercial terms without any public subsidies.

During the latter half of 1999, a top-level committee on health strategies was set up to analyze and discuss options for the future of equitable health care provision in Vietnam. A 10 year plan (2001–2010) for the health sector has recently been submitted by the Ministry of Health to the Prime Minister for approval, stating, as regards health care financing, that "The revenue from social health insurance shall take an increasingly important role in the global budget for health and will gradually take the place of user-fees."

References

Asian Development Bank. 1999. *Health Sector Reform in Asia and the Pacific—Options for Developing Countries.* Manila, Philippines: Asian Development Bank.

Dzung P.H. 1999. *Private Health Services in Vietnam.* Hanoi, Vietnam: World Bank.

LSMS. 1998. Living Standards Measurement Survey, Vietnam 1993 and 1998, Preliminary Results. Hanoi, Vietnam: World Bank.

Phuong D.N. 1999. Efficient and Equity-Oriented Strategies for Health. Presented at the international conference Efficient and Equity-Oriented Strategies for Health, April 1999, Halong Bay, Vietnam.

Saltman R., Figueras J. (eds). 1997. *European Health Sector Reform: Analysis of Current Strategies.* World Health Organization (WHO) Regional Publications, European series No.72. Copenhagen: WHO.

United Nations Development Programme (UNDP). 1999. *Human Development Report 1999.* New York: UNDP.

Vietnam Ministry of Health. 1998. *Vietnam, Health Statistics Yearbook 1998.* Hanoi, Vietnam: Ministry of Health.

Vietnam Ministry of Health. 1997. *Data From the MOH Sentinel Surveillance System 1997.* Hanoi, Vietnam: Ministry of Health.

Vietnam Ministry of Health. 1996. *Strategic Orientation of People's Health Care and Protection in the Period of 1996–2000.* Hanoi, Vietnam: Ministry of Health.

World Health Organization. 1999. *The World Health Report 1999—Making a difference.* Geneva: World Health Organization.

Further Reading

Dung Pham H. 1996. The political process and the private health sector's role in Vietnam. *International Journal of Health Planning and Management* 11:217–230.

Ensor T., San Pham B. 1996. Access and payment for health care: the poor of northern Vietnam. *International Journal of Health Planning and Management* 11:69–83.

Pham Manh Hung, Minas, J.H., Liu, Y., Dahlgren, G., Hsizo, W. 2000. *Efficient Equity-oriented Strategies for Health: International Perspectives—Focus on Vietnam.* Melbourne: The Center for International Mental Health, University of Melbourne.

Sen K., Koivusalo M. 1998. Health care reforms and developing countries—a critical overview. *International Journal of Health Planning and Management* 13:199–215.

Witter S. 1996. Doi Moi and health: the effect of economic reforms on the health system in Vietnam. *International Journal of Health Planning and Management* 11:159–172.

CONCLUSION

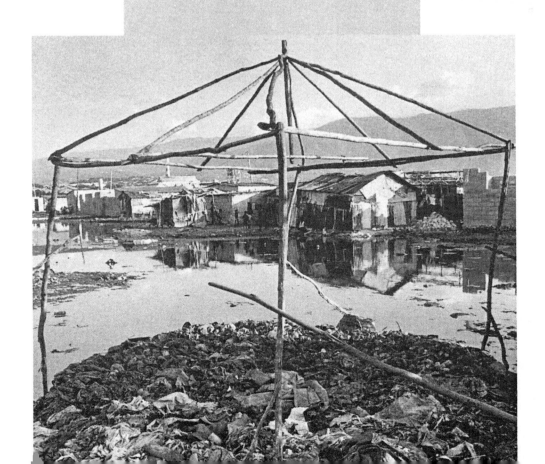

CHAPTER 21

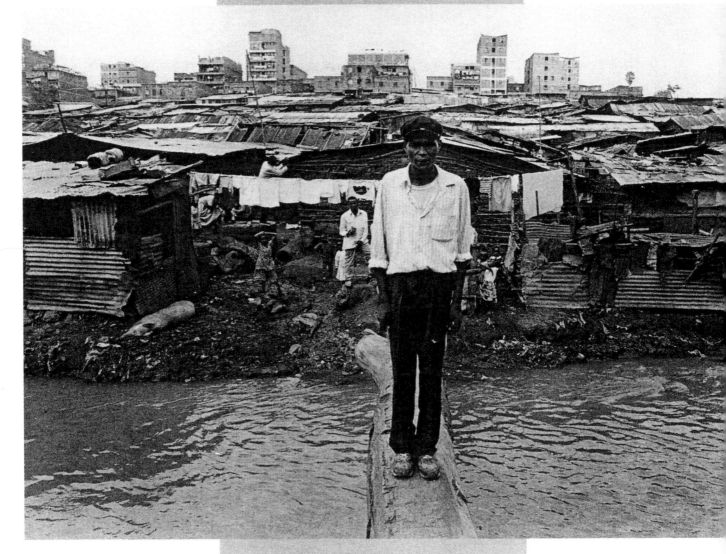

Village One, a notorious slum in Kenya.
Source: Crispin Hughes/Panos.

Developing the Policy Response to Inequities in Health: A Global Perspective

MARGARET WHITEHEAD, GÖRAN DAHLGREN, AND LUCY GILSON

Accumulating evidence across the globe demonstrates that social inequities in health are widespread—in countries of the South as well as the North. The country analyses in this book have provided ample illustrations of this fact. In some cases, the health differences within countries have widened across decades marked out by worsening macroeconomic conditions and increasing socioeconomic crises. At the same time, economic growth in various countries has not necessarily distributed the benefits across all sections of the population. Overall gains in a population's health frequently mask significant and worsening health outcomes for some population groups.

We believe that addressing health inequities is one of the major challenges for policies that aim to promote and sustain population health. The underlying premise of this chapter is that something can and must be done about inequities in health. The evidence that the choice of development policy, for example, makes a significant difference to the heath status of the population as a whole and that differentials in health vary over time and across countries with different policy environments yields the important message that *macroeconomic and social policies do matter* (Radcliffe 1978; Caldwell 1986; Drèze and Sen 1989; Sen 1995;

Dahlgren 1993, 1996; Cornia 1996). In essence, our contention is that it is possible to challenge health inequities with purposeful public policy. Such a challenge is long overdue.

Building a robust and appropriate policy response to health inequities requires action across a broad spectrum of areas: first, establishing values; next, describing and analyzing causes; then, tackling the root causes of inequities; and finally, reducing the negative consequences of being in poor health. This chapter works through these four key elements in turn, drawing lessons from the various analyses presented in this book. A particular effort is made to focus on the practical approaches that address these unacceptable disparities in health. The chapter concludes with some reflections on the opportunities now opening up for a more concerted global response to this major challenge.

Element I: Establishing Shared Values

Any planned response to the gross and pervasive inequities in health must acknowledge right from the start that action involves ethical and political choices—and therefore has to be based on a firm foundation of shared values within a society. Developing value-driven policy action is, however, particularly challenging in the current global context. Economic, social, and health policies have increasingly sacrificed ethical concerns in the race to contain costs and in the pursuit of "efficiency" (Gilson 1998, 2000). Therefore, an essential first step is to demonstrate the injustice and unfairness of present economic and social arrangements while making explicit the values on which proposed action is based. A start can be made by

- Setting equity objectives and targets for policy
- Subjecting existing and proposed developments to health equity impact assessment

Setting Health Equity Objectives

Establishing a consensus on societal values for policy may seem a daunting task, but it is worth remembering that through international agreements many countries have already committed themselves to health and health care policies with common equity objectives. Several international documents, including the seminal 1948 United Nations Declaration of Human Rights and the 1977 World Health Organization (WHO) Health For All Policy, state that social inequalities should be reduced and that access to good quality health services should be increased and provided according to need. Likewise, the International Conference on Population and Development 1994 in Cairo and the Fourth World Conference on Women 1995 in Beijing catalyzed global solidarity in gender equity in health and other social spheres.

Equity objectives tend to be of two types: symbolic, their main purpose being to inspire and motivate; and practical or action targets, to help monitor progress toward equity and to improve accountability in the use of resources (Whitehead et al. 1998). The two types are mutually supportive in shaping policy action. Such targets are instrumental at global, regional, and national levels.

At a global level, the Organization for Economic Cooperation and Development called upon its Development Assistance Committee to establish International Development Targets (IDTs) that articulate economic and social goals to be achieved by all countries by the year 2015. The economic target aims at reducing the proportion of people living in extreme poverty by 50%. Of concern, the health targets are general and therefore lack an equity focus. As Gwatkin (2000) demonstrates, achieving the overall goal of reducing infant mortality by two-thirds in each developing country can

be reached through many different routes. The most likely of these routes will disproportionately improve infant health in the upper and middle income groups, thereby increasing poor–rich gaps in infant mortality. Most concerning is the possibility that the target could be achieved without improving the infant mortality for the poorest quintile of the population. It is argued, therefore, that the IDTs for health should incorporate equity objectives to ensure improving health among the poor (Gwatkin 2000).

The symbolic "Target One" of the WHO European Region's Health for All strategy (first set in 1985, to which all 50 countries in Europe signed up) has done much to focus attention on the equity issues: "By the year 2000, the differences in health status between countries and between groups within countries should be reduced by at least 25%, by improving the level of health of disadvantaged nations and groups" (WHO 1985). Adoption of this symbolic target spurred important developments in the conceptualization, measurement, and articulation of pragmatic equity policies (Dahlgren and Whitehead 1992; Kunst and Mackenbach 1995; Gunning-Schepers 1989).

After years of lobbying from the public health community in the United Kingdom, the latest national health strategy for England has at last acknowledged the centrality of equity for promoting population health and has set one of its two key aims as "to improve the health of the worst off in society and to narrow the health gap" (U.K. Department of Health 1999). In addition, all local statutory agencies are now required to set local targets for reducing health inequalities and to specify plans to meet those targets. Similarly, in January 2000, the U.S. Department of Health and Human Services released national health goals for the decade to 2010, with one of the two overarching goals for the United States being to eliminate health disparities between different segments of the population, including those related to gender, race, education, income, disability, rural location, and sexual orientation (U.S. Department of Health and Human Services 2000).

The uptake of symbolic targets has not been limited to Northern countries. Triggered by the grossly unjust policies that prevailed under the apartheid regime in South Africa, for example, symbolic equity goals are now at the heart of social policy development in that country. The government's White Paper, *The Transformation of the Health System,* states that the overall vision for the health sector includes playing a part in promoting equity within society as a whole by developing a single, unified health system (Republic of South Africa 1997). In addition, the country's new constitution includes a Bill of Rights that encompasses socio-

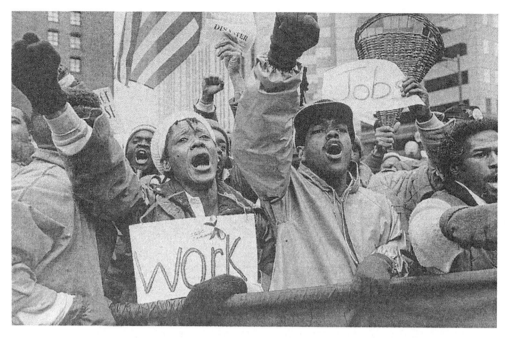

Protests against welfare cuts in Ohio, the United States.
Source: Piet van Lier/Impact Visuals/Picture Quest.

economic rights such as to health care. Likewise, the commitment to gender equity enshrined in the Bangladeshi Constitution has legitimized a groundswell of activities advancing the status and well being of women, thereby challenging pervasive cultural norms. Politically, the potential power of such explicit objectives should not be underestimated. These represent useful tools in the attempts to establish the legitimacy of work toward health equity.

More practical, action-oriented targets have recently been announced for Sweden (SOU 1999), focused on tackling the wider determinants of inequities in health, such as income disparities, poverty, marginalization, and poor working environment. For example, for the stated strategy of strengthening the social cohesion and solidarity of Swedish society by the year 2010, the following targets have been set (SOU 1999):

- Income disparities should not increase beyond the present level of a GINI of 0.25.
- Prevalence of poverty (EU definition) should be reduced to less than 4%.
- Long-term dependence on social welfare should be reduced to under 1% and homelessness should be reduced to under 0.05%.
- Political marginalization should be reduced through increasing voting rates in deprived suburban areas.
- Suicide rates should be reduced by 25% from present level of 21 per 100,000.

Setting equity objectives is only the first step in establishing shared values. There is often a gap between stated objectives and how the policies are implemented on the ground. Both the implementation and outcomes of policy therefore need to be monitored and judged against the original equity objectives. At the heart of the monitoring issue is the definition of effectiveness, defined in our analysis as the degree to which the effort expended, or the action taken, achieves the desired result or objective (Slee et al. 1996). In other words, effectiveness must be related to overall objectives. Consequently, if the equity dimension is explicit, then the central focus is on how to achieve this politically determined objective in the most cost-effective way. This contrasts with the more common approach, which sets equity in conflict—or as a trade-off—with efficiency.

Making Health Equity Impact Assessments

The emphasis on underlying values and recognition of the wider determinants of health inequities carries with it an obligation (or the imperative) to undertake heath equity impact assessments. Policies and programmes in a wide range of sectors must be subjected to such assessments so that "unhealthy policies" can be identified and "healthier" ones developed. The focus of the assessment process should be the impact of policies on the health and circumstances of the most vulnerable sections of society relative to other population groups. The field of environmental impact assessment is instructive with regard to its emphasis on prospectively identifying negative impact on ecosystems (Vanclay and Bronstein 1995).

Similarly, the idea of "gender mainstreaming" that emerged from the U.N. World Conferences on Women provides important insights into and experience with the application of equity lenses (Standing 1999). A parallel means of assessing health impact (Birley 1995; Birley et al. 1998; Lehto and Ritsatakis 1999), and more specifically health *equity* impact, must be defined and accepted as standard practice (Acheson et al. 1998; Scott-Samuel 1998; Whitehead et al. 2000).

One example of a health impact assessment that takes equity into consideration was carried out on the European Union's Common Agricultural Policy—a major policy with a budget of about 40 billion ECU a year (roughly equivalent to US$40 billion), aimed at regulating food and agricultural production in 15 countries in Europe (Dahlgren et al. 1997). This study concluded that the regulations governing the growing and distribution of fruits and vegetables, for example, created a financial barrier for low-income consumers to afford a nutritious diet. Even more striking was the fact that cultivation and production of tobacco—primarily for export to developing countries—was heavily subsidized by scarce public funds (see also chapter 4). Agricultural policies such as these are seen as a significant obstacle to improved health, in particular among disadvantaged groups. It was clear from the analysis, however, that there were practical possibilities for changing the regulations to make the policy more health enhancing (Dahlgren et al. 1997).

In the current context of rapid globalization, with its attendant propensity to generate disparities, there is a rich agenda of issues that urgently need analysis through an equity lens. For example, the effect of global ecological changes on human health (such as climate changes, depletion of resources including food stocks, environmental damage arising from increased economic activity; see chapter 4) are a ripe subject for health equity impact assessment. Furthermore, the World Trade Organization's recent negotiations could have profound implications for the ability of states to maintain equitable health, education, and social services (Price et al. 1999). This development re-emphasizes the need to assess prospectively and retrospectively both the positive and negative effects on health of various policies, interventions, and actions.

This is not an argument for stand-alone health equity impact assessments, but rather a call for an equity-oriented lens—encompassing, among others, health, environment, and gender concerns—for the prospective analysis of economic and development policies.

Element II: Assessing and Analyzing the Health Divide

Describing Inequities in Health

Another key element in any strategy to tackle health inequity is to assess the size and nature of the problem. In this respect we start with the following assertions— first, that health measures based on population averages are not reliable guides to what may be happening to the health of different groups in society; and second, it is *always* possible (and necessary) to make some assessment of the health divide. What is surprising is that such analysis is still not yet routine practice. Many national databases are analyzed by averages only, undifferentiated by gender, area, ethnicity or socioeconomic characteristics. Differentiation by social groupings should be as natural as the current universal practice of describing the health status of different age groups.

Even if data-poor countries are limited to basic descriptions from the available statistics or from more qualitative assessments, these can still be valuable in providing policy-relevant information on the equity situation in a country (see chapter 12 on Tanzania and chapter 15 on Kenya). Regional differences, for example, may be gleaned from health care statistics and hospital records and backed up by population-based surveys to inform resource allocation (as in Mexico; see chapter 19). In sub-Saharan Africa, where reliable data on health are most scarce, a resourceful group— comprising over 20 computer-connected, district demographic surveillance sites—is compiling the best health data for populations that are otherwise invisible and neglected. Recent analyses have disaggregated Demographic and Health Survey (DHS) data, often the most reliable population health data in data-poor countries, into income quintiles derived from a household asset index. This analysis has highlighted dramatic socioeconomic gradients in health across about 50 of the poorest countries in the world using a data source not originally designed for this purpose (Pande and Gwatkin 1999). Analyses by gender should be possible in nearly all cases and are essential to equity studies. Some countries may be able to go further in analyzing health data by ethnic group or by socioeconomic characteristics, such as education and income, while the data-rich countries will be able to add to these descriptions with more sophisticated measures.

It is also important to analyze the prevalence of not only health and disease in different population groups but also *differentials in exposure* to health hazards, in behavioral risk factors, in opportunities and barriers to adopting a healthier lifestyle or to gaining access to essential goods and services, and in the costs and benefits of macroeconomic policies. To do so, monitoring must be improved and socioeconomic variables must be added to health information systems. Conversely, more health information could be added to routine socioeconomic data collection. Chapter 5 on measurement issues outlines a set of principles and indicators that inform the analysis of health differentials within societies.

Analyzing Causes and Understanding Pathways

Many of the causes of inequities in health are social in origin. Considering the magnitude of the problem from a human development and well-being point of view, it is striking how little systematic research has been done on the social causes of ill health. Furthermore, it is equally striking that the now emerging literature on the social determinants of health has been predominantly concentrated in the North. Diderichsen's model (see chapter 2) outlines a valuable framework for understanding how health inequities are generated and maintained in a society. This model provides both a theoretical and a practical tool for analyzing which causes are important for a particular country, at different points in the pathways from social position to disease/disability, and looking both upstream and downstream.

Starting at the "upstream" end of the pathways, with social context and social position and their relationships to health, it is possible to consider the impact of macroeconomic and social policies on life chances and ultimately on health status for different groups in the population. Equally, searching "downstream" is also necessary in order to trace the physiological mechanisms by which specific risk factors or risk conditions actually generate/cause different diseases or poorer health. Not to be forgotten is the imperative of moving back "upstream" to understand how the sick and disabled are dealt with differentially by health and social systems. Above all, the accumulating evidence on the social origins of inequities in health highlights the need to tackle the root causes of poor health, not just the symptoms. In this respect, it should be recognized that

- Determinants of inequities may be different from determinants of aggregate health. For example, in modern-day Sweden, while poor physical working conditions play only a minor role as an influence on the health status of the population as a whole, they explain a large proportion of

the differences in health between different occupational groups in the country. Policies specifically designed to reduce inequities in health in Sweden, therefore, may need to focus more strongly on improving the work environment, while a general health promotion policy may focus on other determinants of health (Dahlgren 1997). In Chile, although cardiovascular disease is the leading cause of death, road traffic accidents actually prove to account for much of the disparity in longevity between the least and most educated (see chapter 10).

- The possible synergy between risk factors needs to be considered, in particular when analyzing social inequities in health, as risks to health tend to accumulate in sections of the population already experiencing disadvantage. The effect of a certain risk factor might therefore be different depending on the social position of an individual. The framework presented in chapter 2 provides the methodology for distinguishing empirically between differential exposure and differential vulnerability in particular circumstances. This methodology is employed in the Anglo-Swedish case in chapter 17, in which the two countries provide an illustration of a "natural experiment," offering the opportunity of carrying out comparative analysis of the different policies in the two countries to help make a more robust health impact assessment.

Element III: Tackling Root Causes

Once the health divide in a country has been described and the causes analyzed, the most critical element of a strategy to promote health equity is to identify points of entry for action on root causes. The main determinants of health *in general* can be thought of as layers of influence (Fig. 1). Individuals have age, sex, and constitutional characteristics that influence their health (largely fixed), but surrounding them are influences that are modifiable by policy. First, there are personal, behavioral factors such as smoking habits, sexual behavior, and physical activity. Second, individuals interact with peers and their immediate community and come under social and community influences, factors represented in the next layer. The wider influences on a person's ability to maintain health (in the third layer) include their living and working conditions, food supplies, and access to essential goods and services. Finally, as an overarching mediator of population health, there are the economic, cultural and environmental conditions prevailing in society as a whole. Figure 1 emphasizes interactions: Individual lifestyles are embedded in social and community networks, and in living and working conditions, which in turn are related to the wider cultural and socioeconomic environment.

Drawing on this general model, below we focus on policy options for those determinants that play a par-

Figure 1 A conceptual model of the main determinants of health—
layers of influence

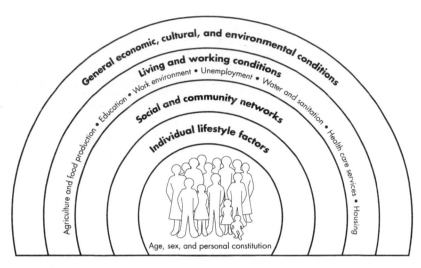

Source: Adapted from Dahlgren and Whitehead 1991.

ticularly major role in generating inequities in health in developing countries, although most are just as relevant to the situation in developed nations. Country-specific analyses are always necessary to take the assessment further, but some general lessons can be gleaned from the Global Health Equity Initiative (GHEI) studies and others about the most effective policy options to tackle root causes (Whitehead 1995; Dahlgren 1997).

Promoting Healthy Macropolicies

The overarching macroeconomic, cultural, and environmental conditions prevailing in a country are of paramount importance in the pathways to inequities in health in developing countries. They are therefore key policy entry points in the promotion of health equity.

First, in relation to macroeconomic policies, it needs to be acknowledged that absolute poverty is still the major risk factor for poor health and premature death globally. The pathways leading from poverty to poor health include inadequate nutrition and lack of access to other prerequisites for health, such a decent housing, sanitation, and clean water. In addition, the evidence on the psychosocial effects of relative poverty, or social inequality, on ill health is also mounting. Wide income inequalities, for example, are associated with indicators of social breakdown and more threatening, stressful environments. Large and increasing income inequities may have a negative effect on health conditions

for the whole population, not just the poorest, as the economic divide promotes social segregation, threatens community values, and thus creates a culture that generates, rather than prevents, violence (Kawachi and Kennedy 1997; Lomas 1998; Kawachi et al. 1999).

Consequently, as discussed above, a health equity impact analysis should inform the articulation of macroeconomic policy. When this is done, it becomes clear that some of the "unhealthy" economic policies are ones based on the widespread view that economic growth should/must occur at any cost, disregarding any adverse impacts on sections of the population. There is now a wealth of experience from around the world on the adverse health effects of macroeconomic policies focused primarily on growth, as eloquently elaborated in the provocatively titled book *Dying for Growth* (Kim et al. 2000). In this respect, a number of the case studies in this volume—on Russia, Chile, and China—bear witness to these adverse effects.

In Russia, the 1992 liberalization of prices and the termination of state subsidies in many sectors of the economy coincided with an acute crisis in the economy. During this period, liberal monetary and macroeconomic measures were not accompanied by compensatory social policies, with disastrous results for the health and welfare of the population, especially the poorer, less educated groups (see chapter 11). Chile and China are both countries that have gone through major economic, political, and demographic transitions over the past 20 years, and both have experienced substantial economic growth, but with widening income inequalities and debates, at least in Chile, about the extent to which the poorer sections of the population have benefited from the economic growth. Although population health on average has improved in both countries, the transition has also been accompanied by increasing inequities in health.

Conversely, the "healthy" economic policies are those that contribute to alleviating poverty and that reduce income inequalities. There is evidence, for example, that it is possible for development strategies to be "pro-growth and pro-poor" by which macroeconomic policies support social policies that deliver services such as primary education and preventive health care, which both have greatest benefit for the poor and high social rates of return (Tanzi 1998). This highlights another important element of macroeconomic policies—their impact on health inequities through their prescriptions on public sector expenditures. Drèze and Sen (1989) emphasize the real potential for a strategy of "support-led security," rooted in direct public support for education, health care, and food, to tackle deprivation even at low levels of income and economic growth.

Second, the overall cultural environment can be improved by pro-equity public policy. The position of women in society or of ethnic minorities, for example, can be greatly influenced by purposeful national action. Countries such as Bangladesh and the Indian State of Kerala, for example, as detailed in chapter 13, have demonstrated this with their dynamic policies of increasing the literacy rate, particularly female literacy, and improving the empowerment and human rights of women, enshrining those rights in the constitution and in law. The role of education in achieving and sustaining greater equity in health is paramount. There are lifelong and intergenerational health benefits arising from the promotion of universal education (Caldwell 1986; see also chapter 8). Furthermore, education may act as a buffer against the adverse health effects associated with increasing economic inequality (see chapters 10 and 11).

Third, hazard control policies in the physical environment are critical at both national and international levels. A poignant example comes from Vietnam, where the country's health system has to deal with the long-term environmental, social, economic, and health problems created by the aftermath of weapons of war, such as Agent Orange. The issue of industrialized countries "exporting" or dumping their toxic waste on the developing world is another example of an environmental cause of injustice. Even within countries, it is noticeable that environmental hazards and degradation are not distributed evenly, but tend to be clustered around where the poorer sections of the population live or work (McLaren et al. 1999). This situation can be a side effect of unhealthy economic policies in which the pursuit of financial profits is given priority over the health of employees and local residents. Recognition of this fact has led in recent years to a growing Environmental Justice movement, advocating policies that redress these excess exposures to environmental hazards.

Improving Living and Working Conditions

The classic public health endeavors to improve living and working conditions and access to essential services, such as education and health care, still have a vital role to play in promoting health equity. Groups experiencing social and material disadvantages are often the ones exposed to the most health-damaging environments. This is painfully obvious in relation to the living conditions experienced in shanty-towns in poor countries, as well as segregated poor urban areas in richer ones. In Mexico, roughly 58% of the indigenous people lack running water and 88% have no sewage facilities. Provision of this basic infrastructure is a prerequisite to reducing the disproportionate burden of diarrheal and other communicable diseases in this group (see chapter 19). Even in a wealthy country like the United States, evidence on the determinants of poor health point to inadequate access of substantial sections of the population to healthy living and working conditions and to essential services, such as an adequate social security system and health care coverage (see chapter 9).

One of the starkest illustrations of the pathways leading from inequitable housing and work policies to disadvantages in many spheres of life, including health, is given in chapter 14, where the apartheid system in South Africa had severe consequences for the nonwhite majority. This resulted in large sections of the population living in poverty, in squalor, and without the basic prerequisites for good health. South Africa is now trying to deal with this legacy of apartheid by implementing policies with explicit equity objectives.

Building Social Cohesion and Mutual Support

Some commentators believe that the most health-damaging effects of social inequality are those that exclude people from taking part in society, denying them self-respect and dignity (Wilkinson 1996; Sen 1999). The negative health effects of social exclusion are increasingly recognized—the exclusion and powerlessness that comes with lack of money, lack of education, and lack of influence.

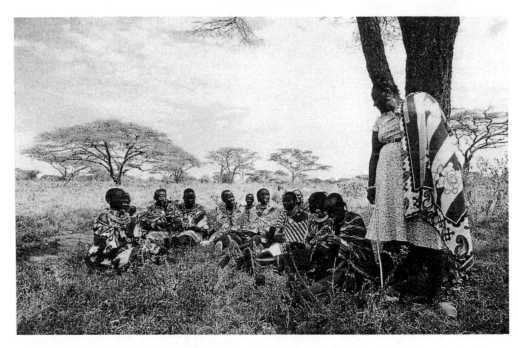

Masai women's co-op meeting, Kenya.
Source: Neil Cooper/Panos.

The challenge is to open up opportunities for everyone in the population, not just for the people who have the loudest voice, at the same time building up conditions in society that offer greater mutual support (Drèze and Sen 1989; Gilson 2000). Policy options at this level include building inclusive social welfare systems (in which everyone contributes and everyone benefits); implementing initiatives to strengthen, and to make it easier for people to participate in, the democratic process; designing facilities to encourage meeting and social interaction in communities; and promoting schemes that enable people to work collectively on their identified priorities for health. These options must give explicit weight to the most disenfranchised, including ethnic and racial minorities, women, and the poor.

The Bangladesh country analysis in chapter 16 provides an example of action on several levels, including strengthening mutual support in communities to promote the rights and status of the poorest women in that society. Development policies in one region in particular, Matlab, have emphasized complementary improvements in access to health care, combined with strategies to reduce poverty and increase the status of women. Among these strategies, participatory microcredit schemes linked to employment for women have been vigorously promoted, together with the provision of more places in schools for the daughters of poor families. The microcredit schemes involve groups of women in poor rural villages meeting together to pool funds. These funds are then used to provide loans at affordable interest rates to members of their group to set up small businesses and stimulate employment opportunities in the community. The scheme is controlled and run by the women themselves—an important aspect of the strategy for improving not only the women's economic position but also their status within the prevailing culture. The chapter provides compelling evidence of a health equity dividend.

Creating Supportive Environments for Behavioral Changes

The pathways linking socioeconomic position to health-damaging behavior highlight the need to take into account the structural barriers to healthier lifestyles and the creation of supportive environments. The research evidence clearly indicates the importance of structurally determined lifestyles, rather than freely chosen lifestyles, among less privileged socioeconomic groups. In short, the evidence reinforces the need for combining structural changes related to economic, living, and working conditions with health education efforts when trying to influence lifestyle factors such as smoking, use of violence, alcohol intake, diet, and sexual behaviors. Furthermore, general policies for health promotion and disease prevention need to be based on the reality ex-

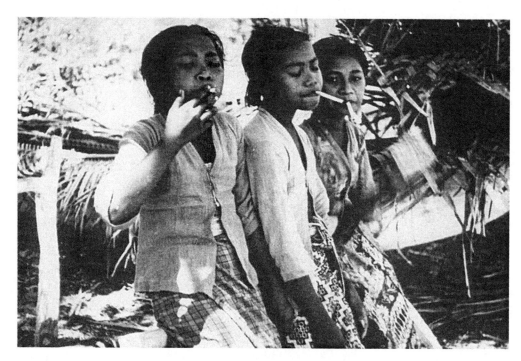

Young girls smoking in Bali, Indonesia.
Source: Culver Pictures/Picture Quest.

perienced by socioeconomically less privileged groups rather than on that of the middle classes (Townsend 1987; Townsend et al. 1993). Tobacco control policies will be of the utmost importance for population health in many developing countries in the coming decade, as the growing opportunities to market tobacco products are aggressively exploited by the major producers in industrialized countries. Once again, it is the poorest countries, and the health of the poor within those countries, that will suffer the most from this trade. Policies will be needed at all levels—from global to local, and from legal and fiscal to community development and individual support—to regulate this threat to health equity.

Another example of the type of policy action relevant to this discussion of behavioral factors is provided by the Kenyan analysis of road traffic accidents in chapter 15. The study demonstrates that taking a broad perspective in developing policy action is important even when the determinants appear to be behavioral. Seeing the reckless behavior of the drivers of *matatus* (i.e., private minibuses) as the major determinant of road traffic accidents previously led policy proposals to a narrow focus on modifying the individual behavior of drivers. The current study, however, revealed the complex linkages between driver behavior and the way the

transport industry is organized, the long hours and employment conditions of drivers, the lack of safer alternatives for low-income passengers, and the role of bribery in the feeble enforcement of road safety laws. The study points to the futility of exacting massive fines on individual drivers. Such action is likely only to exacerbate the problem in the absence of a more comprehensive attempt to address the social and economic context underlying poor driver behavior and traffic accidents.

The Tanzanian country analysis in chapter 12 also illustrates insights from taking into account the lives and livelihoods of vulnerable adolescents rather than the standard approach of scrutinizing their sexual behavior in isolation. It reveals that those who are not in school may face immediate physical health hazards, such as dangerous work environments, unsanitary living conditions, and poor access to food and essential health care. For many there are additional emotional and social health hazards as they attempt to survive in lonely and unprotected circumstances, separated from their families. Their sexual behavior (and related morbidity and mortality), the study argues, has to be seen in the light of these interwoven economic, social, and cultural factors if effective policy responses are to be formulated.

Element IV: Building Equitable Health Care Systems

A critical dimension of social and economic policies for health equity (not mentioned thus far) is, of course, the health care system. There are important welfare issues concerned with improving the quality of life of people who are *already* sick. The issue of how to ameliorate their ill health and reduce the socioeconomic consequences of illness is a concern in all societies. The fourth element of a policy response is therefore concerned with building more equitable health systems, with the dual purpose of removing barriers to access to good quality health care while at the same time preventing the health care system itself from contributing to poverty and other adverse consequences.

Impoverishment and Barriers to Access

The fact that ill health often leads to impoverishment is of major concern. Moreover, the very fact that people experiencing social and economic disadvantage tend to be sicker raises fundamental issues for the organization of health systems. It means, for example, that their need for health care services is greater and would require more resources per capita to meet that need. Despite overwhelming evidence of greater need, a common finding is that health services are sparser and of poorer quality in areas serving populations experiencing disadvantage and access is more difficult—the so-called inverse care law (Tudor Hart 1971). A wide literature proves the tenaciousness of this maxim, showing repeatedly that the lower the level of income, the larger the gap between health needs and utilization of health services (Makinen et al. 2000; Castor-leal et al. 1999). There are several dimensions of access to which the inverse care law can be seen to apply:

- **Financial access:** User charges are often prohibitive. High user fees not only reduce access and utilization of health services but also force people to bypass medical personnel when in need of drugs. Furthermore, economic growth is not enough to increase access to health services. In fact, recent experience in Asia indicates the opposite trend, that is, rapid economic growth tends to generate or spur increasing inequities in access.
- **Geographical or physical access:** There may be uneven distribution between urban and rural areas, most acute in a predominantly agrarian society, or concentration of the system on providing tertiary services that reach relatively few while primary care services that would benefit many are neglected.
- **Cultural access:** Negative attitudes of health workers to poor people often discourage poor people from using the services. Discrimination against girls and women for health

care when resources are scarce (see chapter 13) and against ethnic minorities is also an important issue. Amartya Sen has highlighted a further issue related to "cultural access" concerned with differing perceptions of ill health: an acceptance of one's lot among people experiencing disadvantage, when there is no scientific reason for accepting such poor health from conditions that could be prevented or at least ameliorated by good quality health care (Sen 1999).

All three aspects are vividly illustrated in relation to gender inequities in access to care in the developing world, where women use health services less than men (WHO 1995). Due to a deadly combination of financial, geographical, and cultural barriers, women's access to high quality health care is compromised, often costing them their lives, particularly around the time of labor and delivery (WHO 1998a; Thaddeus and Maine 1994; see also chapter 13).

Building an Equity-Oriented Health System

To address issues of access and impoverishment, there are many factors to consider, including

- How to mobilize financial resources in order to improve access
- How to allocate those resources equitably in relation to need
- How to monitor the use of available resources to ensure that they are being deployed to meet the stated equity objectives.

Mobilizing financial resources

The costs of health care services are paid for by the citizens of a country via taxes, social health insurance, community-based insurance schemes, private health insurance, and/or direct user fees. Foreign aid can also provide health care financing in low-income countries. The mix of these different sources determines to a great extent how the financial burden for health care costs is shared between different age and social groups, as well as how available resources can be utilized. The choice of financing options should be guided by the following equity principles:

- The mobilization of financial resources should be based on contributions from the population as a whole and should be progressive, that is, according to ability to pay
- Financial protection should be optimized by pooling risks among the largest number of people to avoid impoverishment due to high medical expenses.

Despite these clear principles there is no global blueprint for an equitable and sustainable financial system. This is due in part to the multiple stakeholders involved in health care financing, the dynamics of the public–

private mix characterized primarily by increased private sector and reduced public sector presence, and the pervasive trends toward decentralization of health systems. Nonetheless, using the principles outlined above, a set of policy lessons can be drawn from experiences gained in high- as well as in low-income countries:

- Taxes, including payroll taxes and subsidized community health insurance schemes, constitute the fundamental basis of an equitable financial system for health.
- Any shift, at a given level of services, from tax to, for example, direct user fees increases the burden of payment on economically less privileged groups, reduces access, and may generate a serious poverty trap.
- Private, for-profit health insurance schemes, direct user fees for public health services, and direct fees to private for-profit schemes produce substantial, and over time usually increasing, inequities in terms of financing, access, and financial security.

The Vietnamese case study in chapter 20 illustrates how one country has been struggling with such major financing issues and the complexities behind some of the decisions that have to be made when there is so little room for maneuvering. In such circumstances, however, the importance of analyzing the health sector reforms from an equity perspective is greater than ever.

Allocating financial resources according to need

A key equity principle is that resources should be allocated according to need, regardless of ability to pay. In practice, this can be promoted by devising more equitable resource allocation mechanisms for commissioning health care, with need for care assessed not only based on size and age structure of the population but also according to disease burden and socioeconomic characteristics.

- The allocation of available resources *between* different areas should be based on an assessment of need for health services, for example, as related to the age, disease burden, and socioeconomic structure of the population.
- The allocation of available resources for health *within* a specific area should be determined by perceived as well as by professionally defined need for health services, regardless of age, sex, ethnic background, and ability to pay.

Above all, this requires taking into account the identified social gradients in mortality and morbidity that exist and that indicate differential levels of need in different places and for different groups of people. In Britain and Sweden, for example, funds from general taxation are allocated on a geographic basis to official health authorities to cover the health care needs of the residents in each administrative area. Both countries have selected lack of employment and living alone as important indicators of increased need for health care

resources. Sweden has added indicators of housing tenure (Diderichsen et al. 1997), while Britain has taken into account the proportion of households with single parents, as well as direct health indicators (Carr-Hill et al. 1994).

South Africa provides an example of the potential for and problems associated with trying to develop allocation formulas adjusted for need in a data-scarce system (Doherty and van Den Heever 1998). Similar issues arise for other countries introducing reforms in which the function of commissioning services is separated from the provision of care or in which there is decentralization of budgets and control to local areas. The Chinese country analysis in chapter 7, for example, highlights a particular problem of resource allocation in this respect. Administrative areas that were relatively well-off used to be able to subsidize more disadvantaged areas, but this is no longer the case following health sector reform in the country because of decentralization. In the poorer regions, where the tax base is smaller, there is now less money for health services and these services are at risk of serious decline, while the services in the more affluent areas are in a position to expand and improve. Unless mechanisms can be devised to cross-subsidize, the inequities are bound to increase still further. Similar problems arise under user-fee systems where revenues collected at the point of provision cannot be used to improve services elsewhere (Russell and Gilson 1997).

Vigilance in Monitoring and Protecting Equity

The need to maintain equitable health systems has become more pressing since the early 1980s, as many countries have had to face both economic recession and rising unemployment, pushing more people into poverty and ill health (Whitehead 1992). This situation is made worse by cost-containment measures (or budget cuts) in health systems in response to the economic climate and the introduction of market-oriented health sector reforms (Gilson 1998; Whitehead 1994; Dahlgren 1994b). For many countries, though, the pressing task is to maintain the access that has been achieved in the face of mounting forces working against this aim (Dahlgren 1994a; Gilson et al. 1995). It is particularly important to develop tools and approaches for monitoring and protecting equity in such circumstances.

One equity-monitoring approach is provided by the "benchmarks of fairness" concept. This originated in the context of the U.S. health care reform efforts of 1993 as a means of making explicit in a systematic way the ethical dimensions and trade-offs inherent in the health care system (Daniels et al. 1996). In the U.S. context, benchmarks queried the following equity dimensions of health care reform proposals: the provision of universal access to services; the comprehensiveness of services; uniformity of benefits; equitable financing by ability to pay; value for money (clinical and financial efficiency); public accountability; and degree of consumer choice. Interestingly, efficiency was one of the criteria under a broad enquiry into equity. Since this application in the U.S. context, the "benchmarks of fairness" idea has been initiated in several developing countries, including Thailand, Pakistan, Mexico, and Colombia.

In such settings, new benchmarks have been added as different social determinants of health are highlighted in these diverse contexts. The range of benchmarks discussed in Pakistan, for example, includes benchmarks for intersectoral public health; financial barriers to equitable access; nonfinancial barriers to access (including gender); comprehensiveness of benefits and tiering; equitable financing; effectiveness, efficiency, and quality of health care; administrative efficiency; democratic accountability; and, finally, patient and provider autonomy (Khan 1999). In addition to provoking debate about health care systems within particular countries, the benchmarks have potential to be developed into a useful mechanism for comparing the relative equity of different countries' health systems (Daniels et al. 1996; Khan 1999).

South Africa provides a further example of an explicit equity-monitoring approach. As detailed in chapter 14, the paucity and nature of the available data must be addressed within efforts to allow the impact of new programs on the apartheid legacy of inequity to be monitored (Bloom and McIntyre 1998). One monitoring system that is being developed within South Africa is the "equity gauge." This approach engages legislators at national and subnational levels in monitoring the impact of government policy actions on the health system (Ntuli et al. 1999). The "gauge" monitors equity in health and health care and feeds this information into parliamentary and legislative processes related to health policy and resource allocation.

Strategies for a Global Response

Over and above specific policy actions, what could and should a more concerted global effort to redress inequities in health entail in the immediate future? A number of strategies have been effective at creating a climate for policy change, and some new approaches hold promise for the future. It is important to recognize the two-way traffic in ideas and strategies: from global to local and from local to global. On the one hand, policy developments in other countries or agencies can be valuable in raising awareness and stirring political response closer to home. On the other hand, greater understanding of how inequities in health come about, gleaned from experiences gained locally, can provide some of the most powerful ammunition for global advocacy. Most importantly, perhaps, is the recognition that equity in health is a common challenge to all societies and thus requires an integrated global response.

Taking Advantage of Current Experience and Opportunities in Developing Policy Action

Knowledge about research and policy gained from developments around the world could be used much more systematically to gain entry into national debates, although there is always a need to be sensitive to time and context in a particular country when drawing lessons from elsewhere. First, much more could be made of the power of comparison in spurring national action. For example, researchers and public health advocates in Europe have been successful in raising and maintaining awareness of health equity issues among national policy makers through a diversity of approaches—ranging from a careful consensus building approach in the Netherlands, to a more confrontational strategy in the United Kingdom, and to a stance built on arguments of social justice in Sweden (Whitehead 1998). Despite this diversity, what has been most striking about the European developments is the reinforcing effect of events in one country on the situation in the others. Progress in one country has been used to stimulate or legitimize work toward health equity in others. The fact that the Dutch government set up a prestigious national program of research on inequities in health, for example, helped to persuade other governments to follow suit. The Dutch initiative itself had in part been triggered by the interest stimulated by the British *Black Report,* which also set off a spate of investigations around the world, with countries producing their own "Black Reports" on the extent of inequities in health in their society.

The time has come to marshal these experiences, learning from the mistakes as well as the successes, to strengthen the impact of existing efforts. A more critical challenge, however, in keeping with the themes of this volume, is to extend the burgeoning interest in health inequities to developing countries. Encouraging in this regard are the emergence of global efforts aimed at the reduction of poverty broadly defined. The World Bank's explicit focus on the poor—as exemplified in their *World Development Report 2000/2001*—the G-8–supported Highly Indebted Poor Country (HIPC) initiative for debt relief, and the civil society–led protests for greater transparency of global trade and economic policies are enhancing prospects for concerted action toward distributive justice.

Second, collective setting of international standards, targets, and resolutions can improve the political climate within countries providing impetus to local advocacy efforts or even helping to shape national public health strategies. In this respect, the setting of equity targets in the WHO (1998b) renewal of Health For All in 1998 should not be underestimated as a future lever for change. The UN Conference on Population and Development, Cairo, 1994, continues to aid the recasting of population policies in terms of health, empowerment, and rights of women in many developing countries (Sen et al. 1994). As mentioned earlier, it is particularly important to place equity- or distribution-sensitive targets on the international agenda (Gwatkin 2000).

Third, much can be achieved by taking advantage of windows of opportunity that unexpectedly arise. The global wave of democratization represents one such phenomenon. As Amartya Sen points out, "the absence of democracy is in itself an inequality—in this case of political rights and powers." The strengths of democracy—participation, civil rights, and liberties—are tied to a society's ability to stem inequality, provide security and protection for all citizens, and prevent major catastrophes such as famine (Sen 1999: 187). Despite formidable obstacles in the aftermath of apartheid in South Africa, the advent of democratic elections has resulted in an upsurge of political and popular will to build a fairer society. Similarly, transitions from states of conflict and insecurity to peace and responsible governance provide a solid foundation and fresh hope for redressing long-standing inequities.

Developing the Capacity for Monitoring and Advocacy

Awareness of health equity as an international issue has reached the point where sufficient momentum has built up to stimulate the types of collaborative action that are necessary to monitor and advocate for health eq-

uity worldwide. The types of practical initiatives that need to be taken include

- **Enlarging the health equity policy community.** This can be achieved by building or strengthening networks of researchers and advocates. Examples of existing networks that could be expanded, apart from the Global Health Equity Initiative, include Southern Africa's Equinet and the International Society for Equity in Health, as well as the various human rights networks. Sharpening the equity focus of existing research networks such as the Global Forum for Health Research would be valuable, as would building supportive links between established networks, such as the EU Network of Researchers Evaluating Policies and Interventions to Reduce Inequalities in Health (Mackenbach and Droomers 1999) and emerging networks in the South.

- **Building greater capacity to monitor and analyze policies from an equity perspective.** More collaborative work should be encouraged to focus minds on refining methods and tools for monitoring and analysis, particularly for use in low-income and data-poor settings. The South African Equity Gauge, for example, is being adapted to monitor health system changes in other countries. Research and professional training must be supported to develop the new skills and perspectives required. Innovative thinking and pump-priming support is required to investigate the pressing issues surrounding the effects of globalization on the determinants of health and inequalities. Beaglehole and Bonita (2000) have gone a step further and proposed a worldwide cooperative research program that would be the public health equivalent of the human genome project.

- **Encouraging global advocacy.** There are multiple opportunities for synergistic action by statutory organizations, multilateral funders, and charitable foundations. Following the example of the World Health Organization's *World Health Report 1999*, international reports on health and development issues could be identified while still in preparation and encouraged to have a substantive focus on health equity. Strong efforts should be made to inject a consideration for equity into current policy debates, a prominent instance being health sector reform proposals in low-income countries (Gilson 1998; Whitehead and Dahlgren 1991). Other pressing global developments requiring an equity lens include the effects of moving toward ever more deregulated market economies and the World Trade Organization agreements that recently triggered such a violent reaction in Seattle and Washington (Price et al. 1999).

Taking action on all these frontiers requires respected international leadership, as Chen and Berlinguer emphasize in chapter 4. They call for the World Health Organization to assume that role once more, becoming "the world conscience of health." Certainly, we must launch a more concerted effort—beyond the well-meaning, but thus far largely haphazard, development of advocacy in this field. In a time of growth and promise, yawning health divides must not be tolerated. With a "world conscience" playing a leadership role, it is up to a constellation of governments, ministries of health, regional organizations, nongovernmental organizations, researchers, advocacy groups, and individuals to stem the tide of widening inequities in health. We must collectively seize this unprecedented opportunity for global equity in health.

References

Acheson D., Barker D., Chambers J., Graham H., Marmot M., Whitehead M. 1998. *The Report of the Independent Inquiry into Inequalities in Health.* London: The Stationery Office.

Beaglehole R., Bonita R. 2000. Reinvigorating public health. *Lancet* 356:787–788.

Birley M. 1995. *The Health Impact Assessment of Development Projects.* London: Her Majesty's Stationery Office.

Birley M., Boland A., Davies L., Edwards R.T., Glanville H., Ison E., Millstone E., Osborn D., Scott-Samuel A., Treweek J. 1998. *Health and Environmental Impact Assessment: An Integrated Approach.* London: Earthscan/British Medical Association.

Bloom G., McIntyre D. 1998. Towards equity in health in an unequal society. *Social Science and Medicine* 47:1529–1538.

Caldwell J. 1986. Routes to low mortality in poor countries. *Population and Development Review* 12:171–220.

Carr-Hill R., Sheldon T., Smith P., Martin S., Peacock S., Hardman G. 1994. Allocating resources to health authorities: development of methods for small area analysis and use of inpatient services. *British Medical Journal* 309:1046–1049.

Castor-leal F., Dayton J., Demery L., Mehra K. 1999. Public health spending on health care in Africa: do the poor benefit? *World Bank Research Observer* 14(1):49–72.

Cornia G. 1996. *Labor Market Shocks, Psychosocial Stress and the Transition's Mortality Crisis. Research in Progress 4.* Helsinki: United Nations University, World Institute for Development Economics Research.

Dahlgren G. 1993. Economic analyses of health development. *NU News on Health Care in Developing Countries* 7(2):4–7.

Dahlgren G. 1994a. The political economy of health financing strategies in Kenya. In: Chen L., Kleinman A., Ware N. (eds), *Health and Social Change in International Perspective.* Boston: Harvard University Press. pp. 453–470.

Dahlgren G. 1994b. *Health Markets of the Future: Winners and Losers* [in Swedish]. Stockholm: Natur och Kultur.

Dahlgren G. 1996. Sectoral approaches to poverty reduction: health. In: SIDA, *Promoting Sustainable Livelihoods: A Report From the Task Force on Poverty Reduction.* Stockholm: Swedish International Development Agency.

Dahlgren G. 1997. Strategies for reducing social inequities in health—visions and reality. In: Ollila E., Koivusalo M., Partonen T. (eds), *Equity in Health Through Public Policy.* Helsinki: STAKES (National Research and Development Center for Health and Welfare).

Dahlgren G., Whitehead M. 1991. *Policies and Strategies to Promote Social Equity in Health.* Stockholm: Institute for Futures Studies.

Dahlgren G., Whitehead M. 1992. *Policies and Strategies to Promote Equity in Health.* Copenhagen: World Health Organization.

Dahlgren G., Nordgren P., Whitehead M. (eds). 1997. *Health Impact Assessment of the European Union Common Agricultural Policy.* Stockholm: Sweden's National Institute of Public Health.

Daniels N., Light D., Kaplan R. 1996. *Benchmarks of Fairness for Health Care Reform.* New York: Oxford University Press.

Diderichsen F., Varde E., Whitehead M. 1997b. Resource allocation to health authorities: the quest for an equitable formula in Britain and Sweden. *British Medical Journal* 315:875–878.

Doherty J., van Den Heever A. 1998. A needs-based, weighted-capitation formula in support of equity and primary health care: a South African case study. In: Barer M.L., Getzen T.E., Stoddart G.L. (eds), *Health, Health Care and Health Economics: Perspectives on Distribution.* London: Wiley. pp. 271–294.

Drèze J., Sen A. 1989. *Hunger and Public Action.* Oxford: Clarendon Press.

Gilson L. 1998. In defence and pursuit of equity. *Social Science and Medicine* 47(12):1891–1896.

Gilson L. 2000. Re-addressing equity: the importance of ethical processes. In: Mills A. (ed), *Reforming Health Sectors.* London: Kegan Paul (In press).

Gilson L., Buse K., Russell S. 1995. The political economy of cost recovery: towards equitable health financing policy. *Journal of International Development* 7(3):369–401.

Gunning-Schepers L. 1989. How to put equity in health on the political agenda. *Health Promotion* 4:149–150.

Gwatkin D. 2000. Health inequalities and the health of the poor. *Bulletin of the World Health Organization* 78(1):3–17.

Kawachi I., Kennedy B. 1997. Health and social cohesion: why care about income inequality? *British Medical Journal* 314:1037–1040.

Kawachi I., Kennedy B., Wilkinson R. 1999. Crime: social disorganization and relative deprivation. *Social Science and Medicine* 48:719–731.

Khan K.S. 1999. Benchmarks of Fairness in Health Care: Report of a Karachi Workshop. Karachi, India, April 1–5, 1999.

Kim J.Y., Millen J.V., Irwin A., Gershman J. (eds). 2000. *Dying for Growth.* Monroe, ME: Common Courage Press.

Kunst A., Mackenbach J. 1995. *Measuring Socioeconomic Inequalities in Health.* Copenhagen: World Health Organization.

Laflamme L. 1998. *Social Inequality in Injury Risks.* Report 98/33. Stockholm: Sweden's National Institute of Public Health.

Lehto J., Ritsatakis A. 1999. *Health Impact Assessment as a Tool for Intersectoral Health Policy.* Brussels: European Center for Health Policy/WHO Regional Office for Europe.

Lomas J. 1998. Social capital and health: implications for public health and epidemiology. *Social Science and Medicine* 47:1181–1188.

Mackenbach J., Droomers M. (eds). 1999. *Interventions and Policies to Reduce Socioeconomic Inequalities in Health.* Proceedings of the third workshop of the European Network on Interventions and Policies to Reduce Socioeconomic Inequalities in Health, Rotterdam, November 19–20, 1998. Rotterdam: Erasmus University.

Makinen M., Water H., Rauch M., Almagambetova N., Bitran R., Gilson L., McIntyre D., Pannarunothia S., Orieto A.L., Ubilla G., Ram S. 2000. Inequalities in health care use and expenditures: empirical data from eight developing countries and countries in transition. *Bulletin of the World Health Organization* 78(1): 55–65.

McLaren D., Cottray O., Taylor M., Pipes S., Bullock S. 1999. *The Geographic Relation Between Household Income and Polluting Factors.* London: Friends of the Earth.

Ntuli A., Khosa S., McCoy D. 1999. *The Equity Gauge.* Durban: Health Systems Trust.

Pande R., Gwatkin D. 1999. Country-level information on poor–rich differences with respect to health, nutrition and population. Provisional data. Washington, DC: World Bank.

Price D., Pollock A., Shaoul J. 1999. How the World Trade Organization is shaping domestic policies in health care. *Lancet* 354: 1889–1892.

Radcliffe J. 1978. Social justice and the demographic transition: lessons from India's Kerala State. *International Journal of Health Services* 8:123–144.

Republic of South Africa. 1997. *White Paper for the Transformation of the Health System in South Africa: Toward a National Health System.* Government Gazette 382 (17919): Notice 667.

Russell S., Gilson L. 1997. User fee policies to promote health service access for the poor: a wolf in sheep's clothing. *International Journal of Health Services* 27(2):359–379.

Scott-Samuel A. 1998. Health impact assessment—theory into practice. *Journal of Epidemiology and Community Health* 52:704–705.

Sen A. 1995. Mortality as an indicator of economic success and failure. Innocenti Inaugural Lecture, March 3, 1995, Instituto degli Innocenti, Florence.

Sen A. 1999. *Development as Freedom.* New York: Alfred A. Knopf.

Sen G., Germain A., Chen L. (eds). 1994. *Population Policies Reconsidered: Health, Empowerment, and Rights.* Harvard Series on Population and International Health. Boston: Harvard University Press.

Slee V.N., Slee D.A., Schmidt H.J. 1996. *Health Care Terms.* St. Paul, MN: Tringa Press.

SOU. 1999. *Equity in Health—The Second Step Towards National Health Targets.* Stockholm: National Public Health Commission/SOU 1999:137 [in Swedish].

Standing H. 1999. *Frameworks for Understanding Gender Inequalities and Health Sector Reform: An Analysis and Review of Policy Issues.* Harvard Center for Population and Development Studies. Working Paper Series No. 99.06. Cambridge, MA: Harvard Center for Population and Development Studies.

Tanzi V. 1998. Macroeconomic adjustment with major structural reforms: implications for employment and income distribution. In: Tanzi V., Chu K. (eds), *Income Distribution and High Quality Growth.* Cambridge, MA: MIT Press.

Thaddeus S., Maine D. (1994) Too far to walk: maternal mortality in context. *Social Science and Medicine* 38:1091–1110.

Townsend J. 1985. Cigarette tax, economic welfare and social class patterns of smoking. *Applied Economics* 19:335–365.

Townsend J., Roderick P., Cooper J. 1993. Cigarette smoking by socioeconomic group, sex and age: effects of price, income, and health publicity. *British Medical Journal* 309:923–927.

Tudor Hart J. 1971. The inverse care law. *Lancet* i:405–412.

U.K. Department of Health. 1999. *Saving Lives: Our Healthier Nation.* Command White Paper 4386. London: The Stationery Office.

U.S. Department of Health and Human Services. 2000. *Healthy People 2010.* Washington, DC: U.S. Department of Health and Human Services.

Vanclay F., Bronstein D. (eds). 1995. *Environmental and Social Impact Assessment.* Chichester: John Wiley and Sons.

Whitehead M. 1992. The health divide. In: Townsend P., Whitehead M., Davidson N. (eds), *Inequalities in Health: The Black Report and the Health Divide,* 2nd ed. London: Penguin. pp. 214–450.

Whitehead M. 1994. Is it fair? Evaluating the equity implications of the NHS reforms. In: Robinson R., Le Grand J. (eds), *Evaluating the NHS Reforms.* London: King's Fund. pp. 208–242.

Whitehead M. 1995. Tackling inequalities: a review of policy initiatives. In: Benzeval M., Judge J., Whitehead M. (eds), *Tackling Inequalities in Health: An Agenda for Action.* London: King's Fund.

Whitehead M. 1998. The diffusion of ideas on inequalities in health: a European perspective. *Milbank Quarterly* 76:469–492.

Whitehead M., Burström B., Diderichsen F. 2000. Social policies and the pathways to inequalities in health: a comparative analysis of lone mothers in Britain and Sweden. *Social Science and Medicine* 50:255–270.

Whitehead M., Dahlgren G. 1991. What can be done about inequalities in health? *Lancet* 338:1059–1063.

Whitehead M., Diderichsen F. 1997. International evidence on social inequalities in health. In: Drever F., Whitehead M. (eds), *Health Inequalities—Decennial Supplement.* DS Series No. 15. Office for National Statistics. London: Her Majesty's Stationery Office. pp. 44–68.

Whitehead M., Scott-Samuel A., Dahlgren G. 1998. Setting targets to address inequalities in health. *Lancet* 351:1279–1282.

Wilkinson R. 1996. *Unhealthy Societies: The Afflictions of Inequality.* London: Routledge.

Wilkinson R., Kawachi I., Kennedy B. 1998. Mortality, the social environment, crime and violence. In: Bartley M., Blane D., Smith G.D. (eds), *Sociology of Health Inequalities.* Oxford: Blackwell Press.

World Bank. 1993. *Investing in health. World Development Report 1993.* Oxford: Oxford University Press.

World Bank. 2000. *World Development Report 2000/2001.* Oxford: Oxford University Press.

World Health Organization (WHO). 1985. *Targets for Health for All.* Copenhagen: WHO.

WHO. 1995. *Women's Health: Improve Our Health, Improve the World.* Geneva: WHO.

WHO. 1998a. Report of the Technical Consultation on Safe Motherhood, October 18–23, 1997, Sri Lanka. Geneva: WHO.

WHO. 1998b. *Health for All in the 21st Century.* Geneva: WHO.

WHO. 1999. *World Health Report 1999.* Geneva: WHO.

Contributors

MONICA ÅBERG, MPH, MSc in Sociology, is a PhD student in the Department of Public Health Sciences at the Karolinska Institute, working in the area of social epidemiology for the Stockholm County Council. She has been engaged for several years in the comparative Anglo-Swedish project for the Global Health Equity Initiative, and her main interest is the relationship between income and health.

ALAYNE M. ADAMS is an Assistant Professor in the Department of Population and Family Health, Joseph A. Mailman School of Public Health, Columbia University. She received her doctorate from the London School of Hygiene and Tropical Medicine and pursued postdoctoral studies as a MacArthur Fellow at Harvard University. Her current research interests include the social and economic determinants of health and nutrition, the measurement of interpersonal social networks and community-level social capital, participatory methodology, and qualitative research and analysis. In addition to long-standing research activities in Mali, she has been collaborating with the BRAC-ICDDR,B Joint Project in Bangladesh for the past 7 years.

FARUQUE AHMED received his MA in Economics from Dhaka University in 1974 and his MHS from Johns Hopkins University in 1991. He is currently working as an Operations Officer for the Health, Nutrition and Population (HNP) Team of the World Bank office in Bangladesh. His special area of interest is health sector reform, focusing on health care financing issues and institutional arrangements that benefit the poor, women, and children in achieving desired health outcomes to reduce poverty.

SUDHIR ANAND, BPhil, MA, DPhil, is Professor of Economics at the University of Oxford and Fellow of St Catherine's College, Oxford. He is also Adjunct Professor at Harvard University, Cambridge, Massachusetts, where he has served as Acting Director of the Center for Population and Development Studies. He has written widely on inequality, poverty, undernutrition, and the standard of living. Relevant publications include *Inequality and Poverty in Malaysia: Measurement and Decomposition*, Oxford University Press, 1983, and articles in *Journal of Health Economics, Journal of Economic Perspectives, American Economic Review, Journal of Development Economics, Economic Journal, Review of Income and Wealth*, and *World Development*.

EVGUENIY M. ANDREEV is Head of the Laboratory for Analysis and Prognosis of Population Mortality, Centre for Demography and Human Ecology, Institute for Economics Forecasting, Russian Academy of Sciences. His areas of expertise and interest are population projection, analysis of mortality dynamics and differentiation in Russia, and the demographic history of Russia. Recent major publications include "The dynamics of mortality in the Russian Federation" in *Health and Mortality Issues of Global Concern*, United Nations and Flemish Scientific Institute, Belgium, 1999, and *Demographic History of Russia: 1927–1959*, Moscow, Informatika, 1998, with L.E. Darsky and T.L. Kharkova (in Russian).

LISA F. BERKMAN is the Norman Professor of Health and Social Behavior and of Epidemiology, Chair of the Department of Health and Social Behavior, and Chair of the Harvard Center for Society and Health at the Harvard School of Public Health. Dr. Berkman is an internationally recognized social epidemiologist with long-standing experience in research on social networks, social inequality, social engagement, and aging. Her most recent book, *Social Epidemiology*, is the first systematic account of the field. She was a senior Fulbright Fellow at University College, London, and is conducting ongoing research on social networks and integration in France. She has served on several Institute of Medicine committees on health and behavior and on future directions for the National Institute of Health.

GIOVANNI BERLINGUER is currently President of Italy's National Committee of Bioethics as well as Editor of the journal *Qualità Equità* and a member of the International Bioethics Committee of UNESCO. He received his MD from the University of Sassari (Italy) and was Professor of Social Medicine, University of Sassari (1969–1974) and then Professor of Occupational Health, University "La Sapienza," Rome (1975–1999). Dr. Berlinguer holds honorary degrees from Universitiès of Montréal (1996) and Brasilia (1999). In addition to his academic career, he was in charge of the National Health Program (1962–1963) as well as a Member of Parliament elected at the Chamber of Deputies in 1972, 1976, and 1979 and at the Senate in 1983 and 1987. Dr. Berlinguer has served as a member of the Commissions on Health, Education, and the Environment.

ABBAS BHUIYA, MA, PhD, is the Head of the Social and Behavioural Sciences Programme at ICDDR,B's Centre for Health and Population Research in Dhaka, Bangladesh. Dr. Bhuiya has worked extensively in the field of health and mortality, especially on issues of social, economic, and behavioral determinants. Recent endeavors include work on promotion of self-help for health in rural communities and study of the impact of social and economic development programs on health and well being. He has published articles in journals such as *Population and Development Review*, *Population Studies*, *Social Science and Medicine*, and *Health Policy and Planning*.

BO BURSTRÖM, MD, PhD, is a Senior Research Fellow in the Department of Public Health Sciences at the Karolinska Institute in Sweden. He also works on social epidemiology and health policy issues for the Stockholm County Council. Dr. Burström has previously worked for the World Health Organization in Africa, participates in a European network on interventions and policies to reduce social inequalities in health, and is engaged in Anglo-Swedish comparative studies on the influence of social context and social policy on health.

SEBASTIAN CARRASCO is a Sociologist who obtained his degree from the Universidad de Artes y Ciencias Sociales in Chile. He did his postgraduate training in Population and Sustainable Development at the Latin American Center for Demography, where he is currently a consultant to the Population Division. His major area of expertise is in the development of geographic socioeconomic risk maps based on census and household survey data. His main area of interest is in the use of aggregate data to develop public policy at the local level.

LINCOLN C. CHEN, MD, MPH, is Executive Vice President for Strategy with the Rockefeller Foundation. Before joining the Rockefeller Foundation in January 1997, Dr. Chen was the Taro Takemi Professor of International Health at the Harvard University School of Public Health, where he served as the Chair of the Department of Population and International Health and the Director of the Harvard Center for Population and Development Studies. Prior to joining the Harvard faculty in 1987, Dr. Chen was the Ford Foundation representative for Nepal, India, and Sri Lanka, based in New Delhi. Dr. Chen has written extensively on world health, population, and development. He is a member of the World Academy of Arts and Sciences and the American Academy of Arts and Sciences. He serves on the boards of CARE/USA, the United Nations Fund for International Partnerships, the Center of Economic and Social Rights, New York, and the Center for Sciences and the Environment in Washington, DC.

YUDE CHEN, MD, is a Professor at Peking University School of Public Health. Dr. Chen has authored more than 100 publications on issues including the life-table and its applications, health management, health statistics, social medicine, and health policy and management. Dr. Chen is also Vice-president of the China Preventive Medicine Association, Vice-president of the China Health Statistics Association, and Vice-president of China Medical Informatics. He serves as Chief Editor of the *Chinese Journal of Preventive Medicine*, *Chinese Journal of Health Statistics*, and the *Chinese Journal of Hospital Statistics* and has received several awards, including the Rockefeller Fellowship (1983–1984), the Kellogg International Fellowship Program in Health (1986–1989), and the United Nations Development Program/World Bank/World Health Organization Special Program for Research and Training in Tropical Diseases (1999).

MUSHTAQUE CHOWDHURY, MSc, PhD, is with the Research and Evaluation Division, BRAC, Bangladesh. Dr. Chowdhury joined BRAC in 1977 and is now its Deputy Executive Director and Director of Research. BRAC is the largest nongovernmental development organization in the South, and its Research and Evaluation Division is a large multidisciplinary research group working on a broad range of development issues in Bangladesh. Dr. Chowdhury has published extensively in journals and books. In a recent project, Dr. Chowdhury led a team of international experts in assessing the impact of a large social development program for poor women in China.

GÖRAN DAHLGREN is a Visiting Professor at Liverpool University and, since 1998, a Policy Adviser at the Ministry of Health in Vietnam. He has served on international assignments for the World Health Organization, Swedish International Development Cooperation Agency (SIDA), and United Nations Institute for Training and Research (UNITAR) and worked in Sweden as Assistant Undersecretary of State, Ministry of Social Affairs, and Assistant Director General of the National Institute of Public Health. His publications include government reports on "Health and Health Services for the 1990s" and "Markets for Health Care Services—Winners and Losers."

IRIS DELGADO received her MA in Applied Statistics, Mathematics, and Computing from the University of Santiago and her MA in Biostatistics from the University of Chile, School of Public Health. Currently she works at the Social Division within the Ministry of Planning and Cooperation, where she is the global coordinator of the National Survey on Socioeconomic Conditions (Encuesta de Caracterización Socioeconómica Nacional, CASEN). She focuses her work on mathematical and multivariate statistical model building and on the development of summary indexes to measure social inequalities. She has also acted as a consultant on statistical analysis to several agencies including UNICEF, Pan American Health Organization (PAHO), United Nations Development Program, and the Centers for Disease Control and Prevention.

FINN DIDERICHSEN is a Professor in social epidemiology and health policy research at the Karolinska Institute, Department of Public Health Science. He has an MD from Copenhagen University and a PhD in Social Medicine from Uppsala University. He is leading a research group focusing on causal mechanisms of social inequalities in health and developing epidemiological tools for health policy decisions. He has initiated the newly formed Centre for Health Equity Studies in Stockholm and he is chairman of the board for public health training at Karolinska Institute and a member of the National Public Health Commission of Sweden.

TRUONG VIET DZUNG is an Associate Professor of Public Health as well as the Deputy Director of the Planning Department for the Ministry of Health of Vietnam. He is also a Collaborator with the Institute for Health Strategy and Policy. His publications include *Strengthening Management Skills for Provincial Health Managers* (1993), *Primary Health Care Management for District Health Managers* (1998), and *Health Policy*, a textbook for MPH courses, Hanoi Medical College (1999).

TIMOTHY EVANS is Team Director of the Health Equity Division at the Rockefeller Foundation. He was previously Assistant Professor of Population and International Health at the Harvard School of Public Health. Dr. Evans has degrees in agricultural economics (DPhil, Oxford) and clinical medicine (MD, McMaster University) and completed his residency training in Internal Medicine at the Brigham and Women's Hospital. He is currently serving on the Board of the Global Alliance for Vaccines and Immunizations. Dr. Evans has most recently authored a chapter on health as a global public good with Lincoln Chen and Richard Cash in *Global Public Goods* (1999). Previous publications include work on the socioeconomic consequences of disease.

MARK G. FIELD, MA, PhD, is currently an Associate of the Davis Center for Russian Studies, an Adjunct Professor at the School of Public Health, Harvard University, and a Senior Sociologist at the Department of Psychiatry, Massachusetts General Hospital, as well as Professor Emeritus, Boston University. His major interest is medical sociology and comparative health care systems, with a particular focus on health and health care in the former Soviet Union. He served for 12 years as the Chairman of the Research Committee on the Sociology of Health of the International Sociological Association. He is the author, co-author, or editor of 11 books and over 130 papers in the professional literature. Among his books are *Doctor and Patient in Soviet Russia* and *Soviet Socialized Medicine*. He co-authored, with A. d'Houtaud, *Cultural Images of Health* and was co-editor with Judyth L. Twigg of *Russia's Torn Safety Nets: Health and Social Welfare in Transition*, published in May 2000 by St. Martin's Press.

FRANCISCO FRANCO is affiliated with the Mexican Health Foundation (FUNSALUD) and the National

Institute for Respiratory Diseases (INER). He holds an MPHSc from Johns Hopkins University, an MSc in Epidemiology from the School of Public Health of Mexico, and an MD from the National University of Mexico. Dr. Franco is currently Vice-director of Sociological and Medical Research at INER. He has previously served as Consultant for Center Health and the Economy at the Mexican Foundation for Health (FUNSALUD), Associate Researcher for National Institute for Respiratory Diseases of Mexico, Associate Researcher for Unit of Clinical Epidemiology, General Hospital of Mexico, Ministry of Health, and Vice-director of the studies in cost-effectiveness. He is the author of eight original articles and has a special interest in the fields of demography, cancer epidemiology, and burden of disease.

ASHA GEORGE is a Doctoral Candidate in Development Studies at the University of Sussex. As a Research Fellow at the Harvard Center for Population and Development Studies, she has been coordinating the Gender and Health Equity project since 1998. Previously she was a consultant for the United Nations Development Fund for Women (UNIFEM) and the United Nations Population Fund (UNFPA) in Mexico in the national preparation and follow-up the Beijing Women's Conference. Her research interests include political analysis of international health policy, reproductive health, health systems analysis, and participatory approaches in development. She is co-editor with Gita Sen and Piroska Östlin of *Engendering International Health: The Challenge of Equity,* (MIT Press, 2002).

LUCY GILSON, MA, PhD, is an Associate Professor and Deputy Director of the Centre for Health Policy, University of Witwatersrand, South Africa, and a Senior Lecturer in Health Economics, London School of Hygiene and Tropical Medicine, England. Her research has focused on a range of health sector reform issues, including health care financing and organizational policy change, primarily in Eastern and Southern Africa. She has investigated issues of equity, particularly in relation to health care financing, and is published in a wide variety of journals, including *Social Science and Medicine.*

TOSHIHIKO HASEGAWA, MD, MPH, is Director of Health Care Policy, National Institute of Health Services Management, Ministry of Health and Welfare, Tokyo, Japan. His major books or publications (English only) include *International Symposium on Health Transition and Health Sector Reform in Asia* (ed) (1998); *The Japanese Health Care System: A Step-Wise Approach to Universal Coverage* (World Bank 1997);

a comparative study of development of the modern hospital in Japan and the USA (in *History of Hospitals,* 1989); and a comparative study of hospital admission rates between the USA and Japan, in *Containing Health Care Costs in Japan* edited by Ikegami and Campbell. Dr. Hasegawa is a member of the board of the Japanese Society for Clinical Economics and the Japanese Society for Medical Technology Assessment.

PATRICIA HERNÁNDEZ, PhD (Economics), MPH, and MD, is a Health Economist with the Evidence and Information for Policy, World Health Organization. She is also affiliated with the Mexican Health Foundation (FUNSALUD), Mexico City. Dr. Hernández has received several awards for her research, including Academic Citation in Health Systems (NIPH, 1993) and First Prize in Health Economics Research (MCST-CRTE 1999). Dr. Hernández is also the co-founder of the Health Economics Training Program at the National Institute for Public Health, Institutionalization of National Health Accounts in Mexico and co-producer of the first World National Health Accounts (191 countries). She is the author of six books, five chapters, and 20 original articles, including Hernández P., Zetina A., Tapia M., Coria I., Ortiz C., Childcare needs of female street vendors in Mexico City in *Health Policy and Planning,* 1996.

ROLF DIETER HOLLSTEIN, Centro INUS, Universidad Nacional de La Plata, Argentina, received his BA in Biology and Society with a concentration in international health from Cornell University. He received his MPH with a concentration in epidemiology from the University of Chile; for his thesis, he investigated adult and infant mortality by socioeconomic position in Chile. Currently on a 1 year leave of absence from studies at the Case Western Reserve University School of Medicine, he has been working for the International Society for Equity in Health in its Argentine secretariat.

WILLIAM C. HSIAO is the K.T. Li Professor of Economics at the Harvard School of Public Health. His current research focuses on developing a theory of health system economics that could provide an analytical framework for diagnosing the causes of the successes or failures of a system. He has advised many nations on their health sector reforms, including Colombia, Poland, Taiwan, China, Hong Kong, Sweden, Cyprus, and South Africa. Dr. Hsiao has published more than 100 papers and several books. He received his PhD in Economics from Harvard University, and he is also a qualified actuary with extensive experience in health insurance. Dr. Hsiao is a member of the Institute of Medicine, National Academy of Science.

PHAM MANH HUNG, PhD, is the First Vice Minister of Health, Ministry of Health, Vietnam. He has held the following positions: Associate Professor of Medicine, Vice Rector of Hanoi Medical College, Professor of Medicine, and Rector of Hanoi Medical College. Since 1997 he has served as First Vice Minister of Health and has published in the fields of immunology, community health care, and health financing.

ICHIRO KAWACHI, MD, PhD, is the Director of the Harvard Center for Society and Health at the Harvard School of Public Health, where he also holds an appointment as Associate Professor of Health and Social Behavior. Trained as both a physician and epidemiologist, Dr. Kawachi's research and teaching during the past 10 years has been focused on uncovering the social and economic determinants of population health. His current research ranges from the psychosocial predictors of health and illness (job stress, social networks and support, and psychological factors) to the investigation of more distal, societal influences on population health (income distribution, social capital, gender inequality). For this work he received a Robert Wood Johnson Investigator Award in Health Policy Research. He recently co-edited (with Lisa Berkman) *Social Epidemiology*, the first textbook on the subject, published by Oxford University Press in 2000, as well as a *Reader on Income Inequality and Health* with Bruce Kennedy and Richard Wilkinson (The New Press, 1999).

NANCY KRIEGER, PhD, is Associate Professor of Public Health in the Department of Health and Social Behavior at the Harvard School of Public Health, Associate Director of the Harvard Center for Society and Health, and Adjunct Investigator at the Division of Research of the Kaiser Foundation Research Institute (Oakland, CA). Dr. Krieger is a social epidemiologist, with a background in biochemistry, philosophy of science, and the history of public health, combined with 20 years of experience as an activist in issues involving social justice, science, and health. Her epidemiological research focuses on social inequalities in health, especially in relation to breast cancer and hypertension. Examples include studies of appropriate measures of social class (individual, household, and neighborhood), especially for studying the health of women; possible roles of exogenous carcinogens, such as pesticides, in the etiology of breast cancer; and associations between elevated blood pressure and discrimination based on race/ethnicity, gender, and sexual orientation. She is co-editor, with Glen Margo, of *AIDS: The Politics of Survival* (Baywood Publishers, 1994) and, with Elizabeth Fee, of *Women's Health, Politics, and Power: Essays on Sex/Gender, Medicine, and Public Health* (Baywood Publishers, 1994).

LAURA D. KUBZANSKY, MPH, PhD, is an Assistant Professor in the Department of Health and Social Behavior, Harvard School of Public Health. Her research is focused on the role of psychological and social factors in health, with a particular focus on the role of stress and emotion in cardiovascular disease and healthy aging. She has published several major reviews on the role of emotion in coronary heart disease. Other work concerns the relationships between socioeconomic status and other aspects of social structure, psychological factors (control, anxiety, optimism), and health. She is currently working on several projects designed to examine both the biological mechanisms by which emotions may influence health and also the ways in which the social structure shapes the psychosocial resources available to individuals.

YUANLI LIU, MD, PhD, is an Assistant Professor of International Health at the Harvard School of Public Health. He has conducted research studies and taught graduate courses in the areas of health care financing, economics of health policy, and comparative health systems. One of his latest research interests has been health sector reforms in transitional economies. He has worked closely with both the academic community and government policy makers in China to help design and evaluate health sector reform measures, especially rural health care reforms. Dr. Liu received his medical and public health training from Tongji Medical University, graduate training in health policy and management from Harvard University, and his PhD in health economics from the University of Minnesota.

RAFAEL LOZANO, MD, MA, works with both the Mexican Health Foundation (FUNSALUD) and the Epidemiology and Burden of Disease Cluster at the World Health Organization. He holds an MA in Social Medicine from the Metropolitan Autonomy University, Mexico City, and an MD from the National University of Mexico. Dr. Lozano has previously worked as the Health Needs Assessment Coordinator for the Center Health and the Economy at the Mexican Foundation for Health (FUNSALUD), Mexico City, Mexico; a Research Fellow in the International Health Department, Harvard School of Public Heath; a Consultant for the Health Reform in Mexico, Colombia, Uruguay, Chile, and Ecuador; and a Senior Researcher at the National Institute for Public Health, Cuernavaca, Mexico. Dr. Lozano is the author of six books and more than 25 chapters and originals articles. His particular interests lie in health needs assessment, analysis of inequalities and health, and studies of violence and health.

GUILLERMO MARSHALL holds a PhD in Biostatistics from the University of Colorado and is an Associate Professor at Catholic University of Chile (since 1995) as well as a Visiting Associate Professor University of Colorado, HSC (since 1994). He was Assistant Professor of Biostatistics, University of Colorado (1990–1994). Among his nearly 50 recent publications are: Multi-State Markov Models and Diabetes Retinopathy in *Statistics in Medicine,* 1995 (with R.H. Jones); Predictive modeling of prognosis, in *Encyclopedia of Biostatistics*; and Linear discriminant analysis for unbalanced longitudinal data in *Statistics in Medicine,* 2000 (with A.E. Barón).

AUGUSTINE MASSAWE, Muhimbili University College of Health Sciences, University of Dar es Salaam, The Republic of Tanzania, is currently a Consultant Paediatrician and Neonatologist, a Senior lecturer in Paediatrics and Child Health at Muhimbili University College of Health Sciences in Dar es Salaam Tanzania, and Head of the Neonatal Unit at Muhimbili Medical Center. Publications include *Mother to Child Transmission of HIV in Tanzania*; *Guidelines on Infant Feeding and HIV in Tanzania*; and *Prevention of Perinatal and Neonatal Morbidity and Mortality in Tanzania.* He is also currently the president of the Paediatric Association of Tanzania and is engaged in research on interventions to prevent mother to child transmission of HIV.

DI MCINTYRE, BComm, MA, PhD, is Associate Professor and Director of the Health Economics Unit, University of Cape Town, South Africa. Her research includes health sector reform (especially health care financing and public–private mix), resource allocation, and equity issues. She was the team leader and principal author of the first comprehensive review of health care financing and expenditure in South Africa, which was undertaken to inform policy development after the democratic elections. She has also served on a number of governmental health policy advisory committees.

FLORENCE MULI-MUSIIME, Health Equity Theme, Nairobi Office, Rockefeller Foundation, Nairobi, Kenya is a Senior Scientist with the Rockefeller Foundation's, Health Equity program. Florence Muli-Musiime's commitment to equity was born several years back while she was at the Ministry of Home Affairs in the Kenyan Government. Florence then moved to the African Medical and Research Foundation (AMREF) to become director of Special Programs. Here her work involved

monitoring and evaluation of community based health programs/projects, and the undertaking of operations research activities aimed at enhancing the health status of the poor and marginalized. Florence is a founding member and honorary regional secretary of the African Network for the Prevention and Protection against Child Abuse and Neglect (ANPPCAN), a research network operating in severeal African countries with a special focus on marginalized children and child rights. In 1987 she was awarded the "Grand Warrior of Kenya" in recognition of her work in the area of child rights. Florence holds a BA (Hons), (Makerere University), an M.SC (Indiana State University) and a PhD (University of Edinburgh).

LAWRENCE MUNYETTI is currently the Head of Health Systems Research in the Ministry of Health in Tanzania. He is also serving a visiting lecturer on research methods at the University of Dar es Salaam, Medical College and at the Herbert Kairuki Memorial University in Dar es Salaam. Dr. Munyetti received a medical degree in 1980 from the University of Dar es Salaam and holds a Master's degree in medical demography from the London School of Hygiene and Tropical Medicine as well. He has held several positions in the Tanzanian civil service and at university level. His work experience is in medical demography and public health.

VINAND M. NANTULYA, MD, PhD, FRCPath, African Medical and Research Foundation (AMREF), Kenya, is an immunobiologist with a strong interest in public health. Currently, he is Director of Programs at the African Medical and Research Foundation (AMREF), a health development nongovernmental organization based in Nairobi, Kenya, that won the Conrad C. Hilton Humanitarian Prize. Dr. Nantulya has published extensively, authoring original research articles on subjects that include host–parasite and vector–parasite relationships, hepatitis B virus, and primary liver cancer. He serves on the World Health Organization's Expert Committee for Parasitic Diseases and the World Health Organization/Tropical Disease Research Task Force for African Trypanosomiasis. His interests include health equity and related issues.

PIROSKA ÖSTLIN is a Medical Sociologist with a doctorate in Medical Science from the University of Uppsala and is currently a senior researcher at the Karolinska Institute in Sweden as well as Research Fellow at the Harvard Center for Population and Development Studies. Her research is primarily concerned with methodological problems in studies of occupational epidemiology, as well as the significance of the work environment on women's and men's health. Before her current position at the Karolinska Institute, she was the Secretary of the National Public Health Commission, where she was responsible for defining national public health targets and suggesting strategies to reduce social inequalities in health between different segments of the Swedish society. Apart from publishing extensively on issues of occupational health, she is the lead editor of *Kon Öch Ohälsa,* published by the Harvard School of Public Health as *Gender Inequalities in Health: A Swedish Perspective,* and a co-editor with Gita Sen and Asha George of *Engendering International Health: The Challenge of Equity* (MIT Press, 2002).

JUAN C. PEREZ, a Statistician, obtained his MA in Demography from the United Nations Latin American Center for Demography. His main area of expertise is in the analysis of demographic data and population projections. He is currently a Professor at the University of Chile Faculty of Social Sciences, where he teaches at the Master in Sociology Program, and at the Population and Sustainable Development Post-graduate Degree, jointly offered with the United Nations Development Program. He has participated in several courses as an invited professor, including the Demographic Analysis Intensive Course offered by the Latin American Center for Demography. As a short-term Consultant for the United Nations, he has worked extensively in several countries within the African and Latin American Regions.

FABIENNE PETER obtained her PhD (Economics, 1996) from the Department of Economics, University of Basel, Switzerland. She is assistant professor of economics at the University of Basel, Switzerland, and research fellow at the Harvard Center for Population and Development Studies. Research interests include economics and ethics, philosophy of the social sciences, and public health ethics. Dr. Peter is currently involved in editing a volume on public health, ethics, and equity (with Sudhir Anand and Amartya Sen).

TERESITA RAMÍREZ, MA, is currently a Consultant for the Program Health and the Economy at the Mexican Health Foundation (FUNSALUD). She was awarded one of the 1998 Health of the Economy awards by CIDE (Centro de Investigación y Docencia Económicas) for work on national accounts in Mexico, 1992–1995. Her previous positions include associate researcher at the National Institute of Public Health (1984–1995) and coordinator of the Master of Sciences on Health Systems in the National Institute of Public Health. She has authored chapters on willingness to pay and quality of care and written six originals articles on accessibility, coverage and health services utilization, quality of care, and health accounts in Mexico. She has been a member of the board of Consultations on Health Sector Reform in Mexico and a consultant for nongovernmental organizations in Mexico.

KEQIN RAO, MD, MPH, is the Director General of the Center for Health Statistics and Information of the Chinese Ministry of Health. Since 1982 Dr. Rao has been working at the Ministry of Health, collecting, analyzing, and reporting results of regular national health statistics. He designed the 1993 and 1998 national health surveys, participated in many of the government's policy research studies, and is the national authority on regional health planning. Dr. Rao is the Vice-president of the Chinese Association of Health Statistics and has published extensively on epidemiological studies, health services research, and health policy issues. He received his medical and public health training from Tongji Medical University, and he has been a visiting scholar at many international institutions, including Sussex University, Johns Hopkins University, Harvard University, and the U.S. Centers for Disease Control and Prevention.

BEVERLY ROCKHILL is an Instructor in the Department of Medicine at Harvard Medical School. She is based in the Channing Laboratory, a division of Brigham and Women's Hospital. She received her PhD in Epidemiology at the University of North Carolina at Chapel Hill in 1997. In 1997, she won the Society for Epidemiologic Research's award for outstanding student paper, for a manuscript on breast cancer risk based on her dissertation research. Her current research is focused on breast cancer risk modeling and primary prevention of breast cancer. She has published several articles in this area, as well as in the general area of cancer prevention. She is the co-author of a comprehensive chapter on breast cancer epidemiology included in a leading textbook of breast diseases. She is currently working on projects to improve disease risk communication to persons in the general public and to statistically improve accuracy of disease risk prediction.

AVE MARIA SEMAKAFU is a Lecturer at the Institute of Development Studies of Muhimbili, University College of Health Sciences, Tanzania. She received her BA in International Relations (with Honors) and an MA in Development Studies. She has been involved in research since 1986 on sociohealth issues. Since 1991 she has been concerned with issues related to the impact of the implementation of structural adjustment programs on the health of youth. Her most recent work includes the Tanzanian study for the Global Health Equity Initiative and an International Labor Organization-supported study on sugar plantations with M. Mbilinyi. Her primary interest lies in research and participation in the debate on health equity issues relevant to adolescents.

AMARTYA SEN is Master, Trinity College, Cambridge, United Kingdom, and Lamont University Professor Emeritus at Harvard University. Previously, he was Drummond Professor of Political Economy at Oxford University and fellow of All Souls College, and he has taught at the London School of Economics, Delhi University, and Cambridge University. Dr. Sen is past President of the American Economic Association, Indian Economic Association, Development Studies Association, and Social Choice and Welfare Society. His most recent book, *Development as Freedom*, was published in 1999. In 1998 he received the Nobel Prize in Economics.

GITA SEN has a PhD in Economics from Stanford University. She is a Professor of Economics at the Indian Institute of Management in Bangalore, India, and an Adjunct Lecturer at the Harvard School of Public Health and was formerly a visiting professor at Harvard University, Vassar College, and the New School for Social Research. She is the research coordinator on globalization for the feminist network of researchers, activists, and policy makers, DAWN (Development Alternatives with Women for a New Era) and a trustee of HealthWatch (India). In addition to serving on the boards of numerous other organizations, Gita Sen also works with a number of nongovernmental organizations and other institutions in a consultative and/or advisory capacity. Her most recent books are *Engendering International Health: The Challenge of Equity* (MIT Press, 2002) (with Piroska Östlin and Asha George); *Women's Empowerment and Demographic Processes: Moving Beyond Cairo* (with Harriet Presser), Oxford University Press; and *Gender Mainstreaming in Finance—A Reference Manual for Governments and Other Stakeholders*, Commonwealth Secretariat, 1999.

VLADIMIR M. SHKOLNIKOV has a PhD in Population Geography and is Head of the Laboratory for Demographic Data at the Max Planck Institute for Demographic Research in Rostock, Germany. Since 1982 he has studied Russian mortality. He has also been involved in international projects on the reconstruction of cause-of-death statistics in Russia, Ukraine, and Baltic states and in research on the mortality crisis in Russia in the early 1990s, social inequalities in the face of death, and individual-level studies of mortality among adult men in Russia. Dr. Shkolnikov is also

Head of the International Union for the Scientific Study of Population Committee on Emerging Health Threats.

GILLIAN K. STEEL, Department of Health and Social Behavior, Harvard School of Public Health, is Project Director for Axiom Research Company in Cambridge, Massachusetts. She received her BA in Ethics, Politics, and Economics from Yale University in 1995. In 1999, she received her MSc in Health and Social Behavior from the Harvard School of Public Health. Her interests in social epidemiology relate to the relationship between economic infrastructure, popular culture, socioeconomic status, and health outcomes, including obesity and heart disease. She has a particular interest in examining the consumer environment as a possible mediating mechanism. Her current work involves projects that examine the influence of the physical retail environment and product usage environment on individual consumption decisions with immediate and long-term health consequences.

JOSÉ LUIS TORRES, MA, MD, is a Consultant for the Program Health and the Economy at the Mexican Health Foundation (FUNSALUD) and a Professor of Clinical Epidemiology at the National University of Mexico. Dr. Torres has also served as an Advisor to the Sub-Ministry of Prevention and Control of Diseases, Ministry of Health (SSA), an Associate Researcher for the National Institute for Perinatology of Mexico, and a Coordinator of the National Unit of Investigation, Medical Services Management, Mexican Petroleum. He is the author of seven chapters and five original articles and has a special interest in issues of equity, burden of disease, and health and violence. Dr. Torres is a member of the Editorial Committee of the *Epidemiological Bulletin* published by the Ministry of Health.

TRAN TUAN is Executive Director of the Research and Training Center for Community Development (RTCCD), Vietnam. His career has included working for the Hanoi Medical School from 1987 to 1993; he has been Lecturer in Epidemiology, a Founder of the Community Health Research Unit (CHRU); and a Health Program Officer for the U.K. Save the Children Fund from 1991 to 1993. He was Takemi Fellow at Harvard School of Public Health in 1994–1995, and is just completing a PhD program on Medicine and Health Sciences at Newcastle University, Australia.

JEANETTE VEGA, MD, DrPH, is Associate Professor of Public Health at the Faculty of Medicine, Universidad Catolica de Chile. Before coming to the University she was a consultant for Epidemiology at the Pan American Health Organization. She has long-standing experience in research on environmental health and currently focuses her work on social determinants of health. Dr. Vega is a member of several scientific societies, including the Chilean Epidemiology and Public Health Societies and the Chilean Medical Association. Dr. Vega has participated in several workshops on the issue of Equity and Health in Chile, Argentina, the United States, South Africa, and Bangladesh. She has also acted as a short-term consultant to the Pan American Health Organization on Measurement of Health Inequities. She completed her medical training at the University of Chile and received her DrPH from the University of Illinois at Chicago.

MARGARET WHITEHEAD, Department of Public Health, University of Liverpool, United Kingdom, BA, PhD, HonMFPHM, is W.H. Duncan Professor of Public Health, University of Liverpool. She has worked in the field of social inequalities in health in Europe for many years, is a regular adviser to the World Health Organization EURO on the issue and was a member of the recent Independent Inquiry into Inequalities in Health in Britain (the Acheson Inquiry). Her publications include *The Health Divide*, which is published together with the Black Report and has become a Penguin nonfiction best-seller. Her award-winning publications for the World Health Organization on concepts and policies to promote equity in health have been translated into 20 languages.

MEG WIRTH, MPA, has coordinated the Global Health Equity Initiative for the past 2 years while based in the Rockefeller Foundation's Health Equity Division. She has a strong interest in the link between public health research and policy and a specific interest in ethnicity and health equity, gender issues, maternal survival, and social medicine. Her previous work includes the implementation of an integrated Safe Motherhood Initiative in South Kalimantan, Indonesia, with a focus on the monitoring and evaluation systems and the development of a prenatal outreach program in the Appalachian region of the United States.

DEREK YACH, MBChB, MPH, was appointed Executive Director of the newly merged Noncommunicable Diseases and Mental Health cluster in March 2000. He is also the Project Manager of the Tobacco-Free Initiative at the World Health Organization. From July 1995 to May 1998, Dr. Yach was responsible for the design and facilitation of the World Health Organization's global consultative process that resulted in the development of the new global health policy "Health for All in the 21st Century." Prior work includes the establishment of the Center for Epidemiological Research in Southern Africa and development of a Community Health Research Group for the Medical Research Council. He has served on a number of international, continental, and national advisory committees on public health, including the WHO Ad Hoc Committee on Health Research for Future Interventions and the World Bank Environmental Action Plan Expert Committee Member for the Lesotho Highlands Development Project and has published over 200 original articles, editorials, and chapters.

BEATRIZ ZURITA, MA, MD, PhD, is the Executive Coordinator for the Program Health and the Economy at the Mexican Foundation for Health (FUNSALUD), Mexico City, Mexico. In the past, Dr. Zurita has acted as the Health Policy Analysis Coordinator for the Center Health and the Economy at the Mexican Foundation for Health (FUNSALUD), Mexico City (1996–1998) and the Regional Editor of *Quality Assurance in Health Care*, the official journal of the International Society for Quality Assurance in Health Care (1993–1997). She is the author of six books, five chapters, and six original articles. Dr. Zurita's area of expertise includes analyses of quality, costs, productivity of health services, and allocation of resources for the health sector. She has served as a board member for the Forum for Interagency Exchange Health Reform, which includes bilateral, international, and multilateral agencies (1993–1994) and for the Consultations on Health Sector Reform. Dr. Zurita is a founding member and former Academic Coordinator for the Sociedad Mexicana de Calidad de la Atención a la Salud.

Panel of Referees

We greatly appreciate the help we received from our independent referees. Each chapter was reviewed for scientific quality and clarity by at least two referees: one external and one member of the Global Health Equity Initiative. Revisions were made to chapters in response to their insights and comments. The referees, however, carry no responsibility for the end products as the overall responsibility for the contents and comments within each chapter rests with the chapter authors.

External Referees

CELIA MARIA DE ALMEIDA, Department of Health Administration and Planning, National School of Public Health/Oswaldo Cruz Foundation (FIOCRUZ), Rio de Janeiro, Brazil

AMANDA AMOS, Department of Public Health Sciences, University of Edinburgh Medical School, Edinburgh, United Kingdom

SOLOMON BENATAR, Bioethics Centre, Department of Medicine, Faculty of Health Sciences, University of Cape Town, Cape Town, South Africa

ROY CARR-HILL, Centre for Health Economics, University of York, York, United Kingdom

JUAN ANTONIO CASAS, Division of Health and Human Development, Pan American Health Organization/World Health Organization, Washington, DC, United States

NORBERTO DACHS, Program of Public Policy and Health, Division of Health and Human Development, Pan American Health Organization/World Health Organization, Washington, DC, United States

FRANCES DREVER, Social and Regional Division, Office for National Statistics, London, United Kingdom

JEAN DRÈZE, Centre for Development Economics, Delhi School of Economics, Delhi, India

KATRINA ERIKSSON, Department of Sociology, University of Uppsala and National Institute of Working Life, Stockholm, Sweden

JOHAN HALLQVIST, Department of Public Health Sciences, Division of Social Medicine, The Karolinska Institute, Stockholm, Sweden

JANE HUGHES, Health Equity Division and Population/Cairo Agenda, The Rockefeller Foundation, New York, New York, United States

SAIDI H. KAPIGA, Department of Population and International Health, Harvard School of Public Health, Cambridge, Massachusetts, United States

ANTON KUNST, Department of Public Health, Erasmus University, Rotterdam, the Netherlands

LUCIE LAFLAMME, Department of Public Health Sciences, Division of Social Medicine, The Karolinska Institute, Stockholm, Sweden

ANDREW MASON, East-West Center, and Department of Economics, University of Hawaii, Manoa, Hawaii, United States

S. NANTHIKESAN, Harvard Center for Population and Development Studies, Cambridge, Massachusetts, United States

ALEX SCOTT-SAMUEL, EQUAL (Equity in Health Research and Development Unit), Department of Public Health, University of Liverpool, Liverpool, United Kingdom

STAN D'SOUZA, United Nations Development Program, Senior Demographic Advisor/Analyst (retired), International Population Concerns, Brussels, Belgium

ADAM WAGSTAFF, Department of Economics, University of Sussex, Sussex, United Kingdom; Development Economics Research Group and Health, Nutrition and Population Network, World Bank, Washington, DC, United States

Internal Referees

ALAYNE ADAMS, Department of Population and Family Health, Joseph A. Mailman School of Public Health, Columbia University, New York, New York, United States

BENJAMIN AMICK, Houston School of Public Health, University of Texas, Austin, Texas, United States

LISA BERKMAN, Department of Health and Social Behavior, Harvard School of Public Health, Cambridge, Massachusetts, United States

GIOVANNI BERLINGUER, National Committee on Bioethics, Rome, Italy and International Bioethics Committee of UNESCO

BO BURSTRÖM, Department of Public Health Sciences, The Karolinska Institute, Stockholm, Sweden

GÖRAN DAHLGREN, University of Liverpool, Liverpool, United Kingdom; National Institute of Public Health, Stockholm, Sweden; Ministry of Health, Hanoi, Vietnam

ASHA GEORGE, Harvard Center for Population and Development Studies, Cambridge, Massachusetts, United States

LUCY GILSON, Centre for Health Policy, University of Witwatersrand, Johannesburg, South Africa

PATRICIA HERNANDEZ, Evidence and Information for Policy Cluster, World Health Organization, Geneva, Switzerland; Mexican Health Foundation (FUNSALUD), Mexico City, Mexico

DI MCINTYRE, Health Economics Unit, Department of Public Health, University of Cape Town, Cape Town, South Africa

FLORENCE MULI-MUSIIME, Health Equity Division, The Rockefeller Foundation, Nairobi, Kenya

VINAND NANTULYA, African Medical and Research Foundation, Nairobi, Kenya

PIROSKA ÖSTLIN, Department of Public Health Sciences, The Karolinska Institute, Stockholm, Sweden

VLADIMIR SHKOLNIKOV, Max Planck Institute for Demographic Research, Rostock, Germany

JEANETTE VEGA, Faculty of Medicine, Catholic University of Chile, Santiago, Chile

BEATRIZ ZURITA, Mexican Health Foundation (FUNSALUD), Mexico City, Mexico

Glossary

Absolute poverty: A measure of income poverty often defined as the share of the population living on "less than $1 per day" for the purpose of international comparisons. Within a more developed country, absolute poverty, or the lack of the basics for physical survival (food, clean water, clothes, shelter, essential health services) will occur at levels of consumption much higher than $1 per day. Other dimensions of poverty not captured by this measure include health and educational deprivation, vulnerability, voicelessness, and powerlessness. Contrast with *relative poverty*.

AFp (population attributable fraction): See *population attributable risk.*

Agency: The ability to act in a deliberative way and to pursue a variety of goals, including but reaching beyond the pursuit of individual well being.

Age-standardized: See *standardization.*

Alma Ata declaration: A statement made by the World Health Assembly at the International Conference of Primary Health Care in Alma Ata, in the former Soviet Union, September 12, 1978. The aim of this declaration was to commit all member countries of the World Health Organization (WHO) to the inclusion of life-style and behavioral factors and improvement of the environment within the principles of health for all by the year 2000.

Arriaga method: See *component analysis.*

Attainment equality: The comparison of absolute levels of achievement between groups, assuming each group is capable of reaching the same absolute level of a particular health state. This is assessed by comparing the achievement of different socioeconomic groups against a common optimal norm. See Chapter 16. Contrast with *shortfall equality.*

Bamako Initiative: Announced at the WHO Regional Meeting of African Ministers of Health in 1987, this initiative called on WHO and UNICEF to accelerate primary health care implementation at the district level and below, giving priority to women and children, by "revitalizing" health systems.

Black Report: *The Report of the Working Group on Inequalities in Health,* commissioned by the British government, chaired by Sir Douglas Black and published in 1980. A landmark report, it documented inequalities in health, suggesting that material deprivation and poverty were the most likely explanation for them. The report's recommendations, which included the improvement of material conditions of life of poorer groups and increases in social security benefits, were rejected by the new Conservative government for being too costly to implement. Nevertheless, the *Black Report* greatly influenced research and public health debates in many countries.

Capabilities: An approach to quality of life assessments, developed by Amartya Sen, in which what matters is not simply the resources people have, but what they can do with those resources. A person's "capabilities" include a set of "doings and beings" or "functionings" that a person could achieve—for example, being able to read, having enough to eat, having good health, and having self-respect.

Child Mortality Rate (CMR): The number of annual deaths by age 5 per 1000 children who survived the first year of life (i.e. mortality among children aged 1–4 years) based upon the mid-year population.

Cohort study: A type of study that follows a population with a common experience or characteristics (for example, all born in the same week in the same year (a birth cohort) over time. Often used to determine factors in early life that can be subsequently related to later experience and events.

Component analysis: Or Arriaga method. This demographic technique allows one to split a difference between two life expectancies into contributions of differences in age-specific mortality rates. If cause-specific data are available a further decomposition according to causes of death can be performed. See Chapter 5, Appendix B for the mathematical definitions. See Chapters 10 and 11 for examples.

Concentration index: A measure of the degree to which illness is concentrated in different socioeconomic groups. It is positive when illness is concentrated among the higher socioeconomic groups and negative when illness is concentrated among the lower socioeconomic groups. The concentration index is a relative measure in the sense that it is independent of the absolute levels of both (ill) health and income. See Chapter 5, Box 3, and Chapter 18 for more detail.

Cross-sectional study: A study that examines the relationship between health outcomes (e.g., diseases) and other characteristics in a population at one particular point in time.

Disability-adjusted-life-year (DALY): A measure of the burden of disease in a defined population that combines the years lived with a disability (weighted according to severity) with the years of life lost due to premature death. Also used to measure the effectiveness of interventions.

Ecologic(al) analysis: A type of study in which data are collected and correlated at the population level (based upon some defining characteristic such as group membership or area of residence—e.g., aggregate county-level life expectancy). Because the data are aggregate at the group level, relationships at the individual level cannot be empirically determined but are rather inferred from the group level.

Epidemiological transition: A theory about changing disease patterns in countries according to levels of development. It posits that poor countries will typically have high mortality due to infectious diseases (especially in children) but that with development, this pattern will shift to noncommunicable, chronic illnesses, primarily affecting adults.

Equity: A concept equated with fairness in distribution requiring a normative assessment. It can be applied in different "spaces" such as health services, health status, or income. See also *health equity.*

Etiology: Referring to the causes or origins of disease or health problems.

Functionings: A term coined by Amartya Sen to refer to the valuable things a person can do or be, such as being well nourished, living a long life and taking part in the life of a community. This "quality of life" measure may be contrasted with other more narrow assessments such as command over financial resources.

Gender: The social and cultural traits that different societies assign to males and females. Contrast with *sex,* which is biologically determined. (see Chapter 13)

Gender roles: The patterns of behavior, rights, and obligations defined by a society as appropriate for each sex.

Gini coefficient: The Gini index (devised by the Italian sociologist Corrado Gini) is an indicator of the degree of inequality in a population or group (often measured in geographically defined areas such as countries or counties). The greater the degree of inequality, the larger the coefficient will be, varying between a value of zero when there is no inequality) to a theoretical (but practically impossible) high of 1. In this volume, the Gini is usually used to refer to economic inequality but occasionally is used to refer to health inequalities.

Health equity: Opportunities for all social groups to achieve their full health potential through access to, and a fair distribution of, the pre-requisites for health. Conversely, inequities in health refer to differences in health or opportunities for health that are judged to be unfair and avoidable (see Chapter 3).

Health selection (reverse causation): A hypothesis that suggests that the observed association between poor health and low socioeconomic status arises from the wealth-depleting consequences of illness and not from the ill health effects of adverse socioeconomic circumstances.

Horizontal equity: Equal treatment of equals. This would require that all those with similar health care needs be given equal opportunity to access and receive equal treatment. Contrast with *vertical equity.*

Incidence: The number of new cases of disease occurring in a defined population during a specified period of time. The incidence rate is calculated by dividing the number of new cases of illness (numerator) by the total time units each person was observed/at risk before onset of disease (denominator).

Infant mortality rate (IMR): The number of deaths within the first year of life for each thousand live births in a given year. Calculated as the number of children born alive in a given year that died before the age of 1 (numerator) divided by the total live births during that same year (denominator) multiplied by 1000.

Inverse care law: A phrase coined by Tudor Hart (1971) to describe his observation that the availability of good medical care is inversely related to the need for such services.

Kakwani's index of progressivity: A measure of the extent to which the tax burden borne by each income group departs from proportionality. The value of Kakwani's index of progressivity ranges from -2 (most regressive) to zero (payment is proportionate to income) to 1 (most progressive).

Life expectancy: The average number of years an individual of a given age is expected to live if current age-specific mortality rates continue to apply throughout that individual's life course. Most often expressed as life expectancy at birth. Contrast with *temporary life expectancy.*

Longitudinal study: A study in which people are followed over time with continuous or repeated monitoring of risk factors or health outcomes, or both.

Maternal mortality rate: The number of maternal deaths (deaths of women during pregnancy and up to 42 days after delivery) per 100,000 women aged 15–49 per year.

Maternal mortality ratio: The number of maternal deaths (deaths of women during pregnancy and up to 42 days after delivery) per 100,000 live births per year.

Morbidity: A term that refers to nonfatal health outcomes including acute and chronic illness, injury, and other than normal health. Morbidity rates are expressed as the number of people who are ill expressed as a proportion of those at risk during a specified time interval.

Mortality: A term that applies to death. Mortality rates are expressed as the number of people who died ex-pressed as a proportion of those at risk during a specified time interval.

Occupational class: A classification of the population into social groups using the occupation of the individual or head of the household.

Odds: The ratio of the chance of an event occurring to the chance of it not occurring. If 60 heavy drinkers develop a liver disorder and 40 do not, the odds among these 100 heavy drinkers in favor of developing a liver disorder are 60:40, or 1.5.

Odds ratio: A ratio of two odds. The odds of disease in exposed persons (e.g., heavy drinkers) divided by the odds of disease in unexposed persons (e.g., nondrinkers).

Population attributable life loss index (PALL): A measure of the absolute rate of increase in the overall life expectancy that would occur in the case where everyone has the life expectancy of the group with the highest life expectancy. This measure is like the PAR but specific to mortality measurement.

Population attributable risk (PAR): Measures the proportional reduction in the overall rate of illness that would occur if all groups had the same rate of illness as the reference group, the group with the best health status. Also called AFp or population attributable fraction.

Potential years of life lost (PYLL): A measure of the sum of the years of life that a group of individuals would have lived had they not died prematurely (prior to a pre-established expectation for survival, e.g. 65 years) (see Chapters 9 and 19). Also called years of potential life lost (YPLL).

Poverty: See *absolute poverty* and *relative poverty.*

Prevalence: The number of people who have a disease or attribute in a given population during a specified period. The prevalence rate is the number of individuals with a disease or attribute during a specified period (numerator) divided by the number of people at risk of having the disease or attribute (denominator).

Progressive: A term used to describe a health financing system (for example, the taxes or allocation of public funds) that disproportionately benefits the poor. Contrast with *regressive.*

Quality adjusted life years (QALYs): A measure of health status that combines quality and duration of life considerations. In its calculation, overall life expectancy is reduced by amounts that reflect disability and distress caused by chronic conditions.

Quintile: A measure used to divide a population or set of data into five equal parts. Often used to divide a population into different groups according to income such that the top quintile is the fifth of the population with the highest incomes and the bottom quintile is the fifth of the population with the lowest incomes.

Rate: The frequency with which an event occurs in a defined population over a specific period of time. See *mortality rate.*

Rate difference: The absolute difference between two rates. For example, the difference in mortality rate between a population group exposed to a risk factor and a population group not exposed to the risk factor.

Rate ratio: The ratio of two rates. In epidemiological research the ratio of the rate in the exposed population to the rate in the unexposed population. See also *relative risk.*

Ratio scale: A ranking that includes absolute zero as a reference point, and in which there are equal intervals between the items. A tape measure is an example of a ratio scale. With a ratio scale we can say that one point on the scale is so much more or less than another. In such a ranking we would be able to determine that a certain disease state is, for example, two or four times as severe as another disease state.

Regressive: A term used in economics to describe a tax burden, or some other financing source or allocation of public funds, that falls disproportionately upon the poorer segments of the population. Contrast with *progressive.*

Relative index of inequality (RII): A measure that expresses the ratio of the morbidity and mortality rates of those at the bottom of the social hierarchy compared with those at the top of the hierarchy, based on the systematic association between morbidity and mortality and socioeconomic status for all groups. A large score on the RII implies large differences in morbidity and mortality between low and high positions in the social hierarchy.

Relative poverty: A measure that compares the socioeconomic circumstances of individuals or groups against the accepted norm of the society in which they live. By Townsend's well-known definition: "people living in relative poverty have resources so seriously below those commanded by the average individual or family that they are, in effect, excluded from ordinary living patterns, customs and activities (Townsend 1979). Contrast with *absolute poverty.*

Relative risk: The ratio of the risk of disease, disability, or death among those exposed to a factor under investigation (such as low socioeconomic status) to the risk among those not exposed. If the risk is measured as a rate, the relative risk is calculated as a rate ratio *(q.v.).*

Sex: A biological concept that is used to divide the human species into females and males. Contrast with *gender.*

Shortfall equality: In contrast to *attainment equality,* shortfall equality is assessed according to how far the group/individual falls short of a chosen norm, the optimal value that *particular* group can be expected to attain, assuming different norms for different groups (for example, life expectancy norms for men and women will be different). See Chapter 16.

Slope index of inequality (SII): Measures the inequality of a health outcome across the whole population while weighting each class by the proportion of the population in it. It is the absolute version of the *Relative index of inequality* (RII).

Social class: A complex term simply defined here as a group sharing the same status (based on economic or social factors) within a particular society. See, for example, *occupational class.*

Social stratification: The ranking of different social groups in some hierarchical order that leads to differing access to social resources.

Socioeconomic inequalities in health: Differences in the prevalence or incidence of health problems between groups of people of higher and lower socioeconomic status.

Socioeconomic status (SES): A person's relative position in the social class system based on some combination of factors including their level of education, occupation, or wealth.

Standardization: A statistical technique which uses weighted averages to improve comparability between two populations. The most frequently used form of standardization is age standardization, which removes confounding by age when the two or more populations to be compared have different age compositions.

Standardized mortality ratio (SMR): A measure of how much more (or less) likely a person is to die in a given population compared to someone of the same age and sex in a standard population. The SMR is the ratio of observed to expected deaths that would occur if the age-sex specific rates were the same as those of the standard population.

Statistical significance: An estimate of the probability that a phenomenon under study is not caused by random variation or chance.

Structural adjustment: A term that describes the main macroeconomic and policy reforms required of countries receiving loans from the International

Monetary Fund and the World Bank. Broadly summarized, structural adjustment policies of the 1980s and 1990s obligated recipient nations to liberalize their trade and investment policies. More specific examples of reforms include the following: reduction of government spending; the establishment of a more efficient fiscal policy (imposition of new taxes or collection of unpaid taxes); and privatization of state-owned enterprises.

Stunting (being stunted): A measure of chronic child malnutrition and deprivation based upon a child's height relative to the median height for his or her age.

Synergy index: A measure of the effect of two risk factors occurring together. For example, a measure of interaction between two risk factors such as social position and poverty is calculated as a measure of susceptibility. The synergy index expresses the odds among those who are exposed to the two risk factors in relation to the added effect of the two exposures.

Temporary life expectancy: A measure of the life expectancy between two ages; for example, the number of years lived between the ages of 20 and 65 may be used to measure adult life expectancy, a form of temporary life expectancy. This measure allows comparison of adult life expectancies in two populations but avoids bias due to differences in the age distributions of the elderly in the two populations.

Vertical equity: Unequal treatment for unequals. This concept implies equality in service utilization and positive discrimination toward those who are less willing or able to use health services. Thus, those with greater needs (more severe illnesses, inability to pay, and so on) would obtain concessional access. Contrast with *horizontal equity*.

Whitehall Study: A study of a cohort of 17,000 white male British civil servants whose health and socioeconomic circumstances have been followed from 1967 to the present day.

Years of potential life lost (YPLL): See *potential years of life lost*.

References

Arriaga, E. 1984. Measuring and explaining the change in life expectancies. *Demography* 21(1):83-96.

Townsend P. 1979. *Poverty in the United Kingdom*. London: Penguin Books.

Tudor Hart, J. 1971. The Inverse Care Law. *Lancet*. i: 405-412.

Further Reading on Concepts in the Glossary

Armitage, P., Colton, T. (eds). 1998. *Encyclopedia of Biostatistics*. Chichester and New York: J. Wiley.

Atkinson, A.B., Bourguignon, F. (eds). 2000. *The Handbook of Income Distribution*. Amsterdam: North-Holland.

Berkman, L., Kawachi, I. 2000. *Social Epidemiology*. New York: Oxford University Press.

Keyfitz, N. 1985. *Applied Mathematical Demography*. New York: Springer-Verlag.

Kunst, A.K., Mackenbach, M.P. 1994. *Measuring Socio-economic Inequalities in Health*. Regional Office for Europe. Copenhagen: World Health Organization.

Marmot, M.G., Wilkinson, R.G., (eds). 2000. *Social Determinants of Health*. Oxford: Oxford University Press.

Preston, S.H., Heuveline, P., Guillot, M. 2000. *Demography: Measuring and Modeling Population Processes*. Oxford: Blackwell Publishers Ltd.

Rothman, K.J., Greenland, S. 1998. *Modern Epidemiology*. 2nd edition. Philadelphia: Lippincott-Raven.

Sen, A. 1973. *On Economic Inequality*. Oxford: Clarendon Press.

Sen, A. 1994. Objectivity and Position: Assessment of Health and Well-being. In: Chen, L.C., Kleinman, A., Ware, N.C. (eds), *Health and Social Change in International Perspective*. Cambridge, Mass.: Harvard University Press.

Sen, A.K. 1999. *Development as Freedom*. New York: Alfred A. Knopf.

Sen, G., Östlin, P., George, A. 2002. *Engendering International Health: The Challenge of Equity*. Cambridge: MIT Press.

van Doorslaer, E., Wagstaff, A., Rutten, F. (eds) 1993. *Equity in the Finance and Delivery of Health Care: An International Perspective*. Oxford: Oxford University Press.

Whitehead, M. 1990. *The Concepts and Principles of Equity and Health*. Copenhagen: World Health Organization.

World Bank. 2000. *World Development Report 2000/2001: Attacking Poverty*. Washington D.C.: World Bank.

Index

Praise for
CHALLENGING INEQUITIES IN HEALTH

. . . has been awaited several years as a text for international health, health systems, and equity courses; critical reading for researchers in this field; and a reference for program managers and decision makers to absorb as they contemplate the development or progress of their health policies and interventions."
—Adnan A. Hyder, MD, MPH, PhD, in *JAMA*

. . . opens the door to a fundamental debate about how to reduce health inequalities by discussing ethics and policy."
—*New England Journal of Medicine*

"The editors have succeeded admirably in making a largely coherent whole out of disparate material from numerous authors all over the globe . . . Striking photographs provide an additional eloquent touch. Newcomers and seasoned researchers alike will find this collection of studies invaluable."
—Paula Braveman in *Bulletin of the World Health Organization*

ABOUT THE EDITORS

Timothy Evans, D.Phil., M.D., is Team Director of the Health Equity Program at The Rockefeller Foundation, New York. Dr. Evans is currently a member of the Board of the Global Alliance for Vaccines and Immunizations and the Global Forum for Health Research.

Margaret Whitehead, Ph.D., is W.H. Duncan Professor of Public Health at the University of Liverpool, UK. Professor Whitehead is a regular adviser to WHO EURO on the issue of social inequalities in health, and she is currently analyzing equity issues in relation to health sector reforms around the world.

Finn Diderichsen, M.D., Ph.D., is Professor of Social Epidemiology and Health Policy Research at the Karolinska Institute, Department of Public Health Science. He is chairman of the board for public health training at Karolinska Institute and a member of the National Public Health Commission of Sweden.

Abbas Bhuiya, M.A., Ph.D., is the Head of the Social and Behavioral Sciences Program, ICDDRB's Centre for Health and Population Research in Dhaka, Bangladesh. Dr. Bhuiya has worked extensively in the field of health and mortality, especially on issues of social, economic, and behavioral determinants.

Meg Wirth, M.P.A., manages the Global Health Equity Initiative for the Rockefeller Foundation's Health Equity Program. Her previous public health work includes maternal survival in Indonesia and the founding of a health outreach program in the Appalachian region of the United States.

COVER DESIGN BY AIMEE NORDIN
COVER PHOTOGRAPH BY HELDUR NETOCNY/PANOS.

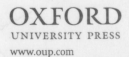

OXFORD
UNIVERSITY PRESS
www.oup.com

90000

ISBN 0-19-513740-X

9 780195 137408